Liver Intra-arterial PRRT with ¹¹¹In-Octreotide

Georgios S. Limouris

Editor

Liver Intra-arterial PRRT with ^{111}In-Octreotide

The Tumoricidal Efficacy of ^{111}In Auger Electron Emission

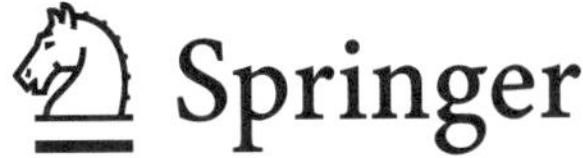

Editor
Georgios S. Limouris
Nuclear Medicine
Medical School
National and Kapodistrian University of Athens
Athens
Greece

ISBN 978-3-030-70775-0   ISBN 978-3-030-70773-6   (eBook)
https://doi.org/10.1007/978-3-030-70773-6

This Springer imprint is published by the registered company Springer Nature Switzerland AG
The registered company address is: Gewerbestrasse 11, 6330 Cham, Switzerland

This book is dedicated to all my patients, for the trust they have shown in me by strengthening and encouraging in doing the best I could for their health.

Preface

The majority of Auger electrons (AEs) have energy lower than 25 keV deposited over short nano- up to micro-meter distances in tissues, whereas yielding high Linear Energy Transfer (LET) are attractive for radiation cancer treatment if emitted in close proximity to DNA. These high LET electrons were first discovered and described 100 years ago, in independent research work by Lise Meitner in 1922 and Pierre Auger in 1923.

[111]In emits on average 14.7 AEs of a broad energy and range spectrum per decay, which varies from 0.0085 to 22.5 keV. The dependence of the direct catastrophic induction of DNA double-strand breaks by them, a prerequisite for cell death and unfeasibility of strand repairing was recently simulated by Piroozfar et al., in 2018. Taking into account the emission probability and the efficiency of the electron energy, AEs of 350 eV generated the maximum number of double-strand breaks. Although the range of 350 eV AEs in water is estimated to be 16.4 nm, the aforementioned simulation data determined a distance of 6 nm to the decay of ^{111}In from the DNA center as a limit value for a significant contribution to the formation of these double-strand breaks.

Assuming a homogeneous intranuclear distribution of ^{111}In-Octreotide reaching the nucleus, the released ^{111}In AE emission would lead to the above-described significant DNA damage which is approved in this book, after a more than 800 intra-arterial infusions in liver neuroendocrine metastasized tumors, in a single Institute.

I believe that there is no one-stop solution to the problem of drug delivery for cancer treatment, and each drug carrier created has its limitations. The same applies in full to the radionuclide supplied. [111]In AE emission should have the greatest influence on the treatment of hard-to-detect micro-metastases and individual cancer cells, only if infused intra-arterially, while its effect in larger than 20 mm tumors is less pronounced and not indicated.

The PRRT in humans with ^{111}In-Octreotide described in this work could be in great demand for intravesical infusion in the treatment not only for neuroendocrine tumors and micro-metastases but also, if incorporated in PSMA, for prostate cancer and in perspective for breast cancer, appropriately built-in, in a specific, not yet established, for the mamma malignancy tracer.

Athens, Greece   Georgios S. Limouris

Acknowledgments

I would like to express my gratitude to the staff of Springer Milan and especially to Mrs Antonella Cerri for their kind support to get this book published. My sincere thanks to Corinna Parravicini for her help during the initial phase of the project. Furthermore, I wish to thank the Project Coordinator Sushil Kumar Sharma and his team for their distinctive patience providing outstanding book production services.

Georgios S. Limouris

Contents

The Efficacy of Auger and Internal Conversion Electron Emission of ^{111}In for Treating Neuroendocrine Tumors

1

Georgios S. Limouris

1.1 Introduction

Treatment modalities using irradiation comprise a potent cornerstone of anti-cancer therapy. Although each malignant tumor type has a different sensitivity profile to radiation, every malignancy, diffuse or solid retreats and succumbs more or less to the applied therapeutic radiation dose. The relatively new evolutionary treatment techniques that protect the radiation-sensitive normal liver parenchyma while still delivering sufficient radiation to malignant cells have dramatically increased the use of liver-tumor-directed radiation (loco-regional) therapy approaches. Being focused on liver tumors and specifically on neuroendocrine ones, these depend on the location of the disease, whether cancer has given metastases and spread to the other areas of the body, i.e. liver, bone, lymph nodes, and if the tumor is secreting hormones, responsible for symptoms. Treatment modalities against primary or metastatic neuroendocrine tumors can be categorised as (a) invasive, i.e. surgical resection, (b) minimally invasive, ablative, or loco-regional, i.e. selective trans-arterial (chemo) embolisation [TA(C)E], radiofrequency ablation [RFA], laser-induced thermotherapy [LIT], selective internal radiotherapy [SIRT] and (c) systemic treatment schemes.

With the development of intra-arterial infusions, the application of radiation to tumors of all origins and in all segments of the liver is a fact. Recent advances in medical oncology (individualised molecular profiling, antiangiogenic drugs and new systemic chemotherapeutics) have resulted in improved response rates, disease-related or progressive survival rates and median survival rates in many solid tumors. However, despite the elimination of the disease elsewhere in the body, the liver often remains a site of tumor resistance and, ultimately, the cause of patient death [1]. In addition, today, qualified interventional radiologists and the development of advanced and specialised catheters can help oncologic patients more than ever, and catheterising the feeding artery of inoperable solid tumors is a routine technique in most radiological centres that treat cancer patients. Nuclear medical devices and imaging agents allow the precise localisation of tumors that have not previously been imaged or irradiated and the detection of active tumors among already destroyed ones. Therapeutic radiation began in the early twentieth century with the successful fight against cancer. Today, patient survival can be predicted, whereas patients with no longer treatment-sensitive tumors or patients who cannot tolerate chemotherapy die. Overall, these data suggest that liver irradiation is not avoided or

G. S. Limouris (✉)
Nuclear Medicine, Medical School, National and Kapodistrian University of Athens, Athens, Greece
e-mail: glimouris@med.uoa.gr

© Springer Nature Switzerland AG 2021
G. S. Limouris (ed.), *Liver Intra-arterial PRRT with ^{111}In-Octreotide*,
https://doi.org/10.1007/978-3-030-70773-6_1

contraindicated, but rather the reverse—thus, why not use radiation for the affected liver? How can we use and optimise trans-arterial endohepatic radiation in favour of liver cancer patients?

1.2 Hepatic Intra-arterial Radiopeptide Flow Dynamics

Most blood of healthy hepatocytes is fed by the portal vein system, whereas a mediocre portion is supplied by the hepatic artery. In liver primary or metastatic tumor cells, most of the blood is delivered via the hepatic artery. Based on this different feeding pathway of benign and malignant cells in the liver, when radiopeptides in high dosage are infused intra-arterially from the hepatic artery, a very large portion of the applied radiation is targeted directly to the tumor cells and additionally attracted from the peptide receptors (Fig. 1.1); in parallel, healthy cells are protected as long as they are protected from radiation damage. There are also minor differences in the distribution of peptide analogues receptor binding due to their different receptor affinities.

According to rheology, there are two distinctly different types of fluid flow: the laminar and the turbulent one. In laminar flow, the fluid particles move along smooth paths in layers with every layer (lamina) sliding smoothly over its neighbour. In turbulent flow, the particles follow very irregular and erratic paths, and their velocity vectors vary repetitively, both in magnitude and direction. The laminar flow becomes unstable at high velocities and breaks down into turbulent flow [2]. Blood flow is laminar when the velocity gradient is smooth and continuous. It is observed that the insertion of a catheter in an artery affects the flow field, disturbs the pressure distribution, and enhances the resistance to flow [3, 4]. Consequently, to maintain the laminar character of flow on the course of ^{111}In-Octreotide infusion either after simple catheterisation of the femoral—iliac arteries—aorta—proper hepatic artery (Fig. 1.2, GS Limouris, Chap. 7) or after the implementation of a drum-port system (IL Karfis, Chap. 8), steady low pressure should be performed by the nuclear physician or, in case the

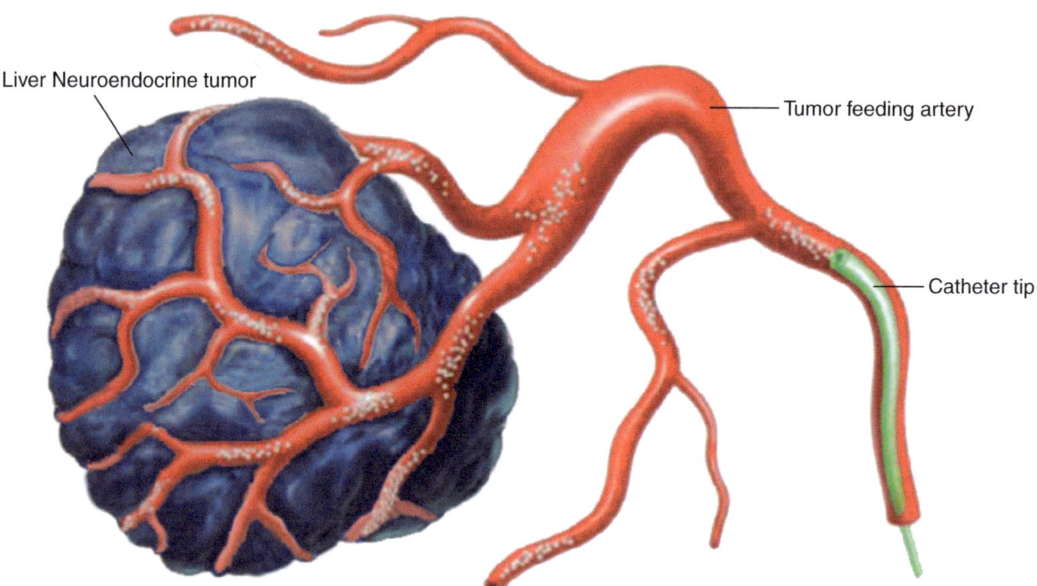

Fig. 1.1 Illustration of radiopeptide molecules released from the terminal endpoint of a micro-catheter overwhelming the tumor

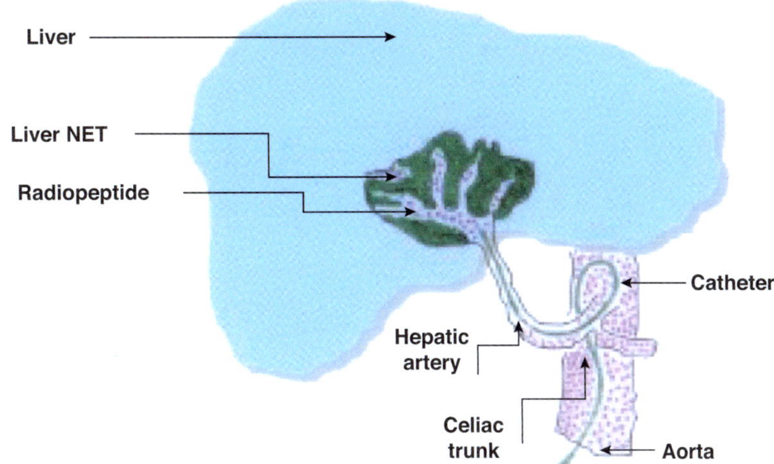

Fig. 1.2 The hepatic artery supplies the tumor and acts as the liver entrance for infusion

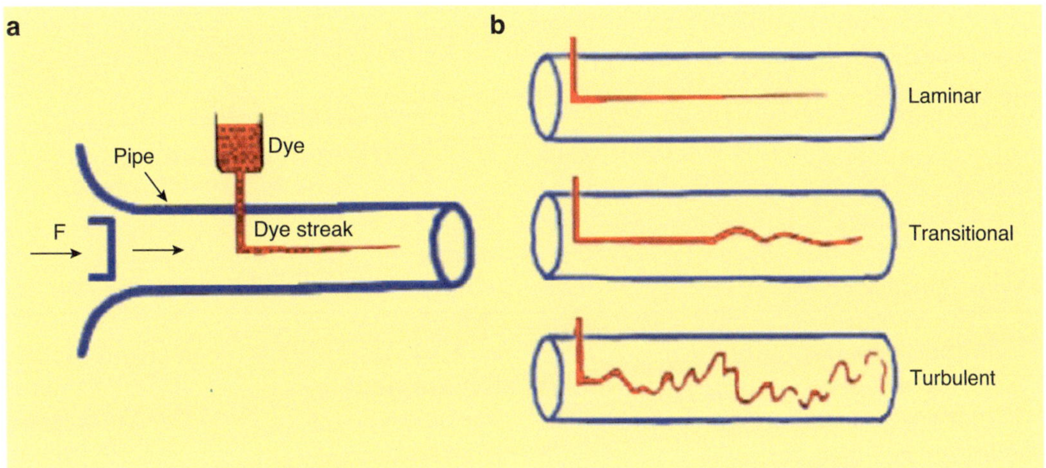

Fig. 1.3 In order to maintain the laminar character of flow against viscosity, a force F is applied to the fluid. Gentle infusion (no excessive pressure) should be done to strictly avoid backflow. (**a**) Reynolds' experiment using water in pipe shows (**b**) the transition of flow from laminar to turbulent [5, 6]

infusion is realised automatically, with the aid of an infusion-pump. Thus, gentle infusion, with steady low pressure, should be used to strictly avoid backflow [5, 6] (Fig. 1.3). Therefore, it is necessary to take into account such flow variables due to catheterisation. The cross-section of the vessel shows the laminate moving at different speeds; when closest to the edge of the vessel, the fluid moves slowly, though when near the centre, it moves quickly.

Thus, patient-specific manoeuvres have to be used. In the case of main hepatic artery injection, radiation is distributed to both lobes of the liver.

If the lesions are limited to one lobe, the catheter can be selectively inserted either into the left or right lobar artery supplying the affected lobe thus sparing the contra-lateral. In selected cases, hyper-selective, single-segment treatments can be considered.

1.2.1 Production and Physical Characteristics of ^{111}In

^{111}In is produced by cyclotron after cadmium-112 (^{112}Cd) collision with protons of a 2.8 MeV

Table 1.1 ^{111}In decay characteristics [5, 6]

Type of decay	Energy (keV)	Emission ratio $(Bq \times s)^{-1}$
Photons	150.8	$3 \cdot 10^{-5}$
Photons	171.3	0.906
Photons	245.4	0.941
Electrons IC[a]	145–170	0.1
Electrons IC[a]	218–245	0.06
Auger electrons	19–25	0.16
Auger electrons	2.6–3.6	1.02
Auger electrons	0.5	1.91

[a]IC: internal conversion

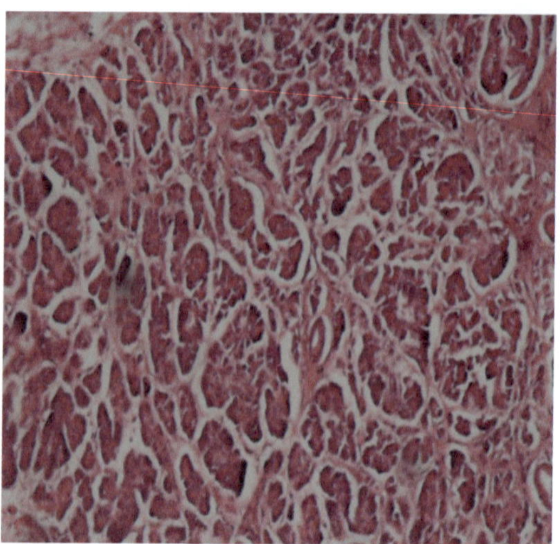

Fig. 1.4 Histological section of a low-grade pancreatic NET metastasised to liver (Haematoxylin-Eosin × 10)

energy according to the nuclear reaction ^{112}Cd (p, 2n) ^{111}In. ^{111}In decays by a physical half-life time of 2.83 days, with emissions displayed in Table 1.1. The purity of the final product of ^{111}In is affected by the undesired isotopes ^{110m}In, ^{110}In and ^{114m}In that are not possible to be spared from ^{111}In due to the similar chemical characteristics of these isotopes with ^{111}In.

Isotopes ^{110m}In and ^{110}In do not affect the dosimetry of radioisotopes labelled ^{111}In, as these undesired isotopes have a minor presence and short half-life time (4.9 h and 1.1 h, respectively). On the contrary, ^{114m}In, which is produced from ^{114}Cd according to a (p, n) nuclear reaction, has 49.51 days half-life time and decays through internal transition (96.9%) and electron capture (3.2%) with the emission of photons at (192, 558 and 725) keV. ^{114m}In affects dosimetry due to its long half-life time [5–7].

In the case of the main hepatic artery injection, radiation is distributed to both lobes of the liver. If the lesions are limited to one lobe, the catheter can be selectively inserted either into the left or right lobar artery supplying the affected lobe thus sparing the contra-lateral. In selected cases, hyper-selective (i.e. single-segment) treatments can be considered.

Patient-specific dosimetry calculations help the physician to optimise the planning of the treatment, avoid side effects to healthy tissue, and assign the administered dose for treatment results.

1.3 Recent Historical Background of Radioactive Infusions for Liver Tumors

The delivery of radioactive isotopes bonded with synthetic peptides to solid tumors dates back to 1994 when, for the first time, Eric Krenning [7] and Dick Kwekkeboom intravenously infused high doses of ^{111}In-Octreotide (Sect. 1.9) to treat liver metastases of an abdominal glucagonoma (Fig. 1.4). Limouris et al. first reported the routine use of intra-arterial infusions of ^{111}In-Octreotide [8] according to a particular protocol of specific bone marrow protective and nephroprotective as well character (Limouris et al. 'Aretaieion Protocol' [9]). Details of the aforementioned novelty were reported by Kontogeorgakos D [10], Troumpoukis N [11] and Karfis I [12] in their Ph.D. theses from the same Institute that published their results, after the catheterisation of the hepatic artery using ^{111}In-Octreotide. In 2014, Pool et al. in a limited cohort of 3 patients, after preclinical, intra-arterial as well intravenous studies in rats observed a two-fold higher ^{111}In-DTPA-TOC tumor uptake after intra-arterial administration than after intravenous injection; the clinical data (of patients) indicated that the intra-arterial administration of radiolabelled somatostatin analogues via the hepatic artery significantly increases radionuclide uptake in gastro-enteropancreatic neuroendocrine tumors (GEP-NETs), sst2-positive, liver metastases up to 72 h post-injection, emphasising that the effect of the intra-arterial administration differs between patients who show a large variability in radioactivity increment in liver metastases [13]. Kratochwil [14, 15] reported on radiopeptide pharmacokinetics in the tumor using, not ^{111}In-Octreoscan, but ^{177}Lu-DOTA-TATE intra-arterially. Although worldwide, most clinical experiences derive from intravenous therapies using ^{177}Lu, inoperable liver metastasised neuroendocrine tumor patients have been treated by our Institution exclusively intra-arterially using ^{111}In-Octreotide with some exceptions where catheterisation was not possible.

[111]*In clinical studies and efficacy*: According to our results in the first cohort of 17 inoperable liver metastasised GEP-NETs, treated with high doses of ^{111}In-Octreoscan [Table 1.2], 1 of 17 (6%) patients achieved a complete response (CR), and 8 of 17 (47%) showed partial response (PR) and 3 (18%) stable disease (SD), whereas in the remaining 5 (29%) patients, the disease progressed, the therapy was discontinued and the patients died shortly thereafter. Consequently, 71% (CR + PR + SD) of the patients showed some radiological benefit from the treatment. Worldwide, only a limited number of authors reported on the efficacy of treatments in GEP-NET-patients using high doses of ^{111}In-DTPA[0] Octreotide. Our results in the CR/PR group (53%), compared favourably with published data (2/26 pts (8%) (Valkema et al. 2002) [16], 2/12 pts (17%) (Buscombe et al. 2003) [17], 2/26 pts (8%) (Anthony et al. 2002) [18], 2/29 pts (7%) (Delpassand et al. 2014)) [19]. Our patients with disease stabilisation (18% (3/17 pts)) differ from previous reports of 58% (15/26 pts) of Valkema et al. [16], 58% (7/12 pts) of Buscombe et al. [17], 81% (21/26 pts) of Anthony et al. [18], and 55% (16/29 pts) of Delpassand et al. [19]. The superiority of our results compared to those of the other authors might be explained by the intra-arterial route of infusions, where the tumor mean absorbed dose per session was estimated to be markedly higher compared to i.v. application (Table 1.3); a finding reported by other authors

Table 1.3 Tumor-absorbed dose comparison between i.v. and i.a. administration of ^{111}In-Octreotide

	Intra-arterial infusion	Intravenous infusion
Liver dose	0.14 (mGy/MBq)	0.40 (mGy/MBq)
Tumor dose	15.20 (mGy/MBq)	11.20 (mGy/MBq)
Tumor/liver dose ratio	108.57[a]	28.00
Tumor/kidney dose ratio	37.07	21.96

[a]The average absorbed dose per session to a tumor for a spherical mass of 10 gr was estimated to be 10.8 mGy/MBq, depending on the tumor histotype

Table 1.2 Experts working on ^{111}In-Octreotide

Author	No. of pts	Cumulative activity (GBq)	CR	PR	SD	PD
Krenning et al. (1994)	1	20.3	–	1(100%)	–	–
Tiensuu Janson et al. (1999)	21	5–18	–	2(40%)	3(60%)	–
Caplin et al. (2000)	8	3.1–15.2	–	–	7(87.5%)	1(12.5%)[a]
Nguyen et al. (2004)	15	21	–	–	13(87%)	2(13%)
Valkema et al. (2002)	26	4.7–160	–	2 (8%)	15 (58%)	9(35%)
Anthony et al. (2002)	26	6.7–46.6	–	2 (8%)	21 (81%)	3(11%)
Buscombe et al. (2003)	12	3.1–36.6	–	2 (17%)	7 (58%)	3(25%)
Delpassand et al. (2008)	19	35.3–37.3	–	2 (7%)	16 (55%)	11(38%)
Limouris et al. (2008)[b]	17	13–77	1(6%)	8(47%)	3(18%)	5(29%

[a]Unrelated to the cause of the tumor
[b]Intra-arterially exclusively

(Pool et al. 2009 [20], Kratochwil et al. 2010 [14], Kratochwil et al. 2011 [15]) too. The results of the clinical evaluation of the Auger electron emitter indium-111 conjugated to the somatostatin analogues that targets and exploits its receptor overexpression on neuroendocrine cells was very encouraging, particularly as it was thereafter proved for the eradication of small volume tumors (Limouris et al. 2008 [8], Reilly 2010 [21]). Summarising the results of previous studies, it might be concluded that the application of ^{111}In-Octreotide leads to disease stabilisation (SD) in previously progressive tumors and clinical symptomatic and biochemical (Cr-A) improvement as well.

1.4 Physics of Radiation Therapy

1.4.1 Radiation Types

The radiant energy causing ionisation in the cell can be categorised into two types: electromagnetic (γ-rays, x-rays) and particulate (α-particles, β-minus and β-plus particles, internal conversion and Auger electrons, ordinary shell electrons). The electromagnetic radiation γ-rays and x-rays of the same energy are indistinguishable, and the only difference is their source; γ-rays are emitted exclusively from the nucleus, whereas x-rays are emitted only from the electron shells.

From the particulate radiation, the most massive α-particles are emitted from the nucleus, with a velocity of about 1/20 that of the speed of light and with energies ranging from 4 to 9 MeV. They consist of two protons (charge +2 as a helium nucleus stripped of its orbital electrons) and have a very high linear-energy-transfer (LET) rate (Quality Factor = 20). The LET is the energy fraction, deposited in an absorber (i.e. tissue) per centimetre of travel. The range of an α-particle in the matter is typically 4–5 μm. Thus, α-particles cannot penetrate a sheet of paper or the epithelial layer of the skin. A single α-particle reaching the nucleus of a cell can deposit up to 1 Gy of radiation.

Ordinary electrons are found only in the electron shells (charge −1), and β-minus particles or negatrons (charge −1) are emitted exclusively from the nucleus. β-plus particles or positrons (charge +1) originate only from the nucleus too. In general, beta particles penetrate up to 3 mm of matter (tissue), while γ-rays and neutron rays completely penetrate the human body and end only in thick walls. Beta-minus particles possess a moderately high LET rate (Quality Factor = 1), allowing them to significantly contribute to the absorbed radiation dose. It is worth noting that there are beta-minus emitters that also emit γ-rays and are useful for both imaging and therapy. Regarding positrons, after having lost all their kinetic energy and having reached their rest mass, they interact with an electron in a process called annihilation, resulting in the total destruction of the positron and the electron and the release of two photons (γ-rays) whose energy is always 511 keV. The angle between the two photons is always 180°. Electromagnetic radiation, either as γ-rays or as x-rays, has an identical interaction with matter. Their LET rates are low, implying that much of the radiation escapes the body following the administration of γ-emitting isotopes. This minimises the radiation dose for patients and permits external imaging. To emphasise, that electromagnetic radiation is only linear and cannot be modified except by collision with tissue.

For photons, electron and proton radiation the damage is done primarily by activated radicals produced from atomic interactions called low linear-energy-transfer (low LET) radiation. On the contrary, the neutrons' radiation is of a high linear-energy-transfer (high LET) and the damage happens primarily by nuclear interactions. If a tumor cell is damaged by low LET radiation, it has a good chance of repairing itself and continuing to grow. Regarding high LET radiation, the possibility of a damaged tumor cell repairing itself is very small. The energy absorbed by the cell can cause DNA/RNA damage, leading to cell death.

Proton beam radiation therapy (PBRT) is a type of external beam radiation therapy (EBRT) that utilises protons precisely targeted to a specific tissue mass. Protons used in the same way as electrons have the ability to penetrate deep into tissues to reach tumors, while delivering less

Table 1.4 Radiation dose damage at cellular level [22]

Radiation dose delivered	Effects
1 Gray (Gy) SI unit or dose	– 1 Joule of energy deposited into 1 kg of tissue (absorbed dose)
	– 100 cGy, (100 'rads' in older terms)
	– Breaks (**usually** lethal to the cell) 40 DNA double-strand bases
	– Breaks (**often** lethal to the cell) 1000 DNA single-strand bases
	– Breaks (**possibly** lethal to the cell) 4000 DNA double-strand bases
1 Gray external beam radiation	>300 cGy/min dose rate

radiation to superficial tissues such as the skin. This may make PBRT more effective for inoperable tumors or for individuals in whom damage to healthy tissue would pose an unacceptable risk (Table 1.4). Furthermore, it is also well known that during proton therapy, neutrons are produced. This has been observed and proved, as protons are used for application in radiation therapy. It is also known that the neutron-absorbed dose is small. However, neutrons are highly biologically effective, and, thus, even a minimal absorbed dose might cause side effects in the patient, the most severe of which is the induction of a second primary cancer [22].

1.4.2 Auger Electrons

Auger electrons discovered in 1922 by the Austrian-Swedish physicist Lise Meitner (Fig. 1.5) [23] and in 1923 by the French physicist Pierre Auger (Fig. 1.6) [24] are formed when the vacancy created in an inner shell is filled with an electron of a higher energy level after electron capture. Most of the excess energy is delivered as X-ray energy, but one part is released as kinetic energy to another electron, which is then called an Auger electron [25–30]. A summary of the properties and characteristics of Auger electron emitters and their emissions can be seen in Table 1.5. Today, the Auger electron emitters mainly used for in vitro or in vivo therapy are ^{125}I,

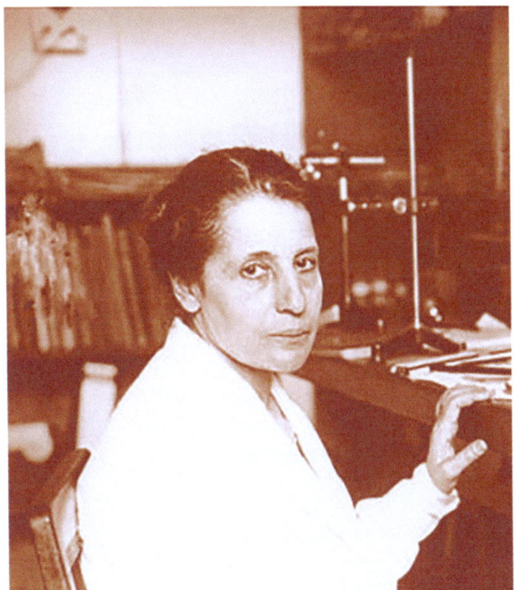

Fig. 1.5 Lise Meitner 1878–1968. [With permission: Archives of the Max Planck Society, Berlin]

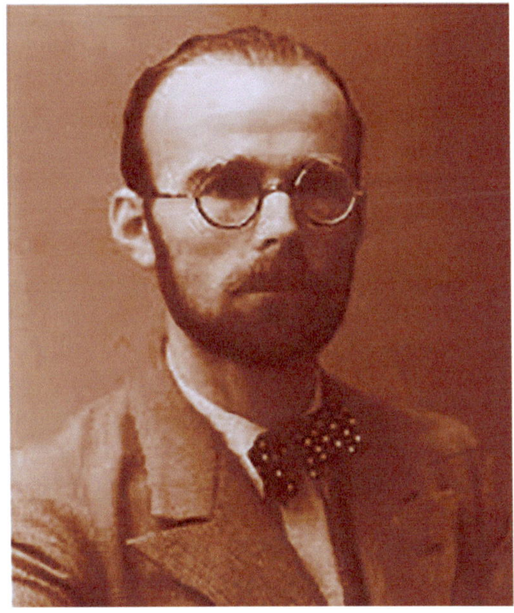

Fig. 1.6 Pierre Auger 1899–1993. [With permission: French Academy of Science-Institut de France]

^{111}In and ^{123}I and to a lesser extent ^{67}Ga, ^{99m}Tc and ^{201}Tl [30, 31]. ^{125}I is the most widely studied Auger electron emitter and has been used in many in vitro experiments to investigate the

Table 1.5 Properties and characteristics of 6 Auger electron emitters [33]

Characteristics	^{111}In	^{125}I	^{123}I	^{67}Ga	^{201}Tl	^{99m}Tc
Half-life (days)	2.80	59.4	0.55	3.26	3.04	0.25
No Auger e$^-$/decay	14.7	24.9	14.9	4.7	36.9	4.0
Auger e$^-$ energy/decay (keV)	6.8	12.2	7.4	6.3	15.3	0.9
Auger e$^-$ energy range (keV)	0.04–25.6	0.02–30.3	0.02–30.35	0.9–9.4	0.07–66.9	0.2–17.8
Conversion e$^-$/decay	0.2	0.9	0.2	0.3	1.1	1.1
Conversion e$^-$ energy/decay (keV)	25.9	7.2	20.2	28.1	30.2	15.4
Conversion e$^-$ energy range (keV)	145–245	3.7–35	127–159	82–291	1.6–153	100–140
Range of Auger e$^-$ in water (nm)	0.25–13.600	1.5–14.000	0.5–13,500	0.1–2700	3–40,000	13–6500
Range of Conversion e$^-$ in water (μm)	205–622	0.7–16	100–130	50–300	0.2–126	70–112
Associated gamma emissions (keV)	171.3 245.4	3535	159.0	9.1, 923 184, 209 300, 393	153.3 167.4	140.5
Total energy/decay (keV)	419.2	61.4	200.4	201.6	138.5	142.6
Total energy deposited per decay (10^{-14} Gy kg/Bq/s)	7.0	1.0	3.2	3.14	2.2	2.3

different effects of low-energy electrons on DNA27 [31–37].

However, its long half-life of 60 days makes it a little less practical for clinical applications. The physical half-life of the radionuclides should preferably be of the same order of magnitude as their biological half-life. A 'too long' physical half-life increases the amount of radionuclides that must be delivered to the tumor cells to allow for a reasonable amount of decay before excretion. On the other hand, a 'to short' physical half-life does not provide enough time for the targeting process. It is reasonable to assume that the most appropriate physical half-lives range from a few hours to a few days when targeting disseminated cells. Longer physical half-lives (up to one or a few weeks) may be desirable when high intakes of solid tumor masses are required.

The use of low-energy electrons has some advantages over the use of high-energy electron beta-emitters. Because of their long range, beta particles will overshoot single disseminated cells and small metastases [23, 31, 38–42] where most of the damage will be done to the surrounding healthy tissues. On the contrary, Auger electron emitters cause much less off-target effects than beta-emitters. On the other hand, for larger tumors, this cross-firing from beta-emitters will result in a more homogeneous deposition of energy in the tumor mass even if the radiopharmaceutical has an inhomogeneous distribution inside the tumor [40–42]. Additionally, for larger tumors, a much larger number of Auger-electron-emitting radionuclides is needed to cause the same cytotoxic effects, unless the Auger electrons are emitted inside the cell's nucleus. In a study by Capello et al., the influence of tumor size on the effectiveness of ^{111}In-Octreotide peptide receptor radionuclide therapy (PRRT) was evaluated [40]. In rats bearing small (<1 cm^3) tumors, complete responses were observed, but only partial tumor regressions were observed in the rats bearing larger (>8 cm^3) lesions. Auger-electron therapy can thus be conceptually compared with alpha- and beta-therapy, based largely on their path lengths and LET. Direct comparison of the various Auger electron-emitting isotopes with each other however is complicated by the diverse electron emission spectra of these isotopes. For example, ^{125}I emits, on average, 12.2 Auger electrons per decay, compared to 6.8 Auger electrons emitted per decay by ^{111}In. However, for ^{111}In the average energy of the AE is higher, and it emits more than threefold higher energy conversion electrons and is accompanied by two gamma-photon emissions that are considerably higher in energy than the 35 keV photon from ^{125}I (Table 1.1) [34, 43].

1.4.3   Radiation Dose

The dose of ionising radiation absorbed by the liver, a solid tumor, or other tissues has been a cornerstone of the design of clinical studies and trials. Earlier reports used the term roentgen (R), which is the ionisation in air, i.e. the exposure of gamma rays. The newer nomenclature uses the SI unit for the absorbed dose in tissue (1 Joule/kg = 1 Gray (Gy) = 100 rads = 100 cGy as the basic unit of measurement).

1.5   Radiobiology

From the turn of the century, attempts to gain an understanding of the effects of radiation in living tissue have been made, with observations reported by Hall [44] on skin reactions, primary erythema and collapse. Since then, clinical experience has been based on observations on normal and malignant tissue reaction and repair due to ionising radiation. The DNA must be damaged, unrepaired or improperly repaired to cause loss of reproductive ability or apoptosis (Fig. 1.7). According to Hall [44] and Kennedy et al. [45], it was estimated that in the presence of sufficient oxygen (>10 mm Hg), any form of radiation (x-rays, gamma rays, beta rays or electron emission in general) potentially interacts with the DNA. About 75% of DNA damage is indirect, with a photon striking a water molecule within 4 nm of the DNA strand (water is 80% of the cell). Kinetic energy from the incident photon is transmitted to an orbital electron of the water molecule and ejects it, which is now called a secondary electron. The energy that is transferred to a water molecule forms a free radical that *is highly reactive,* breaking the bonds of nearby DNA strands. Furthermore, a

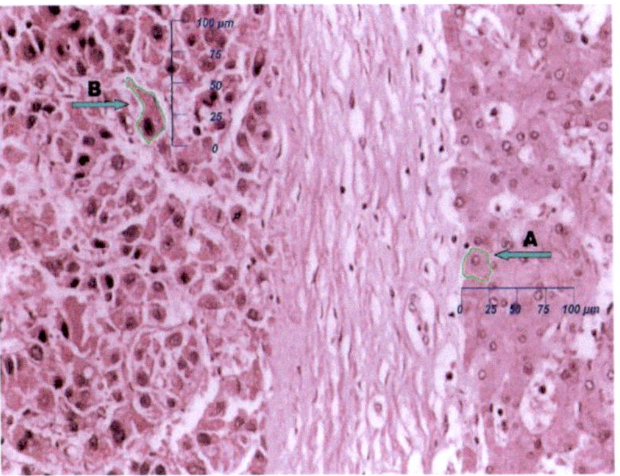

Fig. 1.7 On a histological sample of normal (**a**) and tumor liver cells (**b**), 2μm (*in blue*) are super-imposed. The cellular membrane is delineated *in green* (arrow). The nuclei of normal (**a**) and tumor cells (**b**) are well distinguished. Comparing cell dimensions and distances between cell surface and nuclei obviously can be elicited that DNA lies within the micrometre range of ^{111}In emissions. (Adapted and modified from Limouris et al. [4])

direct interaction of the secondary electron on the DNA strand is expected, which is referred to as a direct effect [44].

Roger Howell in his excellent 'paper-chronical' on Auger elcctrons and their exquisite capacity to finally serve as first-class endocellular radionuclide tumor killers reported on the extreme radiotoxicity of Auger electron emitters that prompted scientists to extensively investigate the radiobiological effects of Auger electron emitters as well as Auger electrons released as a consequence of the photoelectric effect [46]. Their efforts were punctuated by a series of international meetings that focused on the biological aspects of Auger processes. These began with the founding meeting in 1975 that was organised by Ludwig Feinendegen in Jülich, Germany. This meeting was followed by the first one, in 1987 in Charney Basset, UK, the second in 1991 in Amherst, USA, the third in 1995 in Lund, Sweden, the fourth in 1999 in Lund again, Sweden and the fifth in 2003 in Melbourne, Australia. The 2nd–5th proceedings contain a review of the published work of the previous meetings; Kassis [25]. Roger Howell's manuscript [46] continued this tradition. It reviews articles related to the biophysical aspects of Auger processes that were published from 2004 to 2007, excluding articles published in the previous proceedings.

1.5.1 Modifiers of Radiation Response

According to Zeman [47] and Withers [48], oxygen is the most important biological modifier of radiation action at the cellular level and is the main reason for inducing radiation damage caused by free radicals; meanwhile, these damages can be repaired in a hypoxic state. The ratio of the radiation dose without oxygen compared to those with oxygen producing the same biological effect is referred to as the 'oxygen enhancement ratio' (OER). For x-rays, the OER lies between 2 and 3, i.e. a given x-ray image will provoke a 2–3 times stronger burden on the cell in the presence of oxygen than in a hypoxic environment [44]. Other factors affecting radiation efficiency are well known as the 4 'Rs,' i.e. *reoxygenation*, *repair* of radiation damage, *reassortment* (rearrangement) of cells into more or less sensitive sections of the cell cycle (the S-phase is the most resistant to radiation and G2-M the most sensitive) and *repopulation* (rapidly dividing tumor populations), which can be overwhelmed by a continuous low radiation dose delivered for approximately more than 14 days. Repopulation may also become a problem after surgical resection, chemoembolisation, cryotherapy or radiofrequency ablation if hepatic hypertrophy is stimulated in the regional normal cells. The repair of radiation damage or 'sub-lethal damage repair' is improved in low-oxygen environments and with multiple radiation doses (fractionation). The break (typically 24 h) between each fraction of external radiotherapy offers the opportunity to repair DNA strand breaks in normal and malignant cells.

1.6 The Effects of Radiation on the Liver

Until recently, the liver was classified as a radioresistant organ, though it is in fact highly radiosensitive [49]. Thus, it is not surprising that since the early 1960s [50, 51]acute transient effects or long-term (late effects) due to the ionising radiation in the liver have been described in the literature; the former has been described as an increase in liver transaminases, neutropenia and/or coagulopathy and the later as fibrosis, persistent enzyme degeneration, ascites, jaundice, and rarely, radiation-induced liver disease (RILD), and fatal veno-occlusive disease (VOD) [52–54]. RILD is often what is termed 'radiation hepatitis' and has been classically expected within 3 months of initiating radiation, with rapid weight gain, abdominal distension, liver enlargement and occasional ascites or jaundice, with elevation in serum alkaline phosphatase. Clinically, it is similar to the Budd-Chiari syndrome, but most patients survive, though some die of this disease with no evidence of tumor progression. It was reported that the entire liver cannot be treated with radiation above 30–35 Gy in conventional fractionation (1.8–2 Gy/day, 5 days per week), as RILD or VOD may occur [55].

1.7 The Rationale for ^{111}In-Octreoscan Therapy

The unique vascular supply of the liver is well described and understood by radiologists and surgeons but less well by other specialists. A brief review is presented later (Sect. 1.7.1).

1.7.1 Anatomic Vascular Summary

The portal venous system supplies 80% or more of the blood supply to the normal liver [56]. The hepatic artery, with branches to the gallbladder, duodenum and stomach, provides up to 20% of the required blood supply to the normal liver. However, in the presence of tumor growth in the liver, the hepatic artery is the main supplier of blood, from 80 to 100%. The tumor vessel growth is many times more concentrated in the periphery of the tumor compared to the tumor centre and normal liver, in a ratio of 3:1 up to 20:1, and is abnormal in their consistency [57]. These data have been shown to be reliable in many trials [57–59].

1.7.2 Preclinical Reports on Blood Supply in Tumors

Breedis and Young performed a series of animal studies with numerous species, including rabbits, rats, mice and 13 human livers with metastatic solid tumors [56]. They demonstrated that 80–100% of the blood supply to tumors comes from the hepatic artery. The same results were reported by Ackerman et al. [58] and Lien and Ackerman [57] in rat carcinosarcoma liver metastases, using either ^{131}I-tagged human serum albumin (RISA) or resin microspheres labelled with ^{90}Y. Hepatic arterial infusions were compared with those of the portal vein in tumor intake versus normal liver tissue. Results showed that tumors larger than 30 mg received 75% of their blood supply from the hepatic artery, with an estimated tumor-to-normal tissue ratio of 3:1.

1.8 Human Studies with ^{111}In-Octreoscan

Clinical experience with ^{111}In dates back to the early 1990s (Krenning et al. 1994) [7] as reported previously in Sect. 1.3.

1.9 Commercially Available ^{111}In-Octreoscan for Human Medical Use

^{111}**In-Octreoscan** contains ^{111}In-labelled octreotide, which is a somatostatin analogue; it is also known as an OctreoScan®, a brand name for ^{111}In-labelled pentetreotide; pentetreotide is a DTPA-conjugated form of octreotide, originally manufactured by Mallinckrodt Nuclear Medicine LLC, which now is part of Curium. It is particularly useful for the management of neuroendocrine tumors.

References

1. Kennedy S, Dezarn WA, McNeillie. 90Y microspheres; concepts and principles. In: Bilbao J-I, Reiser MF, editors. Liver microembolization with 90Y microspheres. Berlin-Heidelberg: Springer; 2014. p. 1–10.
2. Evans DH, McDicken WN, Skidmore R, et al. Doppler ultrasound: physics, instrumentation, and clinical applications. Wiley; 1989.
3. Taylor KJW, Burns PN, Wells PNT. Clinical applications of doppler ultrasound. Raven: Press; 1987.
4. Zaman A, Ali N, Sajid M, et al. Numerical and analytical study of two-layered unsteady blood flow through catheterized artery. PLoS One. 2016;11(8):e0161377.
5. Lyra ME, Andreou M, Georgantzoglou A, et al. Radionuclides used in nuclear medicine therapy—from production to dosimetry, current medical imaging reviews. Bentham Science Publishers. 2013;9:51–75.
6. Lyra-Georgosopoulou M, Limouris GS. Blood flow and arterial infusion by implanted port in- 111 octreotide therapy. Interv Med Clin Imaging. 2019;2(1):1–8.
7. Krenning EP, Kooij PPM, Bakker WH. Radiotherapy with a radiolabelled somatostatin analogue, [111In-DTPA-D. Phe1]-octreotide; a case history. Ann N Y Acad Sci. 1994;733:496–506.
8. Limouris GS, Chatziioannou A, Kontogeorgakos D, et al. Selective hepatic arterial infusion of In-111-DTPA-Phe1-octreotide in neuroendocrine liver metastases. Eur J Nucl Med Mol Imaging. 2008;35:1827–37.
9. Limouris GS, Karfis I, Chatziioannou A, et al. Super-selective hepatic arterial infusions as established technique ("ARETAIEION" Protocol) of [177Lu] DOTA-TATE in inoperable neuroendocrine liver metastases of gastro-entero-pancreatic (GEP) tumors. Q J Nucl Med Mol Imaging. 2012;56(6):551–8.
10. Kontogeorgakos D. PhD thesis, Medical School, National and Kapodistrian University of Athens-Greece; 2006.
11. Troumpoukis N. PhD thesis, Medical School, National and Kapodistrian University of Athens-Greece; 2016.
12. Karfis I. PhD thesis, Medical School, National and Kapodistrian University of Athens-Greece; 2016.
13. Pool SE, Kam BLR, Koning GA, et al. [111In-DTPA] Octreotide tumor uptake in GEPNET liver metastases after intra-arterial administration: an overview of preclinical and clinical observations and implications for

tumor radiation dose after peptide radionuclide therapy. Cancer Biother Radioph. 2014;29(4):179–87, Mary Ann Liebert, Inc.

14. Kratochwil C, Giesel FL, López-Benítez R. Intra-individual comparison of selective arterial versus venous 68Ga-DOTATOC PET/CT in patients with gastro-enteropancreatic neuro-endocrine tumors. Clin Cancer Res. 2010;16(10):2899–905.

15. Kratochwil C, Lopez-Benitez R, Mier W. Hepatic arterial infusion enhances DOTATOC radiopeptide therapy in patients with neuroendocrine liver metastases. Endocr Relat Cancer. 2011;18:595–602.

16. Valkema R, De Jong M, Bakker WH, et al. Phase I study of peptide receptor radionuclide therapy with [111In-DTPA°] octreotide: the Rotterdam experience. Semin Nucl Med. 2002;32(2):110–22.

17. Buscombe JR, Caplin ME, Hilson JW. Long-term efficacy of high-activity 111In-pentetreotide therapy in patients with disseminated neuroendocrine tumors. J Nucl Med. 2003;44:1–6.

18. Anthony LB, Woltering EA, Espanan GD. Indium-111-pentetreotide prolongs survival in gastroenteropancreatic malignancies. Semin Nucl Med. 2002;32(2):123–32.

19. Delpassand ES, Samarghandi A, Zamanian S, et al. Peptide receptor radionuclide therapy with 177Lu-DOTATATE for patients with somatostatin receptor–expressing neuroendocrine tumors. Pancreas. 2014;43(4):518–25.

20. Pool SE, Kam B, Breeman WAP. Increasing intrahepatic tumor uptake of 111In-DTPA-octreotide by loco regional administration. Eur J Nucl Med Mol Imaging. 2009;36:S427.

21. Reilly MN. Monoclonal antibody and peptide-targeted radiotherapy of cancer, Chapter 9. Hoboken, NJ: Wiley; 2010.

22. Schneider U, Hälg R. The impact of neutrons in clinical proton therapy. Front Oncol. 2015;5:235. https://doi.org/10.3389/fonc.2015.00235.

23. Meitner L. Über die Entstehung der Strahl-Spektren radioaktiver Substanzen. Zeitschrift für Physik A, Hadrons and Nuclei. 1922;9(1)

24. Auger P. Sur les rayons secondaires produits dans un gaz par des rayons X. CRAS. 1923;177:3.

25. Kassis A. The amazing world of auger electrons. Int J Radiat Biol. 2004;80(11–12):789–803.

26. Adelstein SJ, Merrill C. Sosman Lecture. The Auger process: a therapeutic promise? AJR. 1993;160(4):707–13.

27. Kassis A. Cancer therapy with Auger electrons: are we almost there? J Nucl Med. 2003;44(9):1479–81.

28. Kassis A. Radiotargeting agents for cancer therapy. Expert Opin Drug Deliv. 2005;2(6):981–91.

29. Sofou S. Radionuclide carriers for targeting of cancer. Int J Nanomedicine. 2008;3(2):181–99.

30. Boswell CA, Brechbiel MW. Auger electrons: lethal, low energy, and coming soon to a tumor cell nucleus near you. J Nucl Med. 2005;46(12):1946–7.

31. Adelstein SJ, Kassis AI. Strand breaks in plasmid DNA following positional changes of Auger-electron-emitting radionuclides. Acta Oncol. 1996;35(7):797–801.

32. Cornelissen B, Vallis KA. Targeting the nucleus: an overview of Auger-electron radionuclide therapy. Curr Drug Discov Technol. 2010;7(4):1570–638, Bentham Science Publishers Ltd

33. Buchegger F, Perillo-Adamer F, Dupertuis YM, et al. Auger radiation targeted into DNA: a therapy perspective. Eur J Nucl Med Mol Imaging. 2006;33:1352–63.

34. Humm JL, Howell RW, Rao DV. Dosimetry of Auger-electron emitting radionuclides: report no. 3 of AAPM Nuclear Medicine Task Group No. 6. Med Phys. 1994;21(12):1901–15.

35. Adelstein SJ, Kassis AI. Radiobiologic implications of the microscopic distribution of energy from radionuclides. Int J Rad Appl Instrum B. 1987;14(3):165–9.

36. Kassis AI, Harapanhalli RS, Adelstein SJ. Strand breaks in plasmid DNA after positional changes of Auger electron-emitting iodine125: direct compared to indirect effects. Radiat Res. 1999;152(5):530–8.

37. Kassis AI, Harapanhalli RS, Adelstein SJ. Comparison of strand breaks in plasmid DNA after positional changes of Auger electron emitting iodine-125. Radiat Res. 1999;151(2):167–76.

38. Buchegger F, Vieira JM, Blaeuenstein P, et al. Preclinical Auger and gamma radiation dosimetry for fluorodeoxyuridine-enhanced tumour proliferation scintigraphy with [123I] iododeoxyuridine. Eur J Nucl Med Mol Imaging. 2003;30(2):239–46.

39. Carlsson J, Forssell Aronsson E, Hietala SO, et al. Tumor therapy with radionuclides: assessment of progress and problems. Radiother Oncol. 2003;66(2):107–17.

40. Capello A, Krenning E, Bernard B, et al. 111In-labelled somatostatin analogues in a rat tumour model: somatostatin receptor status and effects of peptide receptor radionuclide therapy. Eur J Nucl Med Mol Imaging. 2005;32(11):1288–95.

41. Essand M, Gronvik C, Hartman T, et al. Radioimmunotherapy of prostatic adenocarcinomas: effects of 131I-labelled E4 antibodies on cells at different depth in DU 145 spheroids. Int J Cancer. 1995;63(3):387–94.

42. O'Donoghue JA, Bardies M, Wheldon TE. Relationships between tumor size and curability for uniformly targeted therapy with beta emitting radionuclides. J Nucl Med. 1995;36(10):1902–9.

43. Eckerman K, Endo A, Eds. MIRD (2008) Radionuclide data and decay schemes. 2nd ed. Reston, VA: The Society of Nuclear Medicine.

44. Hall E. Radiobiology for the radiologist. 5th ed. Philadelphia: Lippincott, Williams & Wilkins; 2000. p. 5–16, 80–87.

45. Kennedy AS, Raleigh JA, Varia MA. Proliferation and hypoxia in human squamous cell carcinoma of the cervix: first report of combined immunohistochemical assays. Int J Radiat Oncol Biol Phys. 1997;37(4):897–905.

46. Howell RW. Auger processes in the 21st century. Int J Radiat Biol. 2008;84(12):959–75.

47. Zeman E. Biologic basis of radiation oncology. In: Gunderson L, Tepper J, editors. Clinical radiation oncology. 1st ed. Philadelphia: Churchill Livingstone; 2000. p. 1–41.

48. Withers HR. Gastrointestinal cancer: radiation oncology. In: Kelsen DP, Daly JM, Levin B, Kern SE, Tepper JE, editors. Gastrointestinal oncology: principles and practice. 1st ed. Philadelphia: Lippincott Williams & Wilkins; 2002. p. 83–96.

49. Mornex F, Gérard F, Ramuz O. Late effects of radiations on the liver. Cancer Radiother. 1997;1(6):753–9.

50. Ingold J, Reed G, Kaplan H. Radiation hepatitis. Am J Roentgenol. 1965;93:200–8.

51. Ogata K, Hizawa K, Yoshida M. Hepatic injury following irradiation: a morphologic study Tokushima. J Exp Med. 1963;9:240–51.

52. Lawrence TS, Robertson JM, Anscher MS. Hepatic toxicity resulting from cancer treatment. Int J Radiat Oncol Biol Phys. 1995;31(5):1237–48.

53. Austin-Seymour MM, Chen GT, Castro JR. Dose volume histogram analysis of liver radiation tolerance. J Radiat Oncol Biol Phys. 1986;12:31–5.

54. Dawson LA, Ten Haken RK, Lawrence TS. Partial irradiation of the liver. Semin Radiat Oncol 11. 2001;3:240–6.

55. Fajardo LF, Berthrong M, Anderson RE. Chapter 15, Liver, radiation pathology. 1st ed. New York: Oxford University; 2001. p. 249–57.

56. Breedis C, Young G. The blood supply of neoplasms in the liver. Am J Pathol. 1954;30:969–84.

57. Lien WM, Ackerman NB. The blood supply of experimental liver metastases II: a microcirculatory study of the normal and tumor vessels of the liver with the use of perfused silicone rubber. Surgery. 1970;68(2):334–40.

58. Ackerman NB, Lien WM, Kondi ES, et al. The blood supply of experimental liver metastases I: the distribution of hepatic artery and portal vein blood to "small" and "large" tumors. Surgery. 1970;66(6): 1067–72.

59. Meade VM, Burton MA, Gray BN, et al. Distribution of different sized microspheres in experimental hepatic tumors. Eur J Cancer Clin Oncol. 1987;23(1): 37–41.

Somatostatin

Georgios S. Limouris

2.1 Historical Corner

The first thoughts on a possible link between the hypothalamus and the pituitary gland and further between the central nervous system and the endocrine glands began to be formulated in the late 1940s by the British scientist Geoffrey Wingfield Harris (1913–1971) (Figs. 2.1, 2.2, and 2.3).

Harris proposed the existence of hypothalamic factors, which control the function of the anterior pituitary lobe through the pituitary portal vascular network, and thus lay the foundation of neuroendocrinology. For his contributions, he is rightly regarded as the father of this discipline [4–8]. For a long time, the hypophysiotropic hypothalamic factors, the existence of which was proposed by Harris, remained purely hypothetical entities. Two groups systematically tried initially to isolate and then identify them: (a) one led by the Frenchman Roger Charles Louis Guillemin at the Salk Institute for Biological Studies in California and (b) the Polish scientist Andrew Victor Schally's team at the Veterans Administration Hospital in New Orleans. About 10 years from the initialisation of the aforementioned investigations (1969), the primary structure of the first of the two factors under investigation, i.e. the tri-

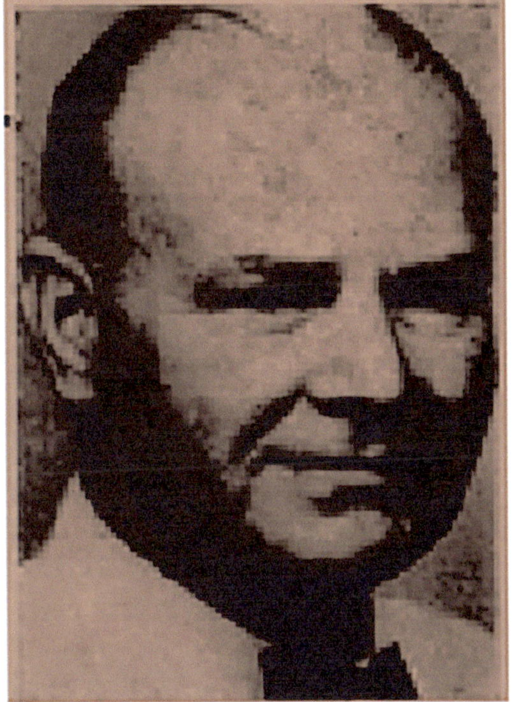

Fig. 2.1 Geoffrey Wingfield Harris (1913–1971) [1]

peptide chloride thyrotropin-releasing factor, was determined almost simultaneously by the two groups [9, 10]. This was a milestone, according to Guillemin and simultaneously received full confirmation from Harris. In 1968, Krulich and colleagues [11], while investigating factors that might govern the secretion of the growth hor-

G. S. Limouris (✉)
Nuclear Medicine, Medical School, National and Kapodistrian University of Athens, Athens, Greece
e-mail: glimouris@med.uoa.gr

© Springer Nature Switzerland AG 2021
G. S. Limouris (ed.), *Liver Intra-arterial PRRT with ^{111}In-Octreotide*,
https://doi.org/10.1007/978-3-030-70773-6_2

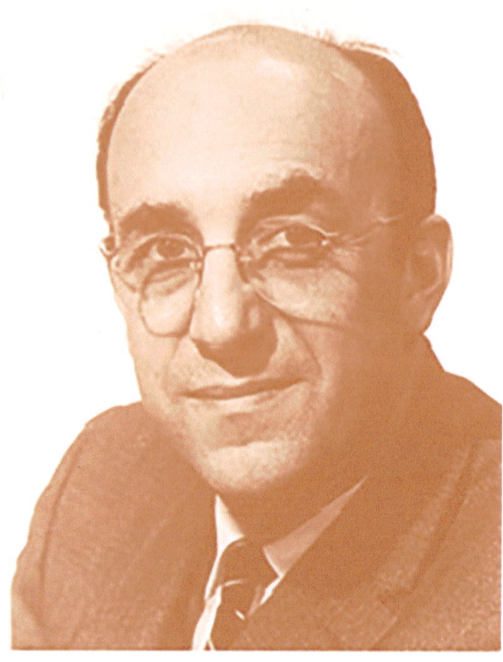

Fig. 2.2 Roger Charles Louis Guillemin (1924–present) [2]

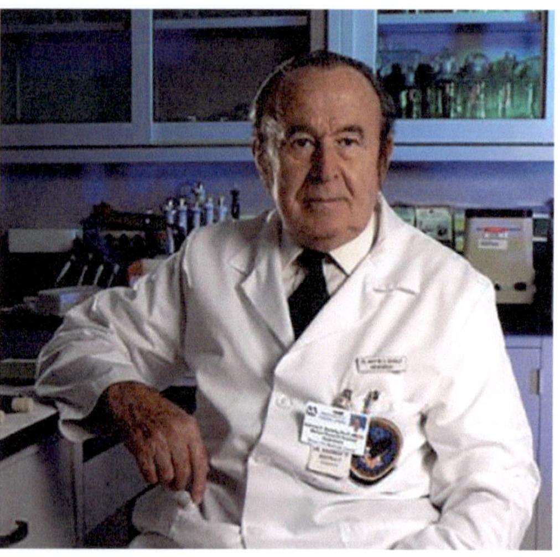

Fig. 2.3 Andrew Victor Schally (1926–present). Caption: Dr. Andrew V. Schally shared the Nobel Prize in Physiology or Medicine for 1977 (with R. Guillemin and R. S. Yalow) for his discovery of the hypothalamic hormones. He heads the Endocrine, Polypeptide and Cancer Institute, Veterans Affairs Medical Center in Miami [3]

mone (GH), isolated from sheep hypothalamic extracts a hitherto unknown substance with inhibiting properties on the secretion of this hormone. The following year, Hellman and Lernmark [12] found a factor in pancreatic islets that also reduced the secretion of insulin. The identity of this compound was determined 4 years later by Guillemin's group and was revolutionary in the field of neuroendocrinology. Adding crude extracts of sheep hypothalamus to in vitro cultures of anterior pituitary cells, Guillemin observed inhibition of GH secretion and even showed a linear correlation between extract concentration and its (GH) inhibition. At that time, a young doctor, Paul Brazeau, and a chemist Roger Burgus, both members of the Guillemin group, isolated the substance responsible, identified as a peptide, from the hypothalamus and discovered in the course of its Edman degradation [13] the sequence of its 14 amino acids (Fig. 2.4). This substance was called 'somatostatin' (SST), a term introduced by Guillemin, who chose it over somatotropin-releasing inhibitory factor or GH-releasing inhibitory factor [14–17].

On 5 January 1973, the paper regarding the discovery of SST was published in *Science* [18], and, a few years later, in 1977, Guillemin and Schally were honoured with the Nobel Prize for Medicine and Physiology, shared with the physicist Rosalyn Sussman Yalow (1921–2011). Yalow perfected and applied for the first time radioimmunoassay methods (Radioimmunoassay, RIA) for the quantification of infinitesimal peptides. Guillemin's contribution in understanding the pathophysiological mechanisms involved in thyrotropic, somatotropic and gonadotropic axes as well as the mechanisms of diabetes was seminal, apart from the discovery of hypothalamic peptides that control pituitary function and of endorphins and endogenous opioid peptides.

A few months after the publication of Brazeau and colleagues' work, it was announced that SST also inhibits the intrinsic function of the pancreas [19], while at that time two almost concurrent

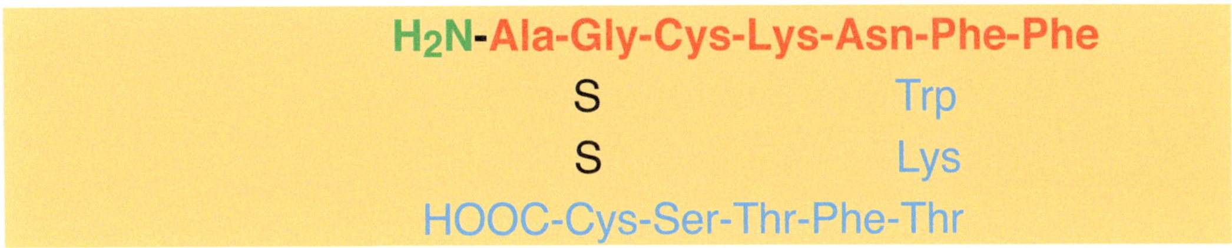

Fig. 2.4 Endogenous (native) SST-14: cyclic peptide of 14 amino acids

studies showed that SST is produced, besides the hypothalamus, from distinct cell populations' islets, named $\alpha1$, or, as finally revealed, δ cells [20, 21].

Scientific papers followed at a staggering rate, expanding the initial consideration of SST as a peptide simply inhibiting the secretion of GH, due to its extensive receptor distribution in biological tissues (healthy or not), to a plethora of regulatory actions and consequently therapeutic applications. To the best of our knowledge, up to the time of writing, according to the PubMed database, the total number of posts related to SST and its analogues (SSTAs) exceeds 27K, with reports at the rate of 800–900 per year!

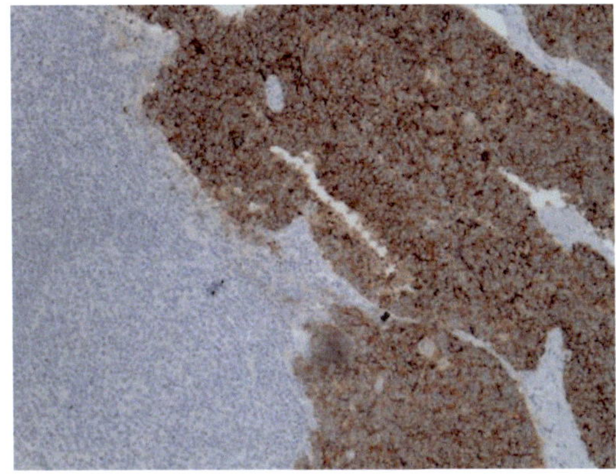

Fig. 2.5 Merkel cell carcinoma of the skin metastatic to lymph node, showing positive immunoreactions to chromogranin (×10)

2.2 Somatostatin Receptors-Tissue Expression [4]

The first description of somatostatin [SST] activity through specific receptors involved in vitro rat pituitary cell cultures (clonal GH4C1calls), whereas later studies showed that they exhibit extensive distribution in a number of tissues, both healthy and neoplastic. Although the existence of more than one SSTR subtype had begun to emerge since the early 1980s, only five SSTR subtypes thus far known were cloned and pharmacologically characterised between 1992 (20 years after the discovery of SST) and 1994. They received the code names sst1, sst2, sst3, sst4 and sst5 based on the chronological order of their discovery. The discovery of SSTRs focused on the research interest in the mechanisms governing SST signal transduction within the target cells, their tissue-dependent expression and their selective ability to bind SST analogues. However,

the possibility of the presence of additional SSTRs remains open (Fig. 2.5).

SSTRs belong to the superfamily of G-protein-coupled receptors (GPCRs); they therefore possess the H2N-terminal extracellular and HOOC-terminal intracellular domain as well as seven hydrophobic α-helical transmembrane domains. All five subtypes necessarily contain, in this seventh transmembrane region, the amino acid sequence [Tyr-Ala-Asn-Ser-Cys-Ala-Ala-Asn-Pro-Iso-Val-Leu-Tyr-], which is also their identity characteristic [22]. Their H2N-terminus has from one to four N-glycosylation sites. Additionally, in the HOOC-terminus, three to eight phosphorylation sites can be observed upon the protein kinases A and C and the calmodulin kinase [22]. Genes encoding hSSTRs are located on a different chromosome for each subtype [22] (Table 2.1).

Regarding somatostatin analogues (SSTAs), their affinity for hSSTRs is variable; octreotide and lanreotide exhibit high affinity for sst2 and somewhat moderate affinity for sst3 and sst5; hSSTRs show wide distribution, being present in the cerebral cortex, cerebellum, hypothalamus, pituitary gland, eye (especially corneal endothelium, iris and retina), thyroid (follicular cells), parathyroid (chief cells), thymus, pulmonary parenchyma, bronchial epithelium, myocardium (myocardial muscle cells express hsst1 and hsst2 receptors, all myocardial fibroblasts express all except hsst3), striated muscles, myenteric plexus (Auerbach) of the gastrointestinal tract, stomach, small and large intestines, rectum, liver, pancreas, spleen, kidneys, adrenal glands, placenta, endometrium, prostate and bone marrow (Table 2.2) [23].

2.3 Somatostatin Analogues

The pharmacokinetics of endogenous SS has some significant disadvantages, such as a short half-life (in healthy populations: 1.1–3.0 s with a renal clearance of 50.3 ± 7.0 mL kg^{-1} min^{-1} for SS-14 [24, 25] and 1.86 s for SS-28 [26, 27]. In particular, endogenous SS-14 undergoes enzymatic catalysis by peptidases at the sites [-Ala01 - GlyO2 -], [- GlyO2 - CysO3 -], [- Phe06 - Phe07 - Trp08-Lys09-] and [-Thr10-Phe11-] [28]. Due to the short half-life of endogenous SS and its limited local paracrine influence, the synthesis of somatostatin analogues with a longer half-life was necessary for feasible and effective action (Table 2.3).

Table 2.1 Characteristics of the five known hSSTRs. Half maximal inhibitory concentration (IC50) [22]

	hsst$_1$	hsst$_{2A/2B}$	hsst$_3$	hsst$_4$	hsst$_5$
Chromosomes	14q13	17q24	22q13.1	20p11.2	16p13.3
No. of amino acids	391	364	418	388	363
Weight (KDa)	53–72	71–95	65–85	45	52–66
IC$_{50}$ (nM): SST-14 SST-28	0.1–2.2 0.1–2.2	0.2–1.3 0.2–4.1	0.3–1.6 0.3–6.1	0.3–1.8 0.3–7.9	0.2–0.9 0.05–0.4
transmembrane domains	7	7	7	7	(4.5) 7

Table 2.2 Distribution of hSSTRs per organ [23]

hsst$_1$	hsst$_{2A/2B}$	hsst$_3$	hsst$_4$	hsst$_5$
Cerebral cortex	Cerebral cortex	Cerebral cortex	Cerebral cortex	–
–	Cerebellum	Cerebellum	Cerebellum	Cerebellum
Hypothalamus	–	–	–	–
Pituitary gland (adult)	Pituitary gland (adult)	Pituitary gland (adult)	–	Pituitary gland (adult)
Eye	Eye	Eye	Eye	Eye
–	Thyroid (2B)	Thyroid	Thyroid	Thyroid
Parathyroid	–	Parathyroid	Parathyroid	Parathyroid
Thymus	Thymus(2A)	Thymus	–	–
Pulmonary parenchyma	Pulmonary parenchyma(2A)	–	Pulmonary parenchyma	–
Bronchial epithelium	Bronchial epithelium (2B)	Bronchial epithelium	Bronchial epithelium	Bronchial epithelium
Myocardium	Myocardium	–	–	–
–	–	–	–	Striated muscles
–	Myenteric plexus (2A)	–	–	–
Stomach	Stomach	Stomach	Stomach	Stomach
Oesophagus	–	–	–	–
Duodenum (Brunner's gland)	Duodenum (Brunner's gland)	Duodenum (Brunner's gland)	Duodenum (Brunner's gland)	Duodenum (Brunner's gland)

Table 2.2 (continued)

hsst$_1$	hsst$_{2A/2B}$	hsst$_3$	hsst$_4$	hsst$_5$
Small intestine, epithelial cell	Small intestine, epithelial cell	–	–	Small intestine
Small intestine, funding gland	Small intestine, funding gland (2B)	Small intestine, funding gland	–	Small intestine, funding gland
Large intestine	Large intestine	Large intestine	–	Large intestine
Rectum	Rectum	–	–	–
Liver, hepatocytes	–	–	–	Liver
Liver, cholangiocytes	Liver, cholangiocytes	–	–	–
Pancreas, islet cells	Pancreas	Pancreas	Pancreas	Pancreas
Pancreas, non-islet cells	–	Pancreas, non-islet cells	Pancreas, non-islet cells	Pancreas, non-islet cells
–	Spleen	–	–	–
Kidneys, glomus	Kidneys	–	–	–
Kidneys, tubule	Kidneys, tubule	–	Kidneys, tubule	Kidneys, tubule
Adrenal glands	Adrenal glands	Adrenal glands	Adrenal glands	Adrenal glands
Placenta	–	–	Placenta	Placenta
–	Endometrium	–	–	–
–	Prostate	–	Prostate	Prostate
–	Bone marrow	–	–	–
–	B and T lymphocytes	B and T lymphocytes	–	–
–	Monocytes, macrophages	–	–	–
–	Parotid gland, acinar cells (2B)	–	–	Parotid gland, acinar cells

Table 2.3 Synthetic somatostatin analogues and their characteristics

	Amino acids	Half-life	Receptors	Application route
Native somatostatin	14 και 28	≤3 min	ss1–5	i.v.
Octreotide [29]	8	2 h	ss2, ss5	acetate: i.v., s.c. LAR: i.m.
Lanreotide [30]	8	2 h	ss2, ss5	Lanreotide: s.c. *Lanreotide PR*: i.m. Lanreotide *AG*: s.c.
Pasireotide [31]	6	12 h	ss1–3, ss5	Pasireotide: s.c. *Pasireotide LAR*: i.m.

AG autogel, *LAR* long acting repeatable, *Lanreotide PR* Lanreotide prolonged release, *Pasireotide LAR* Pasireotide prolonged release

References

1. Obituary notices. Br Med J 1971; 4:628. https://doi.org/10.1136/bmj.4.5787.628.
2. Public domain; http://resource.nlm.nih.gov/101441443
3. CREDIT Phil Jones, GHSU Photographer, usage restrictions none; https://www.eurekalert.org/multimedia/pub/web/40267_web.jpg
4. Karfis I. PhD thesis, Medical School, National and Kapodistrian University of Athens-Greece; 2016.
5. Harris GW. Neural control of the pituitary gland. Monographs of the Physiological Society 3. London: Edward Arnold Publishers Ltd; 1955. p. 298.
6. Green JD, Harris GW. The neurovascular link between the neuro-hypophysis and the adenohypophysis. J Endocrinol. 1947;5:136–46.
7. Harris GW. Humours and hormones. The Sir Henry Dale Lecture for 1971. J Endocrinol. 1972;53:1–23.
8. Raisman G. An urge to explain the incomprehensible: Geoffrey Harris and the discovery of the neural control of the pituitary gland. Annu Rev Neurosci. 1997;20:533–66.

9. Burgus R, Dunn TF, Desiderio D, et al. Molecular structure of the hypothalamic hypophysiotropic TRF factor of ovine origin: mass spectrometry demonstration of the PCA-His-Pro-NH2 sequence. Comptes Rendus Hebdomadaires des Séances de l' Académie des Sci. 1969;269:1870–3.

10. Schally AV, Redding TW, Bowers CY, et al. Isolation and properties of porcine thyrotropin-releasing hormone. J Biol Chem. 1969;244(15):4077–88.

11. Krulich L, Dhariwal AP, McCann S. Stimulatory and inhibitory effects of purified hypothalamic extracts on growth hormone release from rat pituitary in vivo. Endocrinology. 1968;83:783–90.

12. Hellman B, Lernmark A. Inhibition of the in vitro secretion of insulin by an extract of pancreatic alpha-1 cells. Endocrinology. 1969;84:1484–8.

13. Edman P. Method for determination of the amino acid sequence in peptides. Acta Chem Scand. 1950;4:283–93.

14. Guillemin R. Peptides in the brain. The new endocrinology of the neuron. Nobel Lecture; 1977.

15. Guillemin R. Hypothalamic hormones a.k.a. hypothalamic releasing factors. J Endocrinol. 2005;184:11–28.

16. Guillemin R. Somatostatin. The beginnings, 1972. Mol Cell Endoc. 2008;286:3–4.

17. Guillemin R. Neuroendocrinology: a short historical review. Ann N Y Acad Sci. 2011;1220:1–5.

18. Brazeau P, Vale W, Burgus R, et al. Hypothalamic polypeptide that inhibits the secretion of immunoreactive pituitary growth hormone. Science. 1973;179:71–9.

19. Koerker DJ, Ruch W, Chideckel E. Somatostatin: hypothalamic inhibitor of the endocrine pancreas. Science. 1974;184:482–4.

20. Dubois MP. Immunoreactive somatostatin is present in discrete cells of the endocrine pancreas. Proc Natl Acad Sci U S A. 1975;72(4):1340–3.

21. Hökfelt T, Efendić S, Hellerström C, et al. Cellular localization of somatostatin in endocrine-like cells and neurons of the rat with special references to the A1-cells of the pancreatic islets and to the hypothalamus. Acta Endoc Suppl (Copenh). 1975;200:5–41.

22. Patel YC. Somatostatin and its receptor family. Front Neuroendocrinol. 1999;20:157–98.

23. Taniyama Y, Suzuki T, Mikami Y, et al. Systemic distribution of somatostatin receptor subtypes in human: an immuno-histochemical study. Endocr J. 2005;52(5):605–11.

24. Sheppard MC, Shapiro B, Pimstone BL, et al. Metabolic clearance and plasma half disappearance time of exogenous somatostatin in man. J Clin Endocrinol Metab. 1979;48:50–3.

25. Ho LT, Chen RL, Chou TY, et al. Pharmacokinetics and effects of intravenous infusion of somatostatin in normal subjects—a two-compartment open model. Clin Physiol Biochem. 1968;4(4):257–67.

26. Hildebrand P, Ensinck JW, Buettiker J, et al. Circulating somatostatin-28 is not a physiologic regulator of gastric acid production in man. Eur J Clin Inv. 1994;24(1):50–6.

27. Rivier J, Brown M, Vale W. D-Trp^8-somatostatin: an analog of somatostatin more potent than the native molecule. Biochem Biophys Res Commun. 1975;65(2):746–51.

28. Janecka A, Zubrzycka M, Janecki T. Somatostatin analogs. J Pept Res. 2001;58(2):91–107.

29. Mazziotti G, Mosca A, Frara S, et al. Somatostatin analogs in the treatment of neuroendocrine tumors: current and emerging aspects. Expert Opin Pharmacother. 2017;18:1679–89.

30. Caplin ME, Pavel M, Ćwikła JB, et al. Lanreotide in metastatic enteropancreatic neuroendocrine tumors. N Engl J Med. 2014;371:224–33.

31. Vitale G, Dicitore A, Sciammarella C, et al. Pasireotide in the treatment of neuroendocrine tumors: a review of the literature. Endo Related Cancer. 2018;25:R351–64. https://doi.org/10.1530/erc-18-0010.

Georgios S. Limouris

3.1 Syllabus-Classification-Epidemiology

The understanding of the structure and functioning of the neuroendocrine system has engendered impressive developments since the late nineteenth century, along with corresponding changes in its nomenclature [1, 2]. Assumptions about a distinct role began to be expressed, initially by the German physiologist Heidenhain [3–5] (Fig. 3.1) and subsequently by the Russian physician Kulchitsky [3, 6] (Fig. 3.2), after the localisation in the intestine of individual cells or populations of cells having secretory vesicles with chromophilic properties ['chromaffin', potassium dichromate (K2Cr2O7)] staining.

Although these cells were already called Kulchitsky (in honour of the man who discovered them), a few years later, MC Ciaccio (1877–1956) characterised them as entero-chromaffin [8, 9]. Their role remained unclear for a long time, until silverchrom staining ('argenta-chromaffin') [10] and silver staining ('argentaffin') [11] characteristics were observed and the concept of endocrine function was added. Similar cells were also found in the lungs, thymus and thyroid gland. F Feyrter (1895–1973) was the first to formulate the concept of a *diffuse endo-crine system* ('Diffuse Endokrine Epitheliale Organe') that included 'helle Zellen' with local 'paracrine' activity due to the secretion of biologically active peptides [12].

APUD Neoplasms (Apudomas): A few decades later (1966), Antony Pearse observed that some of these cells possess the ability to pick up and decarboxylate precursor amines as well as produce and store peptides in their secretory vesicles. He introduced the term APUD (**A**mine **P**recursor **U**ptake and **D**ecarboxylation cells), which is considered to be the first attempt to determine the neuroendocrine system [13–15]. Moreover, he thought that these were complementary to the autonomic nervous system with regard to the control of organ function and that they had a common embryologic origin from the neural crest as 'misplaced' neuronal cells. Although the use of the term has fallen out of favour,[1] the acronym APUD has demonstrated the connection between neuronal and endocrine

---

[1]This is because there are endocrine cells (parathyroid gland cells) that do not express APUD behaviour and exocrine cells (Lieberkühn's Paneth cells) that surprisingly express APUD behaviour; additionally, it is well known that the neuroendocrine cells of the gastrointestinal tract have an endodermal, rather than exodermal, embryologic origin [20].

G. S. Limouris (✉)
Nuclear Medicine, Medical School, National and Kapodistrian University of Athens, Athens, Greece
e-mail: glimouris@med.uoa.gr

© Springer Nature Switzerland AG 2021
G. S. Limouris (ed.), *Liver Intra-arterial PRRT with* ^{111}*In-Octreotide*,
https://doi.org/10.1007/978-3-030-70773-6_3

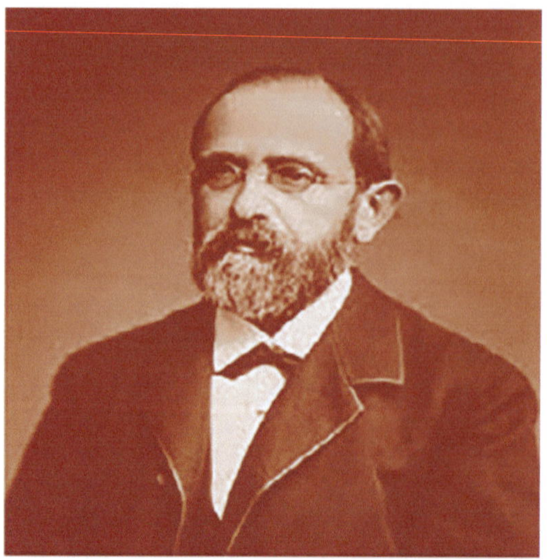

Fig. 3.1 Rudolf P.H. Heidenhain (1834–1897) [3, 5]

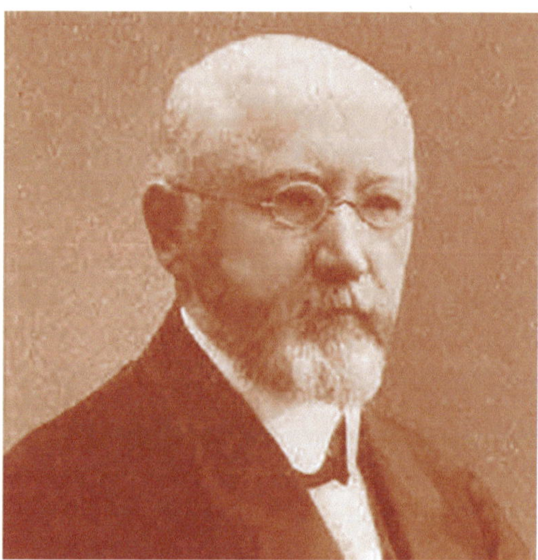

Fig. 3.2 Nikolai K. Kulchitsky (1856–1925) [6, 7]

Table 3.1 The phenotype of a neuroendocrine cell

► The presence of secretory vesicles in the cytoplasm in which they are stored and from which neurotransmitters or neuroregulatory peptides with endocrine, paracrine or autocrine activity are released by exocytosis (after external stimulation). Two types of secretory vesicles have been described so far: (a) dense core secretory vesicles, which consist of the characteristic secretory structures of the endocrine cells and (b) synaptic-like microvesicles, which resemble the synaptic vesicles of nerve endings.

► The expression of a wide range of neuroendocrine immunohistochemical markers: (a) General markers, i.e. chromogranin-A, synaptophysin, enolase, protein gene product 9.5 and (b) Specific markers, i.e. neuroendocrine secretion protein-55, ghrelin.

► The absence of neuro-axial projections or neuronal synapses.

cells, leading to the more relevant determination of these cells as *neuroendocrine* [16–18]. The latter constitutes a population of cells with marked *neuroendocrine* differentiation (Table 3.1), including cells potentially displaying a *neuroendocrine phenotype* after the activation of specific genetic switches [19].

The neuroendocrine system has elements of the central and peripheral nervous system (neuroblasts and paranaglial cells, neurons of the submucosa and myenteric intestinal neural plexus) and endocrine organs (pituitary gland, adrenal medulla, endocrine pancreas, thyroid C cells and parathyroid chief cells) as well as clusters of transiently distributed neuroendocrine cells predominantly localised in the gastrointestinal tract (δ-cells of the mucosa), lungs, skin (Merkel cells) and, less frequently, in the thymus, breasts, larynx, bladder and genital organs [18–21]. In particular, the gastrointestinal δ-cells constitute a broad set of at least 16 different endocrine cells, which produce over 50 different regulatory peptides [22]. They are perhaps the single most important and most complex organ of the endocrine system.

Neuroendocrine Neoplasms (NENs): Neuroendocrine neoplasms (NENs) are neuroendocrine cell tumors. They are a heterogeneous set with different clinical behaviours depending on the organ involved, the size and degree of volume differentiation and whether they are functioning. The identification of these neoplasms as 'neuroendocrine' is controversial. While it does not suggest a common embryological origin [20], it continues to be used mainly because of the common biochemical markers of neuroendocrine cells with nerve cells (chromogranin A, B, C, synaptophysin, neuron-specific enolase). Although there are few who favour this definition of 'endocrine', both names for these tumors are considered equivalent. There is also a

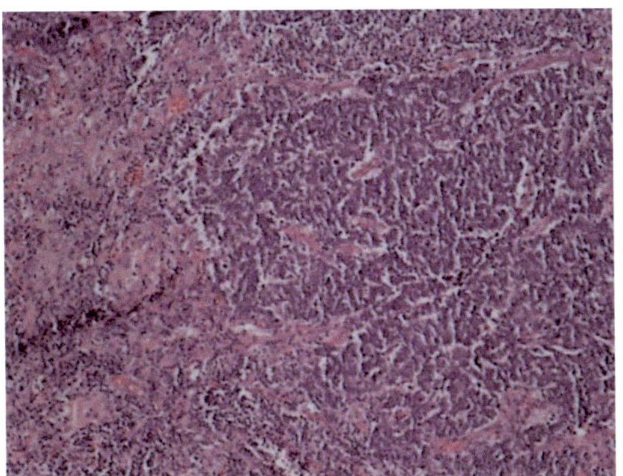

Fig. 3.3 Histological section of a Merkel cell carcinoma of the skin metastatic to lymph node (Haematoxylin-Eosin ×10)

controversy about whether 'tumor' or 'neoplasia' should be used. The latter is more accurate since NENs are potentially malignant; however, the term 'neuroendocrine tumors' dominates internationally, reflecting only the concept of a mass lesion [23, 24].

Gastro-entero-pancreatic Neuroendocrine Tumors (GEP-NETs): Gastro-entero-pancreatic neuroendocrine tumors such as carcinoid tumors and pancreatic tumors (insulinoma, glucagonoma, somatostatinoma, gastrinoma, VIPoma, PPOMa), catecholamine seizures (pheochromocytoma, paraganglioma, neuroblastoma), myeloid carcinoma of the thyroid, adenomas and carcinomas of the pituitary and parathyroid glands, small-cell lung carcinoma and Merkel cell carcinoma (derived from the homonymous cells, (Fig. 3.3)), pheochromocytoma of the adrenals, pituitary adenomas and neoplasms derived from the diffuse neuroendocrine system (DNS)— such as neuroendocrine tumors of the lungs, the gastrointestinal tract and pancreas—are categorised as NENs. GEP-NETs comprise the majority of NENs (about 75%) [25]. Although they account for only 2% of gastric intestinal system tumors [26], given their clinically silent nature, they are the most common neoplasms, after colon cancer, of the digestive system [27]. Reports of

unusual invasive processes in the small intestine, probably GEP-NETs, have existed since the nineteenth century [28–30].

GEP-NETs constitute neoplasms with significant differences in the clinical, laboratory and histological profile as well as in their ability to metastasise. This, coupled with the continuous development of the neuroendocrine system concept and the discovery of neoplasms in the NEN spectrum, has made it extremely difficult to classify them. The first attempt at classification by Williams et al. [31] was based on their embryological segmental origin, morphological idiotype and silverchrom staining ('argenta-chromaffin') and concerned three categories: *'foregut'* for tumors originating from the stomach, duodenum, proximal jejunum, pancreas, lungs and thymus gland, 'midgut' for tumors originating from the distal jejunum, ileum, appendix, cecum, and ascending and proximal half of the transverse colon and 'hindgut' for the tumors of the remaining parts of the colon and rectum. This classification failed to gain widespread acceptance but is still used in everyday clinical practice.

From an *epidemiological* point of view, GEP-NETs are much rarer than adenocarcinomas. Their incidence in the general population is about 2.5–5 cases per 100,000 people, while carcinoid tumors (bronchial-pulmonary and gastrointestinal) generally account for 0.46% of all malignant neoplasms [25]. It is clear however that both the incidence and prevalence of carcinoids have increased significantly in recent decades. The clinical behaviour of GEP-NETs is strikingly diverse in relation to both the manifestation of symptoms and the outcome of the disease. For instance, the 5-year survival rate for all carcinoids is 67.2%, whereas the corresponding survival rate for neuroendocrine pancreatic tumors ranges from 97% (mild insulinoma) to about 30% (on non-functioning, clinically silent endocrine tumors of the pancreas). These data support the need to revise the view of GEP-NETs as relatively benign lesions with slow growth.

3.2 Therapeutic Approaches Towards Neuroendocrine Tumors

In patients, neuroendocrine tumors may appear as a single lesion, with or without regional or distal metastases. The usual location of these metastases is the liver. These tumors, if non-functioning, may remain clinically silent until there is a significant burden to the liver due to the tumor-volume pressure on the hepatic parenchyma. Therapeutic options include surgery, administration of somatostatin analogues (SSA), therapeutic schemes with interferon, chemotherapy, targeting the molecules, loco-regional therapies and peptide receptor radionuclide therapy (PRRNT). Supportive palliative care and pain control play an important role in the management of these patients. These options are not exclusive and are, as a rule, interchangeable in their application. Care options, including PRRNT, should be applied in a correct line strategy by an experienced multidisciplinary team. This approach should provide the maximum benefit, minimising risks and side effects and ensuring the best possible quality of life achievable for the patient.

3.2.1 Interventional Approach

A surgical approach with therapeutic intent should be the method used whenever possible. In selected cases and through a multidisciplinary process, radiopeptide therapy (PRRNT) may be beneficial as an adjuvant treatment to make a patient more accessible to the impending surgery. For functionally active tumors, cytoreductive strategies—such as trans-arterial chemoembolisation (TACE), trans-arterial embolisation (TAE), radiofrequency ablation (RFA)—and other techniques, such as selective internal radiation therapy (SIRT), should be applied with the intention of improving clinical symptoms.

The optimal management of neuroendocrine tumors requires early surgical removal prior to the development of metastases. Unfortunately, there are many patients with metastatic disease whose tumors cannot be completely eradicated. Removing the primaries is indicated to prevent complications, such as bleeding or small bowel obstruction. Even with the presence of liver metastases, the removal of the primary lesion has many advantages and a positive prognostic effect on the survival of these patients [32–35]. Mono- or well-delineated hepatic metastases can be surgically removed, while diffuse hepatic infiltration is best dealt with by applying a loco-regional approach.

Loco-regional approaches or loco-suppressive therapies are mainly applied to hepatic metastases; they aim at controlling the tumor and facilitating the recession of the accompanying functional syndromes. Different techniques are applied according to the associated findings (such as the size and distribution of the number of hepatic lesions), morphology (focal or diffuse), vascularisation, their functioning or non-functioning tumor activity and the therapist's knowledge. In cases of oligo-focal liver localisations with a primary already excised, it is preferable to surgically exclude these few hepatic sites by treating them by RFA application or laser-diathermy suppression. In cases of multiple hepatic localisations or diffuse liver disease of high tumor burden, the application of TACE or TAE would be the best option [36, 37]. Embolisation techniques are particularly useful for treating patients with functionally active liver metastases. After chemoembolisation, a successful response of the symptoms has been reported at a rate up to 60–95%, a biochemical response up to 50–90% and a radiological response up to 33–80% [38–40]. Response time without recurrent symptoms ranged from 18–24 months. Similar responses have been achieved by implementing only TAE [18]. Generally, the procedure requires more than one session to ensure the efficacy and stability of the outcome and to minimise the potential risk of complications. The newly introduced SIRT technique demonstrates varying success rates [41]. Unfortunately, prospective studies on this are missing. In a single prospective study of 34 patients, the objective response was 50% [40]. Given the lack of other comparative studies with other different loco-suppressive applications, the choice of the technique followed depends largely on the physician's experience and skills as well as related criteria such as the number, size, vasculature and distribution of the lesions. In the available medical treatments, octreotide and lanreotide are the two most commonly used somatostatin receptor agonists. They play a key role in controlling both symptomatic and asymptomatic neuroendocrine tumors and should therefore be considered to be first-line therapeutic peptides. Cold somatostatin is to be used in conjunction with the aforementioned therapeutic techniques. Because the majority (87–92%) of neuroendocrine tumors overexpress subtype 2 (sst2) receptors, somatostatin therapy should be offered in parallel with other treatment options to enhance the therapeutic effect. Long-acting somatostatin (SSA-LAR) is characterised by an inhibitory secretory activity and has been shown to reduce the symptoms of carcinoid syndrome, such as flashing, diarrhoea and bronchospasm, and prevent seizures in 40–90% of the patients [42, 43]. Nonetheless, patients may be resistant to the control of the syndrome and require a gradual increase in SSA dosing. Most patients with progressive tumor behaviour resort to PRRNT. A recent PROMID study in Germany demonstrated the efficacy of long-acting SSA as an inhibitory agent in the progression of midgut neuroendocrine tumors [44, 45].

3.2.2 Interferon Alfa (IFN-α)

This has been used to treat patients with neuroendocrine tumors, especially those with carcinoid syndrome, for more than 25 years. It is considered to be the main antisecretory, active drug used for the treatment of functioning tumors [46]. IFN-α effectively reduces hypersecretion in patients with carcinoid syndrome, similar to cold somatostatin analogues (SSAs). A partial response (PR) to tumor growth was also observed in 10–15% of patients with malignant carcinoids and in 39% of patients with disease stabilisation (SD). IFN-α has also been proven effective in treating pancreatic endocrine tumors [47]. Its most common side effect, i.e. 'flu-like' symptoms, limits both the use of higher doses and the duration of treatment as this intolerance causes it to be discontinued.

3.2.3 Systemic Chemotherapy

Systemic chemotherapy is effective in some patients, especially those with low-differentiated NETs (grade 3, WHO, 2010) or progressive NETs of the pancreas. However, in well-differentiated midgut neuroendocrine tumors (NET 1 to 2 WHO, 2010), the response rate to chemotherapy is low (7–20%), without a survival advantage [48–52]. Classical treatment for neuroendocrine tumors (grade 3) is cisplatin in combination with etoposide. The response rate to this combination is 42–67%, and its duration is often short, ranging from 8–9 months [34]. The combination of irinotecan and cisplatin [50] or FOLFOX [Folinic acid + Fluorouracil (5-FU) + Oxaliplatin (Eloxatin)] chemotherapy can be an alternative therapeutic scheme [51]. Streptozotocin-based systemic chemotherapy (Zanosar, STZ) is considered to be the (classical) established therapy for worsening (progressive) neuroendocrine pancreatic tumors, with low or moderate proliferative capacity. A combination of STZ and 5-fluorouracil and/or doxorubicin has been shown to result in a partial response (PR) of the disease at 35–40% [52–54]. Recent Phase II chemotherapy studies have shown efficacy based on temozolomide in combination with antiangiogenic drugs or capecitabine [55, 56]. The standards for patient care in the use of chemotherapy have been extensively defined by the European Society of Neuroendocrine Tumors (ENETS) [57].

In recent years, the efficacy of radio-molecular targeting therapies for treating NETs has been evaluated by clinical trials. These targeting therapies include angiogenesis inhibitors, mono- or poly-inhibitors of tyrosine kinase and the new somatostatin analogue, pasireotide, for which clinical trials are currently in progress. As of now, other drugs with the highest mark of efficacy are sunitinib and everolimus. Both lead to the prolongation of 'progression free survival' (PFS) in patients with advanced pancreatic

NET. Furthermore, there is evidence that everolimus, an mTOR inhibitor, controls NETs, predominantly of pancreatic origin, locally advanced or with metastases accompanied by carcinoid syndrome (most commonly reported with adverse events as stomatitis, anaemia and hyperglycaemia) [58–61]. The most developed antiangiogenic drugs are sunitinib and bevacizumab, the anti-VEGF antibody [58, 59]. The former is used in cases of advanced, progressive, well-differentiated pancreatic NET. Globally, the supportive approach towards PRRNT patients is a key component of care, focusing on diet and pain control. Analgesic therapy in patients with NET follows the general principles performed in adult or minor oncological patients [62]. Effective treatment of neuroendocrine tumors, with PRRNT for instance, can relieve pain, including bone pain. Treatment of depressive bone metastases is also required via the administration of bisphosphonates as supportive therapy.

References

1. Modlin IM, Champaneria MC, Bornschein J, et al. Evolution of the diffuse neuroendocrine system-clear cells and cloudy origins. Neuroendocrinology. 2006;84(2):69–82.
2. Drozdov I, Modlin IM, Kidd M, et al. From Leningrad to London: the saga of Kultschitzky and the legacy of the enterochromaffin cell. Neuroendocrinology. 2009;89(1):1–12.
3. De Herder WW, Rehfeld JF, et al. A short history of neuroendocrine tumours and their peptide hormones. Best Pract Res Clin Endocrinol Metab. 2015; https://doi.org/10.1016/j.beem.2015.10.004.
4. Heidenhain R. Untersuchungen über den Bau der Labdrusen. Arch Mikrosk Anat. 1870;6:368–406.
5. Public domain; http://resource.nlm.nih.gov/101418204
6. Kulchitsky N. Zur Frage über den Bau des Darmkanals. Arch Mikrosk Anat. 1897;49:7–35.
7. Public domain; http://rusk.ru/newsdata.php?idar=175371
8. Ciaccio MC. Sopra speciali cellule granulose della mucosa intestinale. Arch Ital Embriol. 1907;6:498–582.
9. Ciaccio MC. Sur une nouvelle espece cellulaire dans les glande de Lieberkühn. C R Soc Biol (Paris). 1906;60:76.
10. Masson P. La glande endocrine de l'intestin chez l'homme. C R Hebd Seances Acad Sci. 1914;158:59–61.
11. Hamperl H. Was sind argentaffine Zellen? Virchows Arch. 1932;286:811–33.
12. Feyrter F. Über diffuse endokrine epithelial Organe. Leipzig, Germany: JA Barth (Pbls); 1938.
13. Carvalheira AF, Welsch U, Pearse AG. Cytochemical and ultrastructural observations on the argentaffin and argyrophil cells of the gastro-intestinal tract in mammals, and their place in the APUD series of polypeptide-secreting cells. Histochemie. 1968;14(1):33–46.
14. Pearse AG. The cytochemistry and ultrastructure of polypeptide hormone-producing cells of the APUD series and the embryologic, physiologic and pathologic implications of this concept. J Histochem Cytochem. 1969;17:303–13.
15. Pearse AG. The APUD cell concept and its implications in pathology. Pathol Annu. 1974;9:27–41.
16. Langley K. The neuroendocrine concept today. Ann NY Acad Science. 1994;733:1–17.
17. De Lellis RA. The neuroendocrine system and its tumors: an overview. Am J Clin Pathol. 2001;115(S1):S5–16.
18. Kino SR. Ch. 10: Neuroendocrine system and neuroendocrine neoplasia. In: Kini SR, editor. Colo Atlas of differential diagnosis in exfoliative and aspiration cytopathology. 2nd ed. Philadelphia, PA: Wolters-Kluwer Lippincott Williams & Wilkins Section III (Fine Needle Aspiration Cytopathology); 2011. p. 349–69.
19. Day R, Salzet M. The neuroendocrine phenotype, cellular plasticity, and the search for genetic switches: redefining the diffuse neuroendocrine system. Neuroendoc Letters. 2002;23:447–51.
20. Andrew A, Kramer B, Rawdon BB. The origin of gut and pancreatic neuroendocrine (APUD) cells the last word? J Pathol. 1998;186:117–8.
21. De Lellis RA, Tischler AS. The dispersed neuroendocrine cell system. In: Kovacs K, Asa SL, editors. Functional endocrine pathology. 2nd ed. Blackwell Scientific: Malden, MA; 1998. p. 529–49.
22. Modlin IM, Öberg K, Chung DC, et al. Gastroenteropancreatic neuro-endocrine tumours. Lancet Oncol. 2008;9:61–72.
23. Klöppel G. Classification and pathology of gastroenteropancreatic neuro-endocrine neo-plasms. Endoc Rel Cancer. 2011;18(S1):S1–16.
24. Klimstra DS, Modlin IR, Coppola D. The pathologic classification of neuro-endocrine tumors: a review of nomenclature, grading, and staging systems. Pancreas. 2010;39:707–12.
25. Modlin IM, Lye KD, Kidd M. A 5-decade analysis of 13,715 carcinoid tumors. Cancer. 2003;97:934–59.
26. Warner RR. Enteroendocrine tumors other than carcinoid: a review of clinically significant advances. Gastroenterology. 2005;128:1668–84.

27. Schimmack S, Svejda B, Lawrence B, et al. The diversity and commonalities of gastroenteropancreatic neuroendocrine tumors. Langenbeck's Arch Surg. 2011;396:273–98.
28. Langhans T. Über einen Drüsenpolyp im Ileum. Virchow Arch Pathol Anat. 1867;38:550–60.
29. Lubarsch O. Über den primären Krebs des Ileums, nebst Bemerkungen über das gleichzeitige Vorkommen von Krebs und Tuberkulose. Virchow Arch Pathol Anat. 1888;111:280–317.
30. Ransom W. A case of primary carcinoma of the ileum. Lancet. 1890;2:1020–3.
31. Williams ED, Sandler M. The classification of carcinoid tumor. Lancet. 1963;1:238–9.
32. Kerström G, Hellman P, Hessman O. Midgut carcinoid tumors: surgical treatment and prognosis. Best Pract Res Clin Gastroenterol. 2005;19:717–28.
33. Plöckinger U, Couvelard A, Falconi M, et al. Consensus guidelines for the management of patients with digestive neuroendocrine tumors: well-differentiated tumour/carcinoma of the appendix and goblet cell carcinoma. Neuroendocrinology. 2008;87:20–30.
34. Ramage JK, Goretzki PE, Manfredi R, et al. Consensus guidelines for the management of patients with digestive neuroendocrine tumors: well-differentiated colon and rectum tumor/carcinoma. Neuroendocrinology. 2008;87:31–9.
35. Givi B, Pommier SJ, Thompson AK, et al. Operative resection of primary carcinoid neoplasms in patients with liver metastases yields significantly better survival. Surgery. 2006;140:891–7.
36. Steinmüller T, Kianmanesh R, Falconi M, et al. Consensus guidelines for the management of patients with liver metastases from digestive (neuro)endocrine tumors: foregut, midgut, hindgut, and unknown primary. Neuroendocrinology. 2008;87:47–62.
37. Vogl TJ, Naguib NN, Zangos S, et al. Liver metastases of neuroendocrine carcinomas: interventional treatment via transarterial embolization, chemoembolization and thermal ablation. Eur J Radiol. 2009;72:517–28.
38. Kamat PP, Gupta S, Ensor JE, et al. Hepatic arterial embolization and chemoembolization in the management of patients with large-volume liver metastases. Cardiovasc Intervent Radiol. 2008;31:299–307.
39. Ruszniewski P, Malka D. Hepatic arterial chemoembolization in the management of advanced digestive endocrine tumors. Digestion. 2000;62(Suppl 1):79–83.
40. King J, Quinn R, Glenn DM, et al. Radioembolization with selective internal radiation microspheres for neuroendocrine liver metastases. Cancer. 2008;113:921–9.
41. Kennedy AS, Dezarn WA, McNeillie P, et al. Radioembolization for unresectable neuroendocrine hepatic metastases using resin 90Y-microspheres: early results in 148 patients. Am J Clin Oncol. 2008;31:271–9.
42. Ruszniewski P, Ish-Shalom S, Wymenga M, et al. Rapid and sustained relief from the symptoms of carcinoid syndrome: results from an open 6-month study of the 28-day prolonged-release formulation of lanreotide. Neuroendocrinology. 2004;80:244–51.
43. Modlin IM, Pavel M, Kidd M, et al. Review article: somatostatin analogues in the treatment of gastroenteropancreatic neuroendocrine (carcinoid) tumors. Aliment Pharmacol Ther. 2010;31:169–88.
44. Eriksson B, Klöppel G, Krenning E, et al. Consensus guidelines for the management of patients with digestive neuroendocrine tumors—well-differentiated jejunal-ileal tumour/carcinoma. Neuroendocrinology. 2008;87:8–19.
45. Rinke A, Müller HH, Schade-Brittinger C, et al. Placebo-controlled, double-blind, prospective, randomized study on the effect of octreotide LAR in the control of tumour growth in patients with metastatic neuroendocrine midgut tumors: a report from the PROMID Study Group. J Clin Oncol. 2009;27:4656–63.
46. Öberg K. Interferon in the management of neuroendocrine GEP tumors. Digestion. 2000;62(Suppl 1):92–7.
47. Eriksson B, Öberg K. An update of the medical treatment of malignant endocrine pancreatic tumors. Acta Oncol. 1993;32:203–8.
48. Moertel CG, Kvols LK, O'Connell MJ, et al. Treatment of neuroendocrine carcinomas with combined etoposide and cisplatin. Evidence of major therapeutic activity in the anaplastic variants of these neoplasms. Cancer. 1991;68:227–32.
49. Moertel CG, Johnson CM, McKusick MA, et al. The management of patients with advanced carcinoid tumors and islet cell carcinomas. Ann Intern Med. 1994;120:302–9.
50. Mani MA, Shroff RT, Jacobs C, et al. A phase II study of irinotecan and cisplatin for metastatic or unresectable high-grade neuroendocrine carcinoma [abstract]. J Clin Oncol. 2008;26(Suppl)
51. Bajetta E, Catena L, Procopio G, et al. Are capecitabine and oxaliplatin (XELOX) suitable treatments for progressing low-grade and high-grade neuroendocrine tumors? Cancer Chemother Pharmacol. 2007;59:637–42.
52. Kouvaraki MA, Ajani JA, Hoff P, et al. Fluorouracil, doxorubicin, and streptozocin in the treatment of patients with locally advanced and metastatic pancreatic endocrine carcinomas. J Clin Oncol. 2004;22:4762–71.
53. Fjallskog ML, Janson ET, Falkmer UG, et al. Treatment with combined streptozotocin and liposomal doxorubicin in metastatic endocrine pancreatic tumors. Neuroendocrinology. 2008;88:53–8.
54. Moertel CG, Lefkopoulos M, Lipsitz S, et al. Streptozocin-doxorubicin, streptozocin-fluorouracil or chlorozotocin in the treatment of advanced islet-cell carcinoma. N Engl J Med. 1992;326:519–23.
55. Strosberg JR, Fine RL, Choi J, et al. First-line chemotherapy with capecitabine and temozolomide in

patients with metastatic pancreatic endocrine carcinomas. Cancer. 2011;117:268–75.

56. Kulke MH, Stuart K, Enzinger PC, et al. Phase II study of temozolomide and thalidomide in patients with metastatic neuroendocrine tumors. J Clin Oncol. 2006;24:401–6.

57. Eriksson B, Annibale B, Bajetta E, et al. ENETS consensus guidelines for the standards of care in neuroendocrine tumors: chemotherapy in patients with neuroendocrine tumors. Neuroendocrinology. 2009;90:214–9.

58. Yao JC, Phan A, Hoff PM, et al. Targeting vascular endothelial growth factor in advanced carcinoid tumour: a random assignment phase II study of depot octreotide with bevacizumab and pegylated interferon alpha-2b. J Clin Oncol. 2008;26:1316–23.

59. Raymond E, Dahan L, Raoul JL, et al. Sunitinib malate for the treatment of pancreatic neuroendocrine tumors. N Engl J Med. 2011;364:501–13.

60. Yao JC, Lombard-Bohas C, Baudin E, et al. Daily oral everolimus activity in patients with metastatic pancreatic neuroendocrine tumors after failure of cytotoxic chemotherapy: a phase II trial. J Clin Oncol. 2010;28:69–76.

61. Yao JC, Shah MH, et al. Everolimus for advanced pancreatic neuroendocrine tumors. N Engl J Med. 2011;364:514–23.

62. Patrick DL, Ferketich SL, Frame PS, et al. Symptom management in cancer: pain, depression, and fatigue. J Natl Cancer Inst. 2003;95:1110–7.

[^{111}In-DTPA^0-D-Phe^1]-Octreotide: The Ligand—The Receptor—The Label

4

Antonios Zanglis

4.1 The Somatostatin Peptide Family

Almost half a century ago, in the first January 1973 issue of *Science*, the Roger Guillemin group in the Salk Institute (La Jolla, California), published a paper that proved the presence of a bioactive peptide in ovine hypothalamic extracts, with inhibitory effect in the secretion of immunoreactive growth hormone (GH). In the same paper, the structure of this 14-peptide was elucidated and its synthetic form was shown to elicit the same biological response in rats and humans, as well, hence its name: Somatostatin (SST) or Somatotropin-release inhibiting factor" (SRIF) [1]. SST belongs to the homonymous peptide family with cortistatin (CST). CST-17 is the bioactive cleavage product of a CST precursor peptide in humans, being a relatively recent addition. CST-17 shares common structural and functional features with SST (SST: SST-14 and SST-28 are the bioactive peptides, see Fig. 4.1), such as the depression of neuronal activity and some distinct properties as well, such as the activation of cation selective currents, not responsive to SST. It should be emphasized though, that these peptides (SST and CST) are the products of separate genes [3–5].

SST is a phylogenetically ancient peptide that is widely distributed throughout the human body. Besides hypothalamus, SST is secreted by various cell populations interspersed mainly in the central and peripheral nervous system, the gut, and the thyroid, although smaller amounts are synthesized by tumor, inflammatory and immune cells (i.e. lymphocytes or macrophages) upon activation. In the gut, SST is produced in the δ cells encountered either in the submucous/myenteric plexus or in the pancreatic islets, next to other peptide-producing cell populations (i.e. insulin, glucagon, VIP: vasointestinal peptide), while in the thyroid, SST is localized in a subpopulation of calcitonin-secreting cells (C cells). The gastrointestinal tract is the main source for the assayed SST in plasma (picomolar amounts), taking into consideration its rapid proteolytic degradation in the circulation ($t_{1/2} = 1$–2 min). The SST-28 and SST-14 peptides with the GH inhibitory activity, start as part of a larger precursor protein (prepro-somatostatin or prepro-SST), the product of the corresponding gene located at the chromosome 3q28 in humans and consists of 116 amino acid residues. Proteolytic cleavage of prepro-SST yields initially pro-somatostatin (contains 92 amino acids), whose further processing at its C-terminal segment yields SST-28 and SST-14 (see Fig. 4.2). The relative amount of these peptides is a tissue- and species-dependent process [7, 8].

A. Zanglis (✉)
National Health System, Athens, Greece

© Springer Nature Switzerland AG 2021
G. S. Limouris (ed.), *Liver Intra-arterial PRRT with ^{111}In-Octreotide*,
https://doi.org/10.1007/978-3-030-70773-6_4

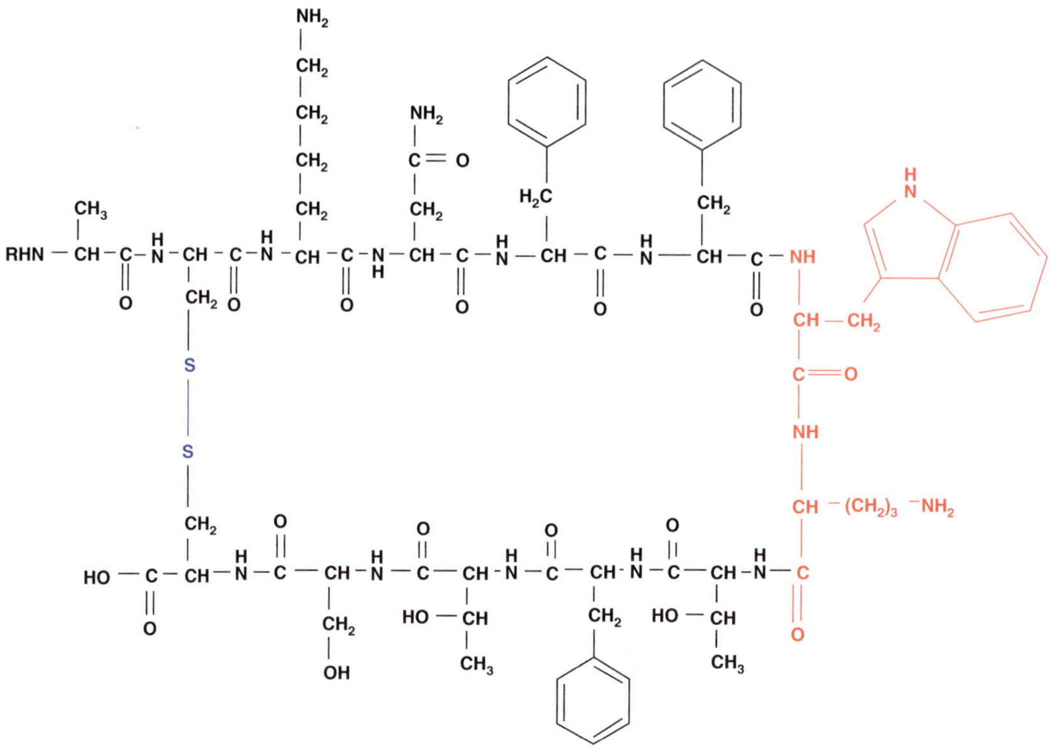

Fig. 4.1 Structure of the natural somatostatin (SST) peptide agonists SST-14 and SST-28. SST-14: R = H and SST-28: R = Ser-Ala-Asn-Ser-Asn-Pro-Ala-Met-Ala-pro-Arg-Glu-Arg-Lys. The pharmacophore (tryptophan and lysine) is highlighted in red [2]

The SST synthesis and release can be stimulated by a variety of hormones, neuropeptides, growth factors, neurotransmitters, cytokines, and nutrients (i.e. GHRH: growth hormone-releasing hormone, neurotensin and CRH: corticotropin-releasing hormone), while other mediators, such as γ-aminobutyric acid (GABA) and opiates generally inhibit SST secretion. In this context, the inflammatory cytokines IL-1, TNF-α, and IL-6 stimulate and TGF-β and leptin inhibit SST synthesis and release. SST acts on various tissues in an autocrine, paracrine, or endocrine fashion [9–11].

The very short biological half-life of somatostatin in the bloodstream, resulting from its vulnerability to the serum peptidases, makes the native bioactive somatostatin molecule (SST-14 or SST-28) unsuitable for imaging or therapy (including radiotherapy) applications. For this reason, the research focused on synthesis of various analogues is devoid of this drawback. The starting point of these efforts was based on the amino acid sequence of the SST-14 molecule and it was soon realized that the central segment of the polypeptide chain (-**Phe**^{7}-**Trp**^{8}-**Lys**^{9}-**Thr**^{10}-) was responsible for the SSTR binding. The main modification of a shortened portion (octapeptide) of the original SST-14 molecule was the substitution of certain key L-amino acids by their D-counterparts (i.e. L-Phe → D-Phe and L-Trp → D-Trp) to render the analogue resistant to the circulating peptidases. In addition, modification of amino acid side chains by incorporation of lipophilic groups (i.e. a 2-naphtalenyl group in place of the methyl group in D-Ala) significantly extended the biological half-life of the synthesized analogues (lanreotide, see Fig. 4.3) and altered its main excretion route (liver vs kidney). The presence of the -**S-S**- bridge between the two cysteine residues is indispensable, since it confers the essential conformational

Preprosomatostatin

H₂N-MLSCRLQCALAALSIVLALGCVTGAPSDP
RLRQFLQKSLAAAGKQELAKYFLAELLSEPN
QTENDALEPEDLSQAAEQDEMRLELQRSAN
SNPMAPRERK**AGCKNFFWTFTSC-COOH**

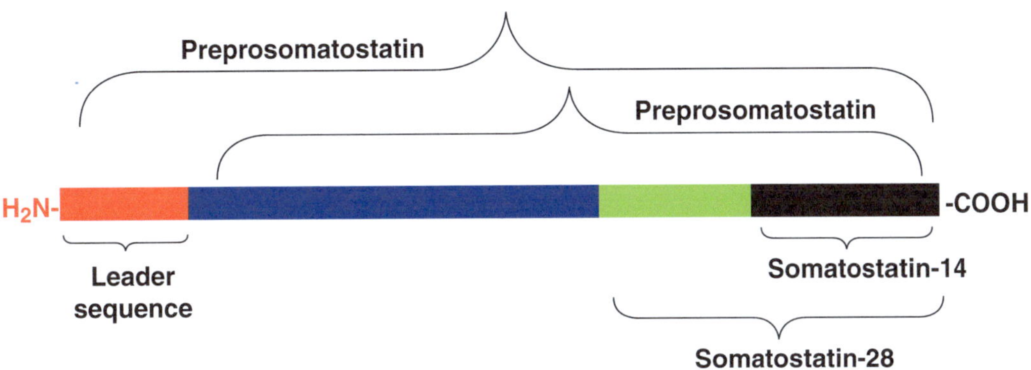

Fig. 4.2 The amino acid sequences of the prepro-somatostatin, pre-somatostatin (biologically inactive), somatostatin-28, and somatostatin-14 (biologically active) peptides (one-letter notation [6]). The biologically active sequences reside in the C-end of the precursor molecule [7]

rigidity to the synthesized peptide analogues, in order to maintain their bioactivity. In Fig. 4.3 the structures of some somatostatin analogues (agonists) are drawn. The peptidomimetic JR-11 is the most potent antagonist known so far [9–14].

4.2 The Somatostatin Receptor Family (SSTRs)

4.2.1 Definitions

Agonists are compounds that activate receptors to produce a characteristic set of biological effects.

Full agonists are compounds that act at receptors to effectively trigger the same signal transduction machinery and regulatory pathways as the native ligand.

Partial agonists are compounds that are less effective than full agonists at producing the downstream signaling and regulatory actions by a receptor.

Biased agonists are compounds that effectively elicit only a subset of multiple actions of a receptor for signaling or for receptor regulation.

Antagonists bind to receptors but do not activate them and hence are characterized by their ability to block agonist binding and action at a receptor. One needs to distinguish between **neutral antagonists**, which have no activity on their own but will block the effects of an agonist, as opposed to **inverse agonists**, which will inhibit receptor activity in the absence of an agonist, if the receptor exhibits constitutive activity. *A neutral antagonist does not distinguish between the active or inactive state of the receptor, whereas an inverse agonist prefers the inactive state.*

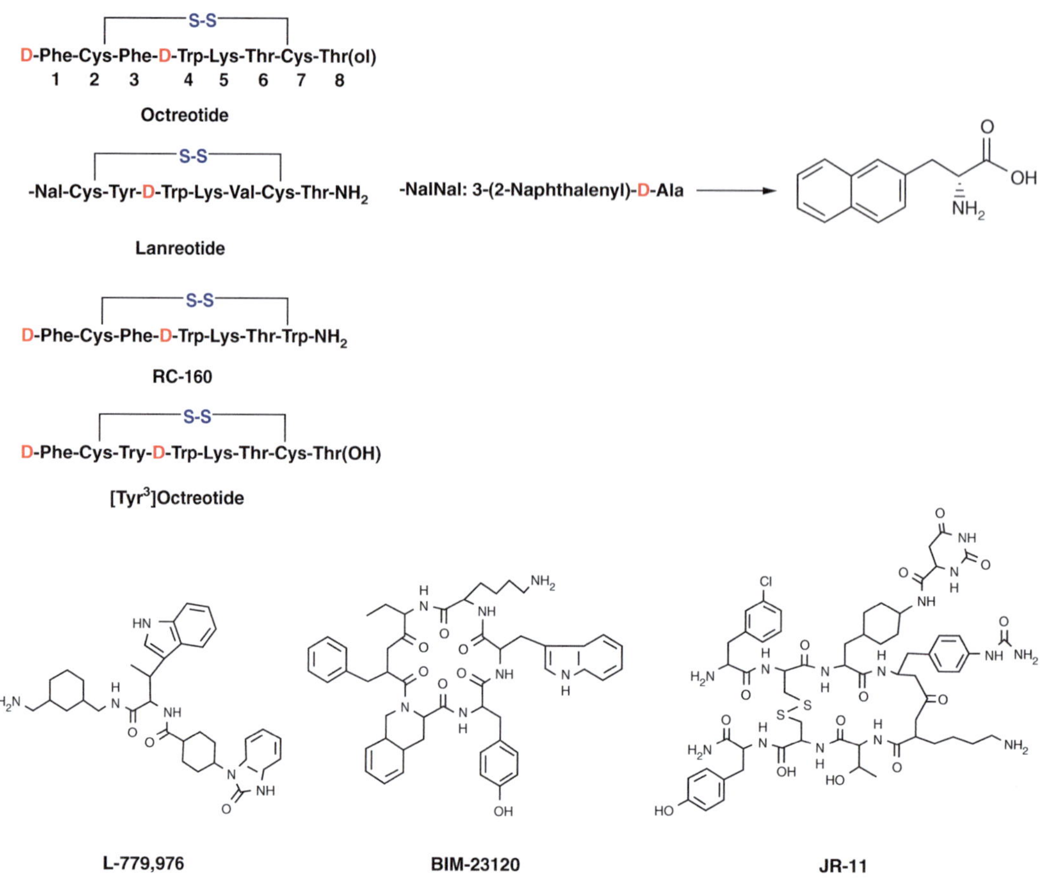

Fig. 4.3 Structures of selected somatostatin analogues (agonists) and antagonists (L-779,976-BIM-2310-JR-11). The presence of D amino acids, the modification of the –COOH end of the molecule (amidation or reduction), and the insertion of a lipophilic group (i.e. 2-naphtalenyl group in lanreotide) have a dramatic impact on the binding of these derivatives by the SSTRs, their solubility, serum half-life, etc. JR-11: Cpa-cyclo[D-Cys-Aph(Hor)-D-Aph(Cbm)-Lys-Thr-Cys]-D-Tyr-NH₂ (Cpa: 4-Cl-phenyl-alanine, Aph(Hor): 4-amino-L-hydroorotyl-phenylalanine, D-Aph(Cbm): D-4-amino-carbamoyl-phenylalanine

Although somatostatin receptor agonists, biased agonists, and neutral antagonists are known, no somatostatin receptor inverse agonists have been described [11].

4.2.2 Somatostatin Receptors: Biological Function

SST is known to exert a broad range of inhibitory behavior in endocrine (i.e. growth hormone, gastrin, insulin) and exocrine (pancreas) secretory processes, by exerting inhibitory neuromodulatory activity acting as neurotransmitter in central and peripheral nervous system, with antiprolifer-ative and proapoptotic behavior in various tissues [15]. These effects are mediated by the initial binding of SST in G-protein coupled receptors (GPCRs) located at the cell surface of the target cells. The somatostatin receptors (SSTRs) constitute a family of six distinct molecules (SSTR₁, SSTR₂ₐ, SSTR₂ᵦ, SSTR₃, SSTR₄ and SSTR₅), originating from five separate genes. SSTR₂ₐ and SSTR₂ᵦ are alternative splicing variants of the same gene and exhibit a somewhat different tissue distribution (SSTR₂ₐ is the prevailing subtype and it is expressed in almost 90% of the various tumors). All SSTSRs are anchored on the cell membrane through seven α-helical transmembrane domains and they are widely distributed in the CNS and peripheral tissues (pancreas, small intestine, etc.). SSTR expression is modulated by various factors, such as thyroid hormones or estrogens, which operate at the transcriptional level [13, 16–19].

There are four known endocytosis mechanisms: macropinocytosis, clathrin-dependent endocytosis, caveola-mediated endocytosis, and caveola/clathrin-independent endocytosis. The SST binding to the SSTRs induces receptor internalization (exception: SSTR₁) and/or uncoupling of the receptor from the G-proteins, thus resulting in receptor desensitization, a typical behavior encountered across the GCPR receptor spectrum. These processes appear to be dependent on molecular mechanisms implying selective phosphorylation of the SST-SSTRs (ligand-activated receptors) by G protein–coupled receptor kinases (GRKs) [18–23]. The phosphorylated SSTRs attract the cytoplasmic β-arrestins (thus terminating the G protein-mediated cellular response), which promote the endocytosis of the β-arrestin-bound receptors by binding to the clathrin-coated pits with the collaboration of adaptors such as adaptor protein AP-2 (see Fig. 4.4). The agonist-induced internalization ability of SSTRs, after binding SST or other analogues, is the key for providing the pathway for the intracellular localization of the various radiolabeled SST-analogues. It is exactly this property that makes the SSTR-targeted radiotherapy with SST-analogues labeled with Auger emitters possible. The affinity of a selected subset of somatostatin analogues (IC₅₀) for the SSTR subtypes is shown in Table 4.1. From this table it becomes evident that even small structural changes in the ligands result in large variations in the SSTR affinity profiles. These structural changes include the binding of

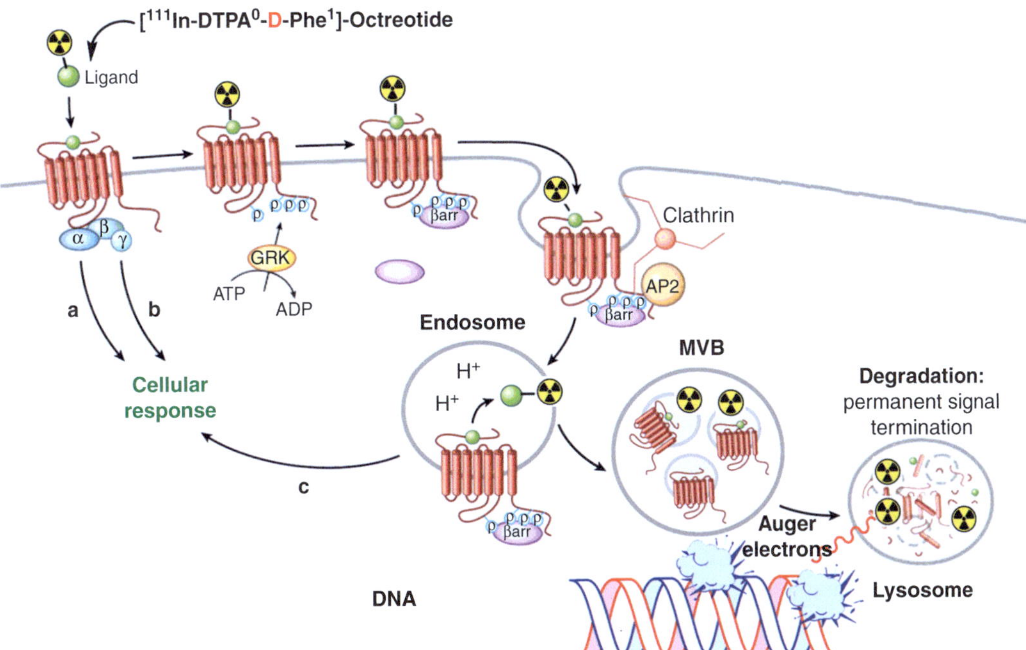

Fig. 4.4 Outline of the receptor-mediated [¹¹¹In-DTPA⁰-D-Phe¹]-Octreotide internalization process, through clathrin-coated pit and endosome formation and finally lysosomal degradation. SSTR phosphorylation promotes the recruitment of β-arrestins from the cytoplasm, preventing subsequent activation of G proteins by receptors and promoting receptor endocytosis via clathrin-coated pits. The receptors are recycled on the cell-surface (resensitization), while the ¹¹¹In-labeled degradation products are trapped in the cell and the emitted Auger electrons in the vicinity of the nucleus are highly radiotoxic (modified from [24]). βarr: β-arrestin, AP2 (adaptor complex): A heterotetramer consisting of two large adaptins (alpha and beta), a medium adaptin (mu) and a small adaptin (sigma), GRK: G protein–coupled receptor kinases, MVB: multivesicular body

Table 4.1 Affinity profiles (IC_{50}, nM) for human SSTRs (1–5 subtypes) of selected SST analogues (agonists) [25]

Peptide	$SSTR_1$	$SSTR_2$	$SSTR_3$	$SSTR_4$	$SSTR_5$
SST-28	5.2 ± 0.3	2.7 ± 0.3	7.7 ± 0.9	5.6 ± 0.4	4.0 ± 0.3
Octreotide	>10,000	2.0 ± 0.7	187 ± 55	>1000	22 ± 6
[DTPA^0-D-Phe^1]-Octreotide	>10,000	12 ± 2	376 ± 84	>1000	299 ± 50
[^{111}In-DTPA^0-D-Phe^1]-Octreotide	>10,000	22 ± 3.6	182 ± 13	>1000	237 ± 52
[DOTA^0-D-Phe^1-Tyr^3]-Octreotide	>10,000	14 ± 2.6	880 ± 324	>1000	393 ± 84
[DTPA^0-D-Phe^1-Tyr^3]-Octreotate	>10,000	3.9 ± 1	>10,000	>1000	>1000
[^{111}In-DTPA^0-D-Phe^1-Tyr^3]-Octreotate	>10,000	1.3 ± 0.2	>10,000	433 ± 16	>1000
[DOTA^0-D-Phe^1-Tyr^3]-Octreotate	>10,000	1.5 ± 0.4	>1000	453 ± 176	547 ± 160

the label (In-111) in the case of [^{111}In-DTPA^0-D-Phe^1]-Octreotide, the type of the aminocarboxylate chelator (DOTA vs. DTPA), a single aminoacid residue substitution (Phe^3 → Tyr^3) or changing the charge of the molecule (Octreotate: carries the –COOH group of threonine residue in the C-terminal of the peptide; Octreotide: reduction of the –COOH group of threonine to –CH$_2$OH) [26]. It is interesting to note from Table 4.1 that no analogue exhibits $SSTR_1$ binding affinity [11, 16, 20, 26, 27].

The SSTR subtypes do not appear to internalize somatostatin or somatostatin analogues with the same efficiency and at the same rate. From an in vitro model based on Chinese hamster ovary (CHO)-K_1 cells, stably expressing one of the five human SSTRs subtypes ($SSTR_2$, $SSTR_3$, $SSTR_4$ and $SSTR_5$), a rapid (within minutes) agonist-dependent internalization of a ^{125}I-labeled SST-28 ligand in a time- and temperature-dependent manner was observed. The maximum of the radioligand internalization was observed 60 min later. In this model, the $SSTR_3$ and $SSTR_5$ expressing cells exhibited the highest degree of internalization (78% and 66%, respectively), followed by $SSTR_4$ (29%) and $SSTR_2$ (20%), while the $SSTR_1$ subtype expressing cells displayed only a negligible amount of internalization (4%). The degree of internalization of the SSTR-ligand complex, besides being the receptor subtype-dependent, has been demonstrated to be ligand-dependent as well. For example, the [^{111}In-DTPA^0-D-Phe^1-Tyr^3]-Octreotate analogue exhibits the highest degree of internalization from the analogues of Table 4.1, an observation that has been confirmed in vivo in rats and humans [2, 14, 16, 18–20, 28].

Besides normal tissues, SSTRs are found on the cell surface of various tumor cells, such as tumors of pituitary, pancreatic, breast, and hematopoietic origin including their metastases. In general, $SSTR_{2a}$ is the most common SSTR subtype found in human tumors, followed by $SSTR_1$, with $SSTR_3$ and $SSTR_4$ being far less common. $SSTR_5$ appears to be more tumor specific with strong expression in some tumors (i.e. breast) and complete absence in others (i.e. pancreatic). The high density and frequency of SSTR expression in human tumors has been widely exploited as a therapeutic target and for imaging. It should be noted that more than one type of SSTRs may be expressed by the same tumor. Table 4.2 summarizes the various tumor types and their respective SSTR expression pattern, which inevitably leads to the wide variations observed in the % uptake of the labeled somatostatin analogues used in imaging or therapy of these neoplasms [19].

A fairly recent development in the field of SSTR targeting was the introduction of SSTR antagonists, which seemed to recognize more receptor binding sites on the cell surface. SSTR antagonists showed favorable pharmacokinetics and better tumor visualization than agonists, despite their very poor internalization rates (internalization is the sine qua non for radiotherapeutic applications of somatostatin analogues labeled with Auger-emitting isotopes). The binding of the SSTR antagonists has been found to be always higher compared to that of somatostatin analogues (agonists) in experiments with human tumor specimens, and this remarkable result can be easily appreciated from the data in Table 4.3. The somatostatin antagonist JR-11 is so far the most potent and selective among the available

Table 4.2 Variation in the expression pattern of SSTR subtypes in some human tumors. Data are based on mRNA, RT-PCR, Northern blotting, and in situ hybridization studies. The values in parentheses indicate the total number of tumors studied [22]. *GEP* Gastroenteropancreatic, *ICT* Islet Cell Tumor, *MCT* Medullary Thyroid Carcinoma

| | SSTR subtype | | | | | | | | | |
| | SSTR$_1$ | | SSTR$_2$ | | SSTR$_3$ | | SSTR$_4$ | | SSTR$_5$ | |
Tumor	mRNA	Protein	mRNA	Protein	mRNA	Protein	mRNA	Protein	mRNA	Protein
Pituitary tumor										
Somatotroph	44% (25)		96% (28)		44% (25)		5% (22)		86% (22)	
Lactotroph	84% (19)		63% (19)		35% 17)		6% (17)		71% (17)	
Nonfunctioning	38% (24)		75% (24)		43% (23)		13% (23)		485 (23)	
Corticotroph	56% (9)		67% (9)		25% (8)		0% (7)		86% (7)	
Neuroendocrine GEP tumors										
Carcinoid	76% (59)	88% (8)	80% (84)	78% (63)	43% (58)		68% (47)		77% (44)	
Gastrinoma	79% (28)	100% (5)	93% (28)	100% (8)	36% (28)		61% (23)		93% (28)	
Insulinoma	76% (21)		81% (21)		38% (21)		58% (19)		57% (21)	
Nonfunctioning ICT	58% (24)		88% (24)		42% (24)		48% (21)		50% (24)	
Renal Ca	85% (13)		100% (13)		0% (13)		50% (12)			
Breast Ca	33% (103)	52% (33)	99% (103)	48% (33)	38% (101)	48% (33)	23% (97)		18% (51)	
Meningioma	46% (24)		100% (24)		33% (24)		50% (12)		71% (14)	
Glioma	100% (7)		100% (7)		67% (6)		71% (7)		57% (7)	
Neuroblastoma	0% (6)		100% (15)		17% (6)					
Colorectal Ca	27% (41)		87% (41)		22% (41)		10% (41)		46% (41)	
MTC	29% (14)		79% (14)		36% (14)		0% (14)		64% (14)	
Pheochromocytoma	100% (11)	80% (5)	100% (11)	90% (20)	73% (11)		73% (11)		73% (11)	

Table 4.3 The extent of the binding in selected tumors expressing SSTR$_2$ of an agonist (^{125}I-Tyr^3-Octreotide vs. an antagonist (^{125}I-JR-11). The superiority of the antagonist binding is obvious [14, 21]. Data are mean ± SEM

Tumor	Samples (*n*)	Antagonist ^{125}I-JR-11 binding (dpm/mg)	Agonist ^{125}I-Tyr^3-Octreotide binding (dpm/mg)	Agonist/ Antagonist ratio
Non-Hodgkin lymphoma	15	3005 ± 499	214 ± 63	14.0
Breast Ca	13	4105 ± 1092	519 ± 156	7.9
Renal Ca	12	3777 ± 582	348 ± 49	10.9
Pheochromocytoma	5	7852 ± 876	446 ± 280	17.6
Medullary thyroid Ca	5	2173 ± 555	100 ± 100	21.8
Ileal NET	4	8470 ± 944	2285 ± 905	3.8
Small cell lung Ca	4	7759 ± 1294	1722 ± 718	4.5
Paraganglioma	2	10,000 ± 0	641 ± 169	15.6

SSTR$_2$ peptide antagonists known (there are non-peptide antagonists as well; see the excellent review of Günther et al. on this subject [16]). Although the SSTR antagonists appear to be in principle superior than the known agonists for imaging and therapy (with **α**- or **β**-emitters), their poor internalization rates preclude the use of Auger electron-emitting labels with these ligands in radiotherapeutic applications [21, 29, 30].

4.2.3 Somatostatin Receptors: Signal Transduction

The SSTRs modulate cellular function through multiple pathways, coupled to G-protein-dependent signaling avenues. The different signaling pathways activated by the various SSTR subtypes vary according to the receptor subtype and tissue localization. The enzyme adenyl cyclase is inhibited in all SSTR subtypes, thus leading to a decrease in c-AMP production, upon ligand binding. A second signaling pathway that is activated following engagement of almost all SSTR subtypes (exception: SSTR$_1$) is the activation of G-protein-regulated inward rectifier K$^+$ channel. The K$^+$ channel activation depolarizes the cell membranes, followed by a decrease in the intracellular Ca^{2+} concentration through a decrease of Ca^{2+} efflux via the voltage-dependent Ca^{2+} channels. The reduction of the intracellular c-AMP and Ca^{2+} concentrations explains the inhibitory effects of SST in neurotransmitter and hormone secretion. A third pathway linked to SST signaling is the regulation of protein phosphatases. Upon binding to its receptor, SST activates a number of protein phosphatases from different families including serine/threonine phosphatases, tyrosine phosphatase (i.e. SHP-1 and SHP-2), Ca^{2+}-dependent phosphatases (i.e. calcineurin), and protein kinases (i.e. MAP kinase). An overview of the SST bioactivity through the various receptor subtypes can be seen in Table 4.4.

SST inhibits various secretory processes in most cases and these antisecretory effects on hormones (i.e. growth hormone, adrenocortico-tropin, glucagon, and insulin), IFN-**γ**, and gastric acid are to a large extent mediated by the SSTR$_{2a/2b}$ subtype, although the SSTR$_5$ subtype inhibits the secretion of amylase. An exception to the SST antisecretory activity is the stimulation of IgM secretion (SSTR$_{2a/2b}$ subtype mediated). These effects occur within seconds to minutes after the SST-SSTR interaction. Finally (Fig. 4.5), the SSTRs mediate either the cellular antiproliferative activity through blocking degradation of the cyclin-dependent kinase inhibitor p27kip1, leading to cellular growth arrest or proapoptotic behavior (i.e. through the BAX/caspases induction).

A common theme that accompanies the GPCR-ligand interaction is its internalization, depending on the ligand concentration, the exposure time, and the parallel operation of other signaling systems. The SSTR$_{2-5}$ subtypes are internalized more efficiently than SSTR$_1$, and since SSTR$_{2a/2b}$ are the major subtypes in various tumors, this fact is of utmost importance in the design of appropriate radiotherapy (with Auger/internal conversion electron-emitting radionuclides) or chemotherapy (SST analogues linked to cytotoxic agents) approaches. The observed SSTR downregulation that accompanies the administration of SST/SST-analogues (agonists) is of critical importance in determining the amount of tumoral uptake of radiolabeled SST-analogues, and besides imaging, it has an adverse effect on tumor therapy (including radiotherapy). The time frame for the desensitization and therapy resistance occurrence (tachyphylaxis) usually ranges from hours to weeks, although the development of tumor resistance to therapy with various somatostatin analogues can take years. In experimental models of tumors treated with either continuous infusion or with b.i.d. dosing of the somatostatin analogue, the SSTR expression was dependent on the administration conditions, leading to either upregulation or downregulation respectively. A summary of the mechanisms that lead to tachyphylaxis and resistance to somatostatin analogues therapy of SSTR-expressing tumors is shown in Table 4.5.

Table 4.4 Summary of the receptor family subtypes, their localization, and their biological effects mediation [2, 9, 11]

Receptor	$SSTR_1$	$SSTR_{2a/2b}$	$SSTR_3$	$SSTR_4$	$SSTR_5$
# of amino acids (MW: kDa)	**391 (42.7)**	**369/356 (41.3)**	**418 (45.9)**	**388 (41.9)**	**364 (39.2)**
Gene location	**14q13**	**17q24**	**22q13.1**	**20p13.3**	**16p13.3**
Signalling pathways					
G-protein coupling	+	+	+	+	+
Adenyl cyclase activity	↓	↓	↓	↓	↓
Phosphotyrosine phosphatase activity	↑	↑	↑	↑↓	↑
MAP kinase activity	↑	↑↓	↑↓	↑	↓
K^+ channels	−	↑	↑	↑	↑
Ca^{2+} channels	↓	↓	−	−	−
Na^+/H^+ exchanger	↓	−	↓	↓	−
AMPA/kainate glutamate channels	↑	↓	−	−	−
PLC/IP_3 activity	↑	↑	↑	↑	↑↓
PLA_2 activity	−	−	−	↑	−
Secretion					
GH	↓	↓	−	↓	↓
Insulin	−	↓	−	−	−
Glucagon	−	↓	−	−	−
ACTH	−	↓	−	−	−
Ghrelin	−	↓	−	−	−
IFN-γ	−	↓	−	−	−
IgM	−	↑	−	−	−
Amylase	−	−	−	−	↓
Gastric acid	−	↓	−	−	−
Cellular effects					
Proliferation	↓	↑↓	↓	↑↓	↓
Apoptosis	−	↑	↑	−	−
Tissue distribution SSTRS 1–4 are almost ubiquitous in their cellular expression	Brain, pituitary, pancreas, stomach, liver, kidneys	Brain, pituitary, pancreas, stomach, lymphocytes, liver, kidneys VSMC	Brain, pituitary, pancreas, T-cells, stomach	Brain, pituitary, pancreas, stomach, placenta, lungs	Lymphoid cells, pituitary, pancreas, stomach

4.3 An Overview of Atomic/Nuclear De-excitation: Internal Conversion and Auger Electrons

The established model describing the atomic structure dictates the presence of an electron cloud surrounding a positively charged nucleus. These constituents of atoms occupy discrete energy levels and can exist in either an excited or a ground state. The excited states originate from either exogenous processes (i.e. particle or radiation bombardment) or this can be an inherent property of certain isotopes (radioactive decay) [3, 31–33].

In the majority of cases, the excited state of a daughter nucleus, formed by α- or β-decay of a parent radionuclide, rapidly proceeds via electromagnetic processes to states of lower energy (eventually to the ground state) in the daughter.

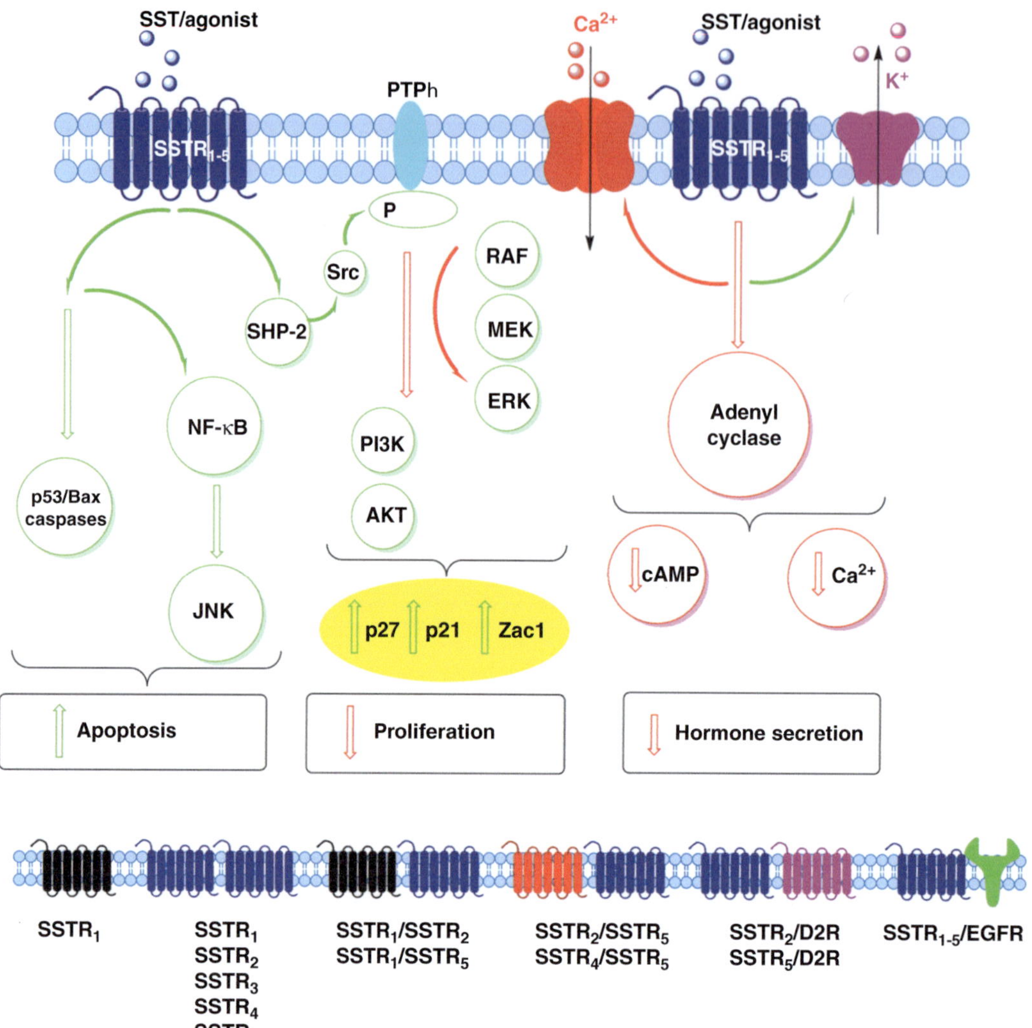

Fig. 4.5 The SST-SSTR-mediated modulation of signaling cascades leading to changes in hormone secretion, apoptosis and cell growth. In most cells, SST inhibits hormone as well as other secretions. SST cell growth and apoptosis are G protein-mediated. Phosphotyrosine phosphatases, such as SHP-1, are activated, leading to dephosphorylation of signal-transducing proteins. SST-induced inhibition of ERK blocks the degradation of the cyclin-dependent kinase inhibitor p27, leading to growth arrest. In rare cases, SST can stimulate proliferation (modified from Barbieri et al. [2, 9, 11]). AC: adenyl cyclase; PI3K: inositol trisphosphate kinase

Table 4.5 Proposed mechanisms of tachyphylaxis and resistance to SST-analogue therapy in patients with SSTR-positive tumors [2, 31]

1. Downregulation: Decrease in the number and/or affinity of SSTRs
2. Desensitization: Decrease in responsiveness due to receptor uncoupling from secondary messenger activation
3. Nonhomogeneous expression of SSTRs in tumors: outgrowth of SSTR (−) cell clones
4. Resistance due to the absence of SSTRs subtypes with high affinity for octapeptide SST analogues
5. Resistance due to tachyphylaxis of the inhibitory effect of SST analogues on direct tumor growth-promoting mechanisms (i.e., GH or gastrin secretion)
6. Mutations on SSTRs genes leading to the absence of functional receptor proteins

This de-excitation process results in the emission of either γ-rays or conversion electrons. Long-lived isomeric states may also decay to lower energy states in the same nucleus via electromagnetic transitions. The energy of the γ-ray emitted by a nucleus in a transition from a higher to a lower energy level equals to the energy difference between the two levels minus the nuclear recoil energy, which is considered negligible, except for the case of high-energy transitions of light nuclei. The emitted conversion electrons are orbital electrons of the *same* atom (internal conversion), and this de-excitation mechanism competes with the electromagnetic de-excitation process (γ-ray emission). In the internal conversion, the energy difference between the initial and final states in the nucleus is transferred *directly* (without a real intermediate γ-ray emission) to a bound orbital electron of the *same* atom, which is then ejected from its orbit, leaving an electronic vacancy behind. The ejected conversion electrons have discrete energies (linear spectrum) and this is another important difference from the electrons of the beta decay, which originate in the nucleus of the atom and have a continuous energy spectrum up to a maximum (E_{max}).

The internal conversion process should not be confused with the superficially similar photoelectric effect, which also results in an inner shell electronic vacancy. In this context, when a γ-ray emitted by an excited nucleus (in this case the emitted γ-ray photon is real!) hits a *neighboring* atom, occasionally it gets absorbed (photoelectric effect), thus producing a photoelectron of well-defined energy (this process is also known as *"external conversion"*). During the radiative transitions, the created electronic vacancy moves stepwise to a higher major shell, with no change in the number of vacancies. However, during the nonradiative transitions the number of vacancies increases by one in each step. Hence, as the innermost vacancy percolates toward the valence shell, a cascade phenomenon develops with corresponding vacancy multiplication and emission of numerous low energy electrons, collectively referred to as Auger electrons [33].

For a particular transition, the ratio of the probability for emission of an X-shell electron (X: K, L, M, etc.) to the probability for emission of the competitive γ-ray is called the X-shell internal conversion coefficient α (**α = # of de-excitations via electron emission/# of de-excitations via γ-ray emission**). The internal conversion coefficients for the different atomic shells and subshells depend on the transition energy, the atomic number of the nucleus, and the so-called transition multipolarity, which is determined by the spin-parity change between the initial and final states in the nucleus (Weisskopf rules). In general, the internal conversion coefficient for a particular atomic shell or subshell increases with decreasing transition energy (as long as the particular internal conversion process is energetically allowed), increasing atomic number, and increasing transition multipolarity. Internal conversion is often negligible for transitions in light nuclei but may occur with nearly 100% probability in isomeric transitions with high multipolarity or in low-energy transitions in heavy nuclei [3, 33].

Usually, the internal conversion coefficient for a given transition is largest for the innermost shell, for which internal conversion is energetically possible and decreases for each higher shell. Exceptions occur, however, for transition energies slightly greater than the binding energy of an atomic shell. If the spins of the initial and final states are both zero, the quantum mechanical rules (conservation of angular momentum) prohibit this electromagnetic transition ($\Delta I = 0$) and therefore the de-excitation via a *single* γ-ray emission is strictly forbidden (emission of two γ-rays is a possibility though, but this de-excitation mechanism is insignificant). In this case, if the energy difference of the two states (ΔE) is <1.022 MeV, the internal conversion is the only de-excitation mechanism. However, if ΔE is ≥1.022 Mev, then the de-excitation via a positron-electron pair production is also feasible [3, 33].

The nuclear decay processes of electron capture (EC) and the production of conversion electrons (CE) always produce a vacancy in an inner atomic orbital, thus leaving the atom (*not the nucleus*) in an excited state and positively charged. The relaxation to the ground state is a rapid process, via either radiative (through emission of characteristic X-rays) or nonradiative processes, known collectively as Auger processes. Auger processes result in the emission of Auger, Coster-Kronig (CK), and super-CK electrons, as their ejection leaves the atom highly charged (positive). These are distinguished by the shells involved in the transition and the ejected electrons are often collectively referred to as Auger electrons [3, 33].

Although the Auger emission process was initially observed and published in 1922 by Lise Meitner, it was also independently discovered by the French physicist Pierre Victor Auger in 1923. In his experimental work, high-energy X-rays were used to ionize gas particles (argon) and the emitted photoelectrons were studied using a Wilson cloud chamber. It was observed that the emitted Auger electrons always originated from the same point (orbital vacancy) that the photoelectron generated from the interaction of the incident X-ray photon and the argon atom. If the Auger effect were a two-step phenomenon, requiring the prior emission of an X-ray photon *before* the Auger electron emission, the emitted X-ray (originating from the argon atom) should have to travel a finite distance, and in this case the Auger electrons would appear at some other point along its track. However, this was not observed to be the case and the concept of a radiationless process was invoked to explain the mechanism of the Auger electron generation [3, 33, 34].

The Coster-Kronig transition is a special case of the Auger process in which the ejected electron carries the energy of a transition within the *same shell* (same principal quantum number $\mathbf{n}$), but it is ejected from a *higher subshell* (with different orbital quantum number $\boldsymbol{\ell}$). Furthermore, the super Coster-Kronig transitions occur within the *same subshell* (same principal quantum number $\mathbf{n}$ and same orbital quantum number $\boldsymbol{\ell}$) and the energy difference is imparted on the ejected electron originating from the *same subshell*. It is understood that this cascade of events continues

until the only remaining vacancies are in the outermost electron shell. The above described processes are competitive processes, with radiative relaxation being more probable for K-shell vacancies and nonradiative relaxation being more probable for vacancies in the L-shell and above (see Fig. 4.5). Most of these Auger electrons have very low energies (20–500 eV) with ranges (1–10 nm) in living tissues and like the internal conversion electrons, the Auger electrons have also discrete energies, resulting in a sharp energy peak spectrum. The entire Auger electron cascade is completed within 1 fs (10^{-15} s) [33] (Fig. 4.6).

The explanation of the Auger effect and the internal conversion processes stems from the quantum-mechanical description of the atomic world. From this perspective, due to the fact that the wave functions of the nuclei and electrons are allowed to overlap (the nonlocality principle), the *direct* energy transfer (quantum-mechanical coupling) to the ejected Auger or conversion electrons is feasible without the prior emission of a photon (X-ray or $\boldsymbol{\gamma}$-ray respectively).

The observation that the Auger electrons are highly radiotoxic, by pioneers in the field like Feinendegen [35] and Howell [36], took approximately two decades to mature for applications in tumor radiotherapy. The Auger electron radiotoxicity, summarized by their high-LET (LET: Linear Energy Transfer: 4–26 keV/µm), low-energy ($\leq$1.6 keV), and short-range ($\leq$150 nm electrons), is caused by multiple ionizations in the immediate vicinity (within a few nanometers) of the decay site. In contrast to $\boldsymbol{\alpha}$- and $\boldsymbol{\beta}$-particles, the Auger electrons, despite their high LET, are much less radiotoxic to healthy cells, while circulating in blood or bone marrow, but they become highly radiotoxic when incorporated or decay near the DNA of target cells (see Table 4.6 and Fig. 4.7).

The Auger electron's range in water varies from a nanometer to several micrometers, comparable with that of subcellular structures and the highly localized energy deposition (10^6–10^9 cGy) in a very small volume near the nucleus can be as cytotoxic as the $\boldsymbol{\alpha}$-particles of a Po-210 atom emitted from a point at the cell surface [33–35, 38].

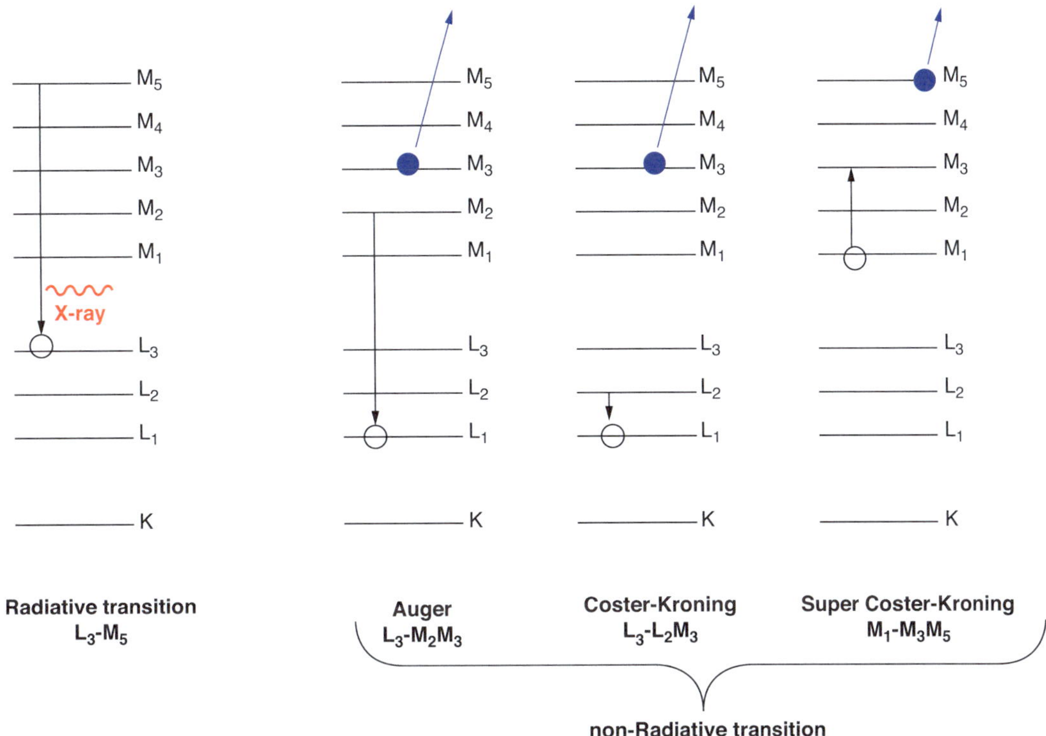

Fig. 4.6 Schematic diagram for radiative and nonradiative transitions. The ejected Auger electrons are shown in blue. In the nonradiative transitions the first two letters refer to the observed transition and the third letter refers to the subshell origin of the Auger electrons [3, 33]

Table 4.6 Radioisotope characteristics for radiotherapeutic applications [31]. *LET* Linear Energy Transfer, *EC* Electron Capture, *IC* Internal Conversion

Decay mode	Emitted particles[a]	$E_{min} - E_{max}$	Range	LET
α-decay	Helium nuclei (1)	5–9 MeV[b]	40–100 μm	≈80 keV/μm
β-decay	Energetic electrons (1)	50–2300 keV[c]	0.015–12 mm	≈0.2 keV/μm
EC/IC	Nonenergetic electrons (5–30)	ev-keV[b]	2–500 nm	≈4–26 keV/μm

[a]Number of particles
[b]Monoenergetic
[c]Average energy (continuous energy spectrum up to a maximum E_{max})

DNA is the principal target responsible for radiation-induced biologic effects of the Auger electrons. The Auger electrons-DNA interaction results in number of different DNA lesions, such as single-strand breaks (SSB), double-strand breaks (DSB), base damage, DNA-protein cross-links, and multiply damaged sites (MDS). These changes may be produced by either the direct ionization of DNA (direct effect) or by the DNA interaction with free radicals (indirect effect), comprised mostly of hydroxyl free radicals (OH•) originating from the radiolysis of the nearby abundant water molecules and whose range is several nanometers (Figs. 4.7 and 4.8). Most of these lesions are repaired with high fidelity, the exceptions being DSB and MDS. Additional damage is caused from the charge neutralization of the de-excited atom, which acquires a high positive charge as the result of the Auger emission cascade [40–42].

The ideal Auger emitter for radiotherapy applications must fulfill certain criteria which are

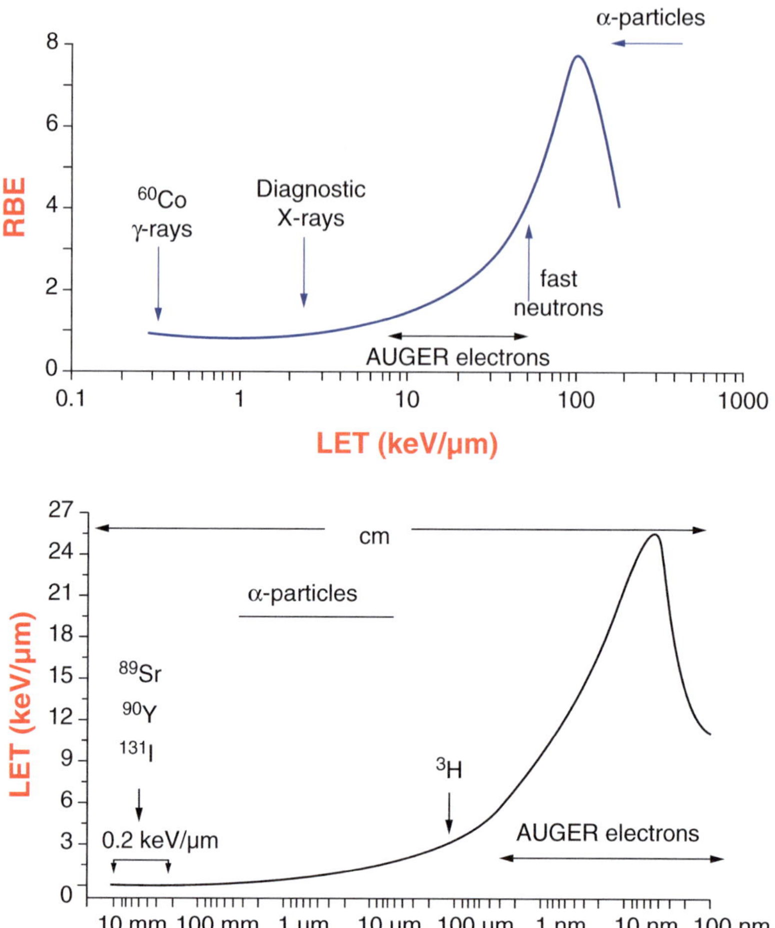

Fig. 4.7 *Upper*: Relative biological effectiveness as a function of LET (*LET* linear energy transfer) expressed in keV/μm of tissue. *Lower*: LET as a function of distance (LET refers to the *energy* absorbed by the media per unit of distance travelled by the ionizing radiation) [3, 31]

summarized in Table 4.7. The first criterion is absolutely essential to ensure the Auger emission process. The half-life range (second criterion) is based on the need for long $t_{1/2}$ in case of slow tumor uptake kinetics. Thus, a much shorter $t_{1/2}$, combined with slow tumor uptake, will rather irradiate the surrounding normal tissues during the circulation, than the tumor. In his context, a much larger $t_{1/2}$ results in a lower radiation dose to the tumor, since the number of receptors on the tumor cells is finite and the occupancy by an appreciable number by non-emitting ligands will result in a suboptimal irradiation of the tumor cells, especially if they exhibit a rapid proliferation rate. The third criterion is needed to avoid the normal tissue irradiation and especially the rapidly dividing bone marrow cells. However, a low-intensity photon emission in the 100–200 keV range is desirable for dosimetry calculations. The last three criteria (4–6) are essential to minimize the presence of radionuclidic impurities, originating from either the same element as the desired therapeutic radionuclide (for example, the presence of In-114m during the In-111 production) or from the radioactive decay products that could expose the normal tissues to undesirable radiation burden. The (p, n) nuclear reaction offers the opportunity for the local production of radionuclides with cyclotrons during the development and clinical trial phases. For practical reasons (availability), the isotopes Ga-67, In-111, I-123, and I-125 are currently

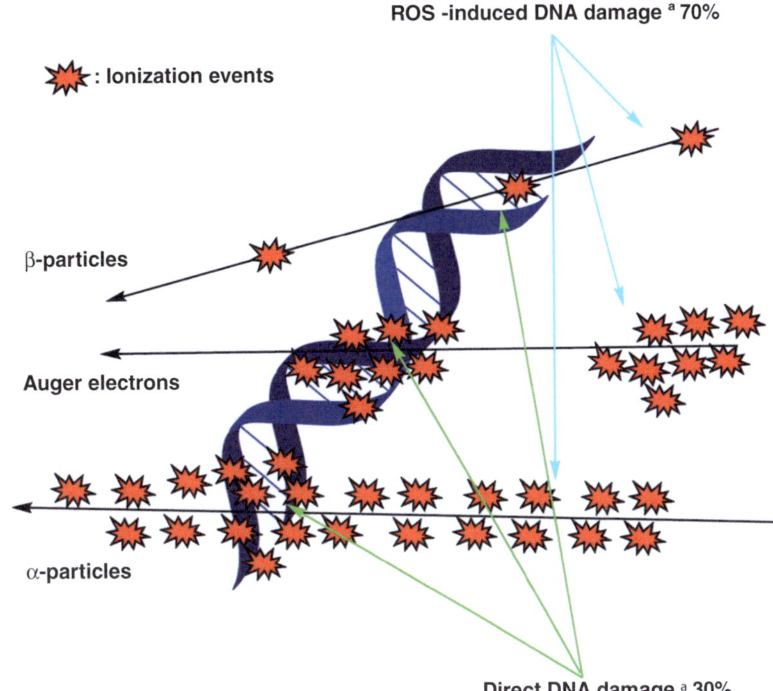

Fig. 4.8 Schematic representation of ionization density along the path of **α**-, **β**-particles, and Auger electrons (**α**-particles are considered densely-ionizing radiation, **β**-particles are sparsely ionizing and Auger electrons form clusters with a high density of ionization [37, 39–41]. *ROS* Reactive Oxygen Species

Table 4.7 A tabulation of the most important characteristics of Auger-emitting radionuclides for tumor therapy applications

Desirable properties of Auger-emitting radionuclides
1. Radioisotope must decay either via EC or IT (IT: internal transition) decay
2. $3\,h < t_{1/2} < 5$ days
3. Low abundance of emitted γ-photons
4. Production via the (p, n) nuclear reaction
5. Preferably no other co-existing nuclear states of the isotope
6. Stable or very long half-life of daughter nuclide
7. Chemical properties for easy synthesis of the appropriate labeled vectors

considered for Auger electron radiotherapy applications, despite the fact that they do not fulfill all the above criteria [32, 43, 44].

Many radionuclides decay by electron capture and/or internal conversion and therefore inevitably emit Auger electrons with energies ranging from a few eV to a few keV. In Table 4.8 the internal conversion and Auger-emitting parameters are listed for a few of commonly used radioisotopes. From this table, it is obvious that the total energy deposition per decay is the highest for In-111, thus making this isotope appropriate for tumor therapy applications, despite its limitations, mostly appropriate for the treatment of micrometastases or small-volume metastatic foci. It has been shown that in therapy of neuroendocrine tumors with [^{111}In-DTPA^0-D-Phe^1]-Octreotide, it is the Auger electrons that are responsible for the observed tumoricidal effects and not the high-energy conversion electrons (145–245 keV) [25, 32].

The ongoing research effort has been exploring the potential of other CE/AE-emitting isotopes for radiotherapeutic applications, such as Pt-193m/Pt-195m, Sb-119, and Cu-64. However, radioisotope availability (for example, Pt-195m is not available in carrier-free form, although with 33 emitted electrons/decay, it has the highest Auger electron yield known), lack of convenient and/or appropriate chemistry or cost-related considerations, have hampered these efforts so far, leaving as practical choices In-111 (8 Auger electrons/decay), I-125 (21 Auger electrons/decay), and I-123 (11 Auger electrons/decay) and

Table 4.8 Auger (AE) and conversion electron (CE) emission parameters of some commonly used radionuclides

Parameter	I-125	In-111	I-123	Tc-99m	Ga-67	Tl-201
Half-life (days)	59.4	2.80	0.55	0.25	3.26	3.04
Number of AE/decay	24.9	14.7	14.9	4.0	4.7	36.9
AE energy/decay (keV)	12.2	6.8	7.4	0.9	6.3	15.3
AE energy range (keV)	0.02–30.3	0.04–25.6	0.02–30.35	0.2–17.8	0.9–9.4	0.07–66.9
Range of AE in water	1.5 nm–14.0 μm	0.25 nm–13.6 μm	0.5 nm–13.5 μm	13 nm–6.5 μm	0.1–2.7 μm	3 nm–40 μm
Number of CE/decay	0.9	0.2	0.2	1.1	0.3	1.1
CE energy/decay (keV)	7.2	25.9	20.2	15.4	28.1	30.2
CE energy range (keV)	3.7–35	145–245	127–159	100–140	82–291	1.6–153
Range of CE in water (μm)	0.7–16	205–622	100–130	70–112	50–300	0.2–126
Associated γ-emissions (keV)	35	171.3, 245.4	159.0	140.5	9.1, 9.3, 184, 209, 300, 393	135.3, 167.4
Total energy/decay (keV)	61.4	419.2	200.4	142.6	201.6	138.5
Total energy deposited/decay ($\times 10^{-14}$ Gy kg/Bq/s)	1.0	7.0	3.2	2.3	3.14	2.2

even Ga-67. It has to be emphasized though, that there are significant differences in the Auger yields reported in the literature and most of these difference can be attributed to the lack of detailed knowledge of the relevant atomic transition rates, most prominently in the outer (M, N, etc.) shells. In addition, another important consideration for the Auger emitter choice is not only the number of emitted electrons per decay but also the residence time of the Auger emitter inside the cell, so that the energy deposition from its decay would have the expected tumoricidal effect [41–46].

4.4   The In-111 Decay Pathway

Indium (In-111) is a cyclotron-produced radio-isotope (Curium, France, formerly Mallinkcrodt BV, the Netherlands) by the proton irradiation of a cadmium (Cd-112)-enriched target, via the reaction: [^{112}Cd (p, 2n) ^{111}In]. This production path is preferred over the alternative reaction

[^{111}Cd (p, n) ^{111}In], which is accompanied by the co-production of high levels of In-111m as an undesirable radionuclidic impurity [47, 48]. At the time of calibration, the preparation contains not less than 99.925% In-111 and not more than 0.075% In-114m and Zn-65 combined. At the time of expiration, it contains not less than 99.85% In-111 and not more than 0.15% In-114m and Zn-65 combined. At the time of calibration, the no carrier added (n.c.a.) Indium (In-111) Chloride sterile solution in dilute HCl acid (0.02– 0.05 N) contains not less than 95% of the Indium present in the In^{3+} ionic form, while any metal impurities (tested: Cu, Fe, Cd, Pb, Zn, Ni, Hg) are below ppm levels. Indium (In-111) decays by electron capture (EC) to cadmium (Cd-111), a stable isotope, with a physical half-life of 67.32 h (2.8049 days). A detailed In-111 decay map is shown in Fig. 4.9.

The In-111 decay to the ground state of Cd-111 (stable) proceeds not directly, but through three intermediate steps, since the direct transition

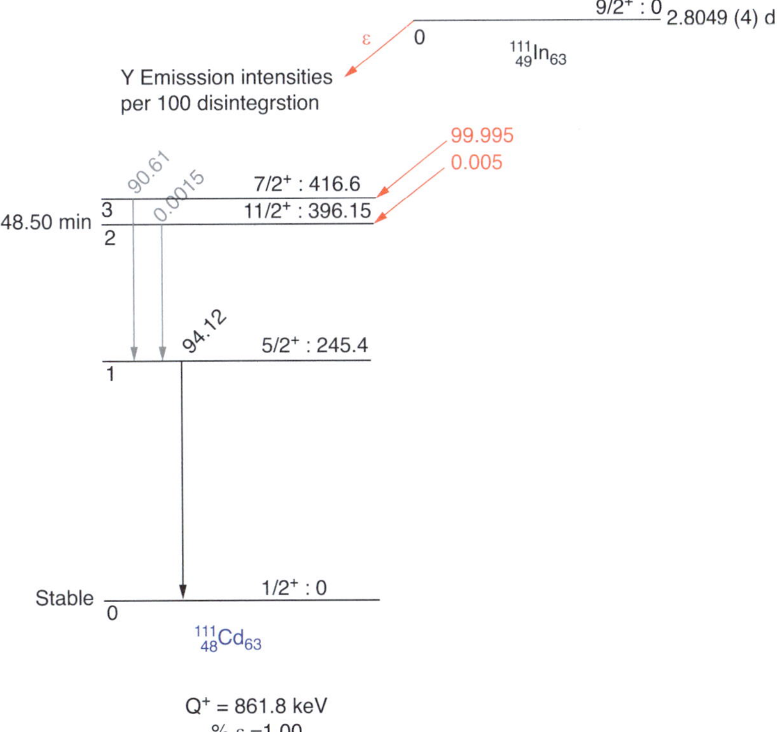

Fig. 4.9 The decay diagram of In-111 by EC. Note the nuclear spin changes of the transition levels [35, 49]

Table 4.9 Energy, yield, and range of photons and particles emitted by decaying In-111 nuclei. Very low energy photons and electrons are omitted [35, 45, 46]

Radiation	E (keV)	Yield/ decay	Range (μm)
Auger electrons			
Auger KLL	19.1	0.1030	8.21
Auger KLX	22.3	0.0394	10.8
Auger KXY	25.5	0.0036	13.6
Auger LMM	2.59	0.835	0.287
Auger LMX	3.06	0.190	0.375
Auger LXY	3.53	0.109	0.473
Auger MXY	0.35	2.09	0.0164
Auger NXY	8.47×10^{-3}	7.82	2.51×10^{-4}
Coster-Kroning electrons			
CK-LLX	0.183	0.151	8.69×10^{-3}
CK-MMX	0.125	0.915	6.35×10^{-3}
CK-NNX	0.0183	2.54	2.50×10^{-3}
Conversion electrons			
IC 1 K	145	0.0824	2.05×10^{-3}
IC 1 L	167	0.0100	2.72×10^{-3}
IC 1 M, N, …	171	0.0140	2.83×10^{-3}
IC 2 K	219	0.0521	5.20×10^{-3}
IC 2 L	241	0.0091	6.09×10^{-3}
IC 2 M, N, ….	245	0.0019	6.22×10^{-3}
X-rays			
X-ray K_{a1}	23.2	0.4630	–
X-ray K_{a2}	23.0	0.2400	–
X-ray $K_{\beta 1}$	26.1	0.0788	–
X-ray $K_{\beta 2}$	26.6	0.0186	–
X-ray $K_{\beta 3}$	26.1	0.0382	–
X-ray $K_{\beta 5}$	26.3	0.0011	–
X-ray L	3.23	0.0499	–
X-ray M	0.356	0.0030	–
γ-Rays			
γ-1	171	9.06×10^{-1}	–
γ-2	245	9.37×10^{-1}	–

from In-111 → Cd-111 ($I = 9/2^+ \rightarrow I = 1/2^+$) with a single γ-ray emission is strictly forbidden on quantum mechanical grounds ($\Delta I = 4$).

- **Step1:** The transition from the energy level of Indium-111 to the 416.6 keV excited state of Cd-111 via an electron capture process, accompanied by K X-ray emission in 71.7% of the transitions, with the other 28.3% consisting of conversion and Auger electrons and low energy photons.
- **Step 2: The** transition from the 416.6 keV excited state of Cd-111 to its 245.4 keV excited state; in the 90.6% of these transitions 171 keV γ-rays are emitted. In the other 9.4% of transitions, a conversion electron is produced, followed either by K X-rays (71.7% of the transitions) or by Auger electrons and low-energy photons (in 28.3% of the transitions).
- **Step 3: The** transition from the 245.4 keV excited state of Cd-111 to its ground state; 94.1% of these transitions consist of 245.4 keV γ-rays. In the other 5.9% of transitions, a conversion electron is produced and that is followed either by K X-rays (in 71.7% of cases) or by Auger electrons and low-energy photons (in 28.3% of the transitions).

The 171.3 and 245.4 keV γ-rays of Cd-111 de-excitation are used for imaging; the energy, range, and yield per decay of Auger and the conversion electrons emitted and responsible for tumor radiotherapy effects are shown in Table 4.9.

4.5 A Brief Reminder of Indium Chemistry

Indium is a group (IIIA), p-block metal like Gallium (Ga) and Thallium (Tl) and its most stable oxidation number is +3. In^{3+} is a Lewis acid and according to the Pearson HASB (HASB: Hard Acid-Soft Base) classification it is considered a hard acid ($I_A = 6.30$ for In^{3+}). In^{3+} exhibits marked similarities with Fe^{3+}, although Fe^{3+} is a harder acid ($I_A = 7.22$ for Fe^{3+}) than In^{3+} (the larger the parameter I_A, the harder the acid). The radiochemistry of indium is fairly straightforward and it deals with the metal ion in its stable In^{3+} form and in complexes with coordination numbers usually 6 or 7 (range: 4–8). There is generally little π-bonding to stabilize the indium–ligand bond and in the presence of monodentate ligands (i.e. acetate) there is a tendency for these complexes to undergo rapid ligand exchange reactions. The desired kinetic stability for the synthesis of radiopharmaceuticals can be achieved only through the use of polydentate ligands, preferably those with substituents that provide steric shielding [50–56].

In acidic aqueous solutions, for example in aqueous HCl solution (0.1 M HCl), the mixed octahedral indium In^{3+} complexes [In (H$_2$O) $_4$Cl$_2$] $^+$ and [In (H$_2$O)$_5$Cl]$^{2+}$ prevail. These species are weak complexes with small affinity constants (logk_a = 3.84 and logk_a = 2.58 respectively) and highly labile, since the H$_2$O and halide ligands are exchanged rapidly moving from the inner coordination sphere of the indium ion to the solution and vice versa. In the case of the complexation of In^{3+} by citrate in acidic conditions, a complex mixture of species is formed. Taking into account the very low [In^{3+}]/[citrate] ratio during the preparation of various radiopharmaceuticals, the labile citrate complex [InH$_2$Cit] $^+$ with logk_a = 5.20 (logk_a = 6.80 has also been reported, although both values are of questionable validity) is the most likely species. It is reminded that the magnitude of the affinity constant reflects the ΔG change of the reaction (for $\Delta G < 0$, $k_a > 1$) [57, 58]. It should be kept in mind that ΔG is a thermodynamic parameter, while the lability or inertness of the formed complex is a kinetic parameter and it reflects the magnitude of the activation energy (E_a) of the rate-limiting step of the reaction mechanism. In radiochemistry, besides the thermodynamic stability, the kinetic inertness of the radiopharamaceutical is the other parameter of utmost importance. In the case of the Indium-DTPA complexes, their kinetic stability dictates their behavior in vivo (after the IV administration), where these complexes encounter transferrin, an iron-binding blood plasma glycoprotein with a high plasma concentration (0.25 g/100 mL). Transferrin has two Fe^{3+} binding sites (respective affinity constants: log K_{a1} = 30.5 and log K_{a2} = 25.5), and it is normally saturated only by 20–30% with iron ions, therefore, it is capable of sequestering any other radiometal present that can form complexes with, including In^{3+} [59].

Fortunately, the sequestering of In^{3+} from its Indium-protein conjugates to transferrin at physiological pH is a quite slow process. Being otherwise, these complexes would be useless for radiopharmaceutical applications. In fact, Yeh et al. [60] showed an In-111 label transfer rate from a ^{111}In-DTPA-HSA conjugate to transferrin of 1.6% per day at physiological pH and 37 °C (HSA: Human Serum Albumin), which was only slightly lower (2.6%) than the transfer rate of the In-111 label from the ^{111}In-DTPA complex to transferrin. In the case of benzyl-EDTA-HSA and phenyl-EDTA-HSA, which are sterically hindered ligands for the ^{111}In^{3+} complexation and more lipophilic, the transfer rate of the In-111 label from these complexes to transferrin drops to 0.11% and 0.060 respectively. The exceptional stability of ^{111}In-DTPA-fibrinogen towards transferrin transchelation of the ^{111}In^{3+} label was also shown from 24 h incubation experiments of this compound in serum at 37° C [61].

As mentioned before, Indium ion is a hard acid; therefore it forms complexes with a wide variety of organic ligands, especially with nitrogen, oxygen, or charge-carrying oxygen atoms (hard bases). Indium complexes of interest in the radiopharmaceutical field are based on the N$_3$O$_5$ or N$_4$O$_4$ motif of aminocarboxylate ligands (i.e. DTPA, DOTA), which exhibit very high affinity or formation constants (logk_a = 28.4 for the In-DTPA complex). It should be noted though that even S-containing ligands (i. e. aminothiol: **-N-CH$_2$-CH$_2$-S$^-$**) have been prepared with even higher affinity constants (log$k_a > 33$), despite the "softness" of the sulfur atom (sulfur has a larger atomic radius than oxygen and it is polarizable, hence its "softness") [62–64].

The In^{3+} ion is also known for its amphoteric character, and for this reason it hydrolyzes easily in aqueous solutions, forming insoluble hydroxides/colloids at pH > 3.4 (in dilute concentrations, In(OH)$_3$ does not actually precipitate). Since the In-hydroxy colloid formation occurs more rapidly than the complexation with aminocarboxylate ligands in acidic solutions (pH: 4.0–5.5), this problem is avoided through the rapid formation of an intermediate weak (and labile) complex with an appropriate chelator, such as citrate followed by a transchelation reaction with the aminocarboxylate ligand. The citrate use is preferred, instead of an acetate-based buffer, since Indium does not precipitate or forms

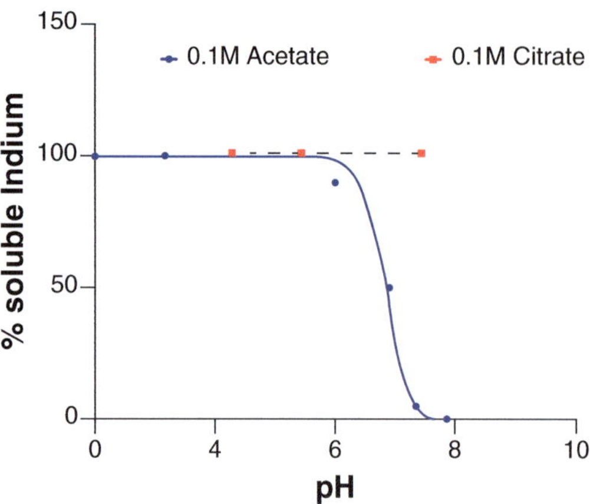

Fig. 4.10 The percentage of soluble Indium in citrate and acetate buffers, as a function of pH. Note that acetate ions are monodentate ligands, while citrate (4-dentate ligand) can form kinetically labile chelate complexes [55]

colloids at the slightly acidic solutions (pH: 4.0–5.5, see Fig. 4.10) of various radiopharmaceutical preparations [65]. Once prepared, the thermodynamically stable DTPA-Indium complexes are relatively inert, with minimal in vivo transfer of the In-111 label to transferrin [57, 61, 66, 67].

Cadmium is a ubiquitous environmental contaminant that can be encountered in syringes or vials and is also the unavoidable decay product of the In-111 label, thus competing with In^{3+} in its complexation reactions (i.e. with the DTPA moiety, $\log K_a = 19.1$ for the Cd^{2+}-DTPA reaction). The time delay between the production of In-111 and its incorporation to the appropriate radiopharmaceutical (usually 7–11 days later), before their administration to patients, contributes to the increase of the undesirable cadmium levels in the $^{111}InCl_3$ solutions (Cd^{2+} in growth). Another problem encountered in the In^{3+} handling is its tendency to get adsorbed on glass vial walls (even a 20–30% of the dose can get adsorbed). As a result, the number of In-111 labeled DTPA-Octreotide molecules available for receptor binding is substantially decreased with adverse impact on its use as imaging or therapy agent. Therefore, it is imperative to take precautions such as use of appropriate containers and syringes during the radiopharmaceutical preparation and the use of ultrapure $^{111}InCl_3$ solution. Ideally, the purification of the $^{111}InCl_3$ solution should be done imme-

diately prior to the complexation reaction. Such a purification method relies on column chromatography with a strong anion exchange resin (DoweX-1-chloride, 8% X-linking, 100–200 dry mesh), preconditioned with the successive passage of 10 mL of HCl (0.1 N), 10 mL of a 0.9% NaCl (for IV use) solution, and 10 mL of water for injection. Then, the crude $^{111}InCl_3$ solution is loaded on top of the resin bed and the purified $^{111}InCl_3$ eluate is collected in a sterile polypropylene vial. Since Indium-111 is commercially available in dilute hydrochloric (HCl) acid (0.2–0.5 N), the Cd^{2+} contaminant to be removed is present as an *anionic* tetrahedral complex $[CdCl_4]^{2-}$, which is retained by the column [68].

An interesting approach to maximize the $^{111}In^{3+}$ incorporation in various In-111 complexation reactions was through the use of either MES (MES: 2-(N-morpholino)ethanesulfonic acid) or HEPES (HEPES: 4-(2-hydroxyethyl)-1-piperazineethanesulfonic acid) as buffers. With these buffers, high specific activities of ^{111}In-labeled peptides are achieved (see Fig. 4.10), possibly due to their weak complex formation tendency with the In^{3+} ions (the HEPES and MES structures are shown in Fig. 4.11; the presence of electron-donating atoms is obvious). Moreover, when the labeling was performed in MES- and HEPES-based buffers, the labeling efficiency of ^{111}In-labeled peptides was not adversely affected by Cd^{2+} concentrations up to 0.1 nM (see Fig. 4.12). Therefore, with the use of HEPES or MES in place of citrate or acetate buffers, the time-consuming purification step of $^{111}InCl_3$ described previously can be safely avoided [69].

4.6 The Preparation of [^{111}In-DTPA^0-D-Phe^1]-Octreotide

4.6.1 The Kit Components

Octreoscan™ is a commercial kit used for the preparation of [^{111}In-DTPA^0-D-Phe^1]-Octreotide, a radiopharmaceutical (CURIUM™, France; formerly Mallinckrodt Nuclear Medicine BV, the

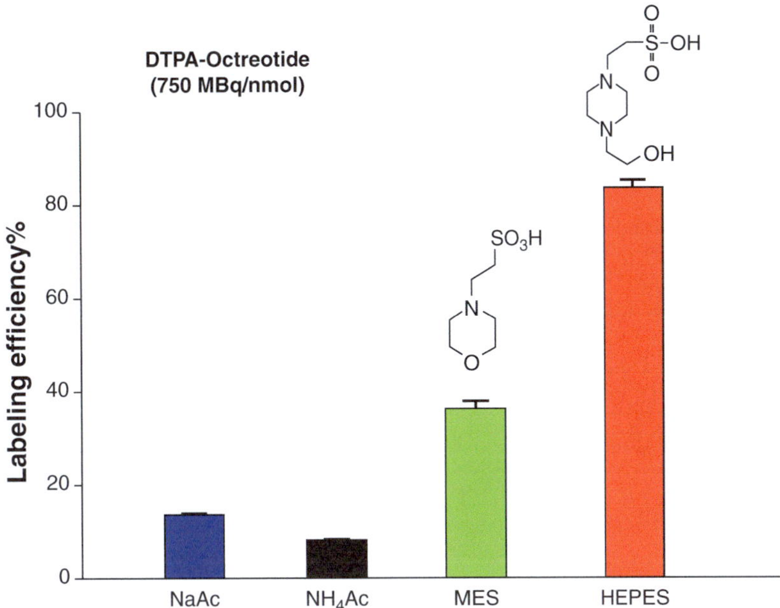

Fig. 4.11 The % ^{111}In-labeling efficiency of DTPA-Octreotide in 0.1 M NaAc, NH$_4$Ac, MES and HEPES buffers [69]. MES: 2-(N-morpholino) ethanesulfonic acid), HEPES: 4-(2-hydroxyethyl)-1-piperazineethanesulfonic acid)

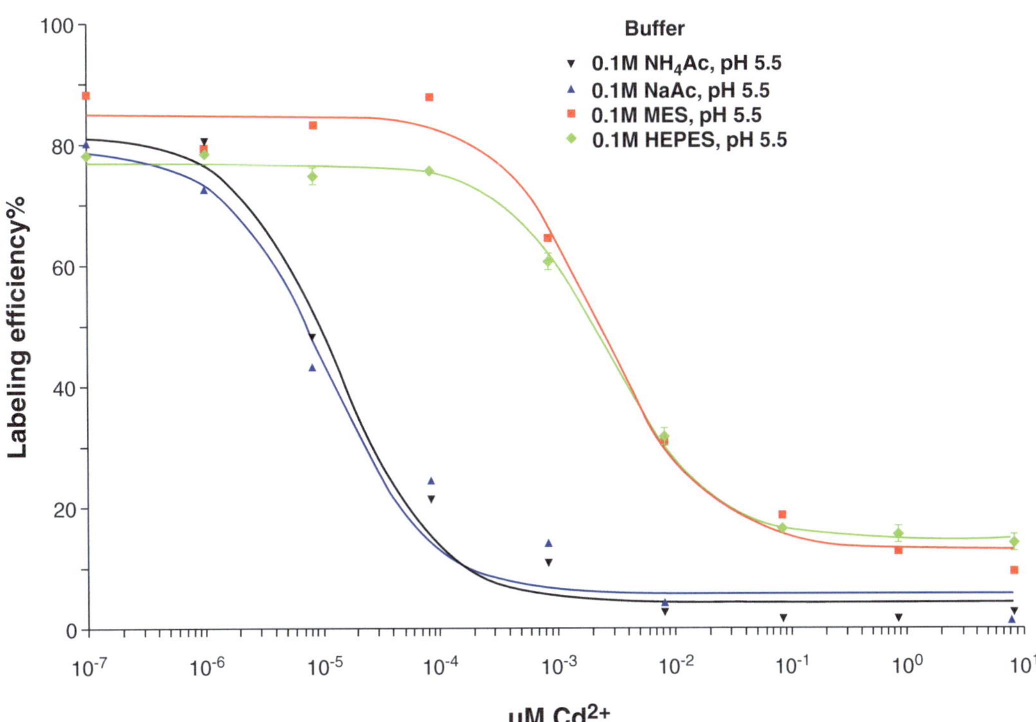

Fig. 4.12 The effect of [Cd^{2+}] on the labeling efficiency of ^{111}In-DTPA-exendin-3 in 0.1 M NaAc, NH$_4$Ac, MES and HEPES buffers (pH: 5.5) [69]. MES: 2-(N-morpholino) ethanesulfonic acid), HEPES: 4-(2-hydroxyethyl)-1-piperazine ethanesulfonic acid)

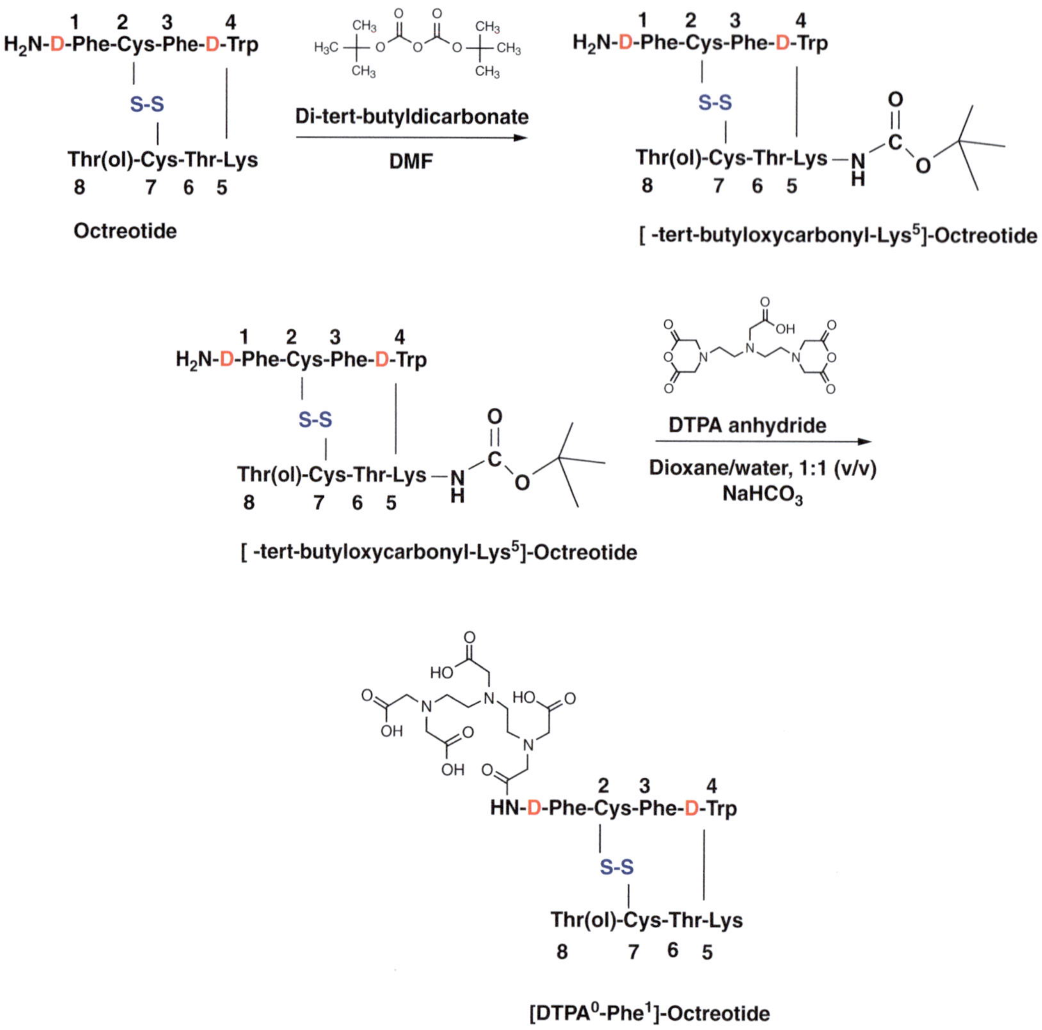

Fig. 4.13 Reaction scheme for the synthesis of [DTPA⁰-D-Phe¹]-Octreotide. Replacement of Phe³ in Octreotide by Tyr³ (which can be easily radioiodinated) leads to an analogue with improved SSTR₂ affinity, but the SSTR₃ and SSTR₅ affinity is reduced; the C-terminal presence of Thr instead of Thr(ol) results in a SSTR₂-selective ligand with a sevenfold improvement of SSTR₂ affinity [73]

Netherlands) approved for diagnostic applications. The same kit can be also used for radiotherapeutic applications, although in this case, much higher total doses must be administered [70, 71]. This kit consists of two components:

Vial 1: The 10-mL Octreoscan™ Reaction Vial 1 contains a lyophilized mixture of:

1. 10 μg [DTPA⁰-D-Phe¹]-Octreotide [*N*-(diethylenetriamine-*N*,*N*,*N*′,*N*″-tetraacetic acid-*N*″-acetyl)-D-phenylalanyl-L-hemicystyl-L-phenylalanyl-D-tryptophyl-L-lysyl-L-threonyl-L-hemicystyl-L-threoninol cyclic (2 → 7) disulfide], also known as pentetreotide,
2. 2.0 mg gentisic acid [2, 5-dihydroxybenzoic acid] as antioxidant,
3. 4.9 mg trisodium citrate, anhydrous as transfer ligand,
4. 0.37 mg citric acid, anhydrous, for buffering and
5. 10.0 mg inositol as bulking agent.

Prior to lyophilization, sodium hydroxide or hydrochloric acid is added for pH adjustment. The vial contents are sterile and nonpyrogenic, without bacteriostatic preservatives present (the information presented about the Octreoscan™ kit was obtained from the CURIUM™/Mallincrodt package insert [72]).

Vial 2: The 10-mL vial 2 of Indium In-111 Chloride sterile solution contains:

1. 1.1 mL or 111 MBq/mL (3.0 mCi/mL) of indium In-111 chloride (^{111}InCl$_3$) in 0.02 N HCl, at the time of calibration.
2. Ferric chloride (FeCl$_3$) at a concentration of 3.5 µg/mL ([Fe^{3+}] = 1.2 µg/mL), as a labeling efficiency augmenter. The vial contents are sterile and nonpyrogenic, without bacteriostatic preservatives present.

For radiotherapeutic applications, 4–5 vials of the diagnostic kit were used, with a total peptide amount 40–50 µg and total added radioactivity of ^{111}InCl$_3$ ranging between 110–160 mCi (4070–5920 MBq).

4.6.2 Synthesis of [DTPA^0-D-Phe^1]-Octreotide

The synthesis of the "cold" ligand ([DTPA^0-D-Phe^1]-Octreotide) is a three-step reaction (see Fig. 4.13) [73]:

First step: Reaction of Octreotide (Sandostatin™) with di-ε-*tert*-butyldicarbonate (Boc)$_2$O in dimethylformamide (DMF) for the protection of the ε-NH$_2$ group of lysine.

Second step: The Lys^5 protected product ([ε-*tert*-butyloxycarbonyl-Lys^5]-Octreotide) reacts with *N,N'*-diethylenetriaminepentaacetic acid (DTPA). DTPA dianhydride is then coupled to the selectively protected octreotide. The [ε-*tert*-butyloxycarbonyl-Lys^5]-Octreotide is dissolved in dioxane/water (1/1, v/v) and after addition of 20 equivalents of NaHCO$_3$, 1.1 equivalents of the DTPA-dianhydride are added. After 5 min, the dioxane solvent is removed under reduced pressure and the remaining aqueous solution is lyophilized. Purification of the product is achieved by silica gel chromatography (Silica Gel 60) with chloroform/methanol/acetic acid 50% (7/3/1, v/v/v), in order to separate the desired [DTPA^0-D-Phe^1-Boc-Lys^5]-Octreotide from the contaminating double-substituted DTPA-derivative and the unreacted starting material ([ε-*tert*-butyloxycarbonyl-Lys^5]-Octreotide).

Third step: Deprotection of the ε-NH$_2$ group of lysine with trifluoracetic acid, with subsequent sequential purification on Silica Gel 60, Duolite™ ES-861 and a weak basic anionic exchanger AG4-X4 (BioRad). The eluted desired product [DTPA^0-D-Phe^1]-Octreotide is then lyophilized. The purity of the preparation can be checked either by reverse phase HPLC [mobile phase: solvent A = H$_2$O/CH$_3$CN/H$_3$PO$_4$ (85%)/TMAH (tetramethylammonium hydroxide, 10% in water), 90/10/0.2/4 (v/v/v/v), (pH = 2.9) and solvent B = H$_2$O/CH$_3$CN/H$_3$PO$_4$ (85%)/TMAH (tetramethylammonium hydroxide, 10% in water), 30/70/0.4/4 (v/v/v/v), (pH 4.0); gradient 5–95% B in 20 min; column temperature: 45 °C; flow rate: 1.5 mL/min; detection wavelength: 205 nm) or by HPTLC on Silica Gel 60 HPTLC plates.

4.6.3 Labeling of [DTPA^0-D-Phe^1]-Octreotide with ^{111}In^{3+}

The [^{111}In-DTPA^0-D-Phe^1]-Octreotide (see Fig. 4.14) was prepared by combining the two kit components. An aliquot of the supplied Indium In-111 chloride solution was added to the vial containing the "cold" ligand [DTPA^0-D-Phe^1]-Octreotide molecule to form the [^{111}In-DTPA^0-D-Phe^1]-Octreotide labeled complex (the added radioactivity was the total radioactivity divided by the number of vials used (4 or 5). The pH of the resultant [^{111}In-DTPA^0-D-Phe^1]-Octreotide solution was between 3.8 and 4.3. No bacteriostatic preservative was present. The labeling yield of [^{111}In-DTPA^0-D-Phe^1]-Octreotide of the pooled preparations was determined prior to the administration to the patient. A method recommended for determining the labeling yield of the preparation will be described in the Sect. 4.6.4 [70, 72, 73].

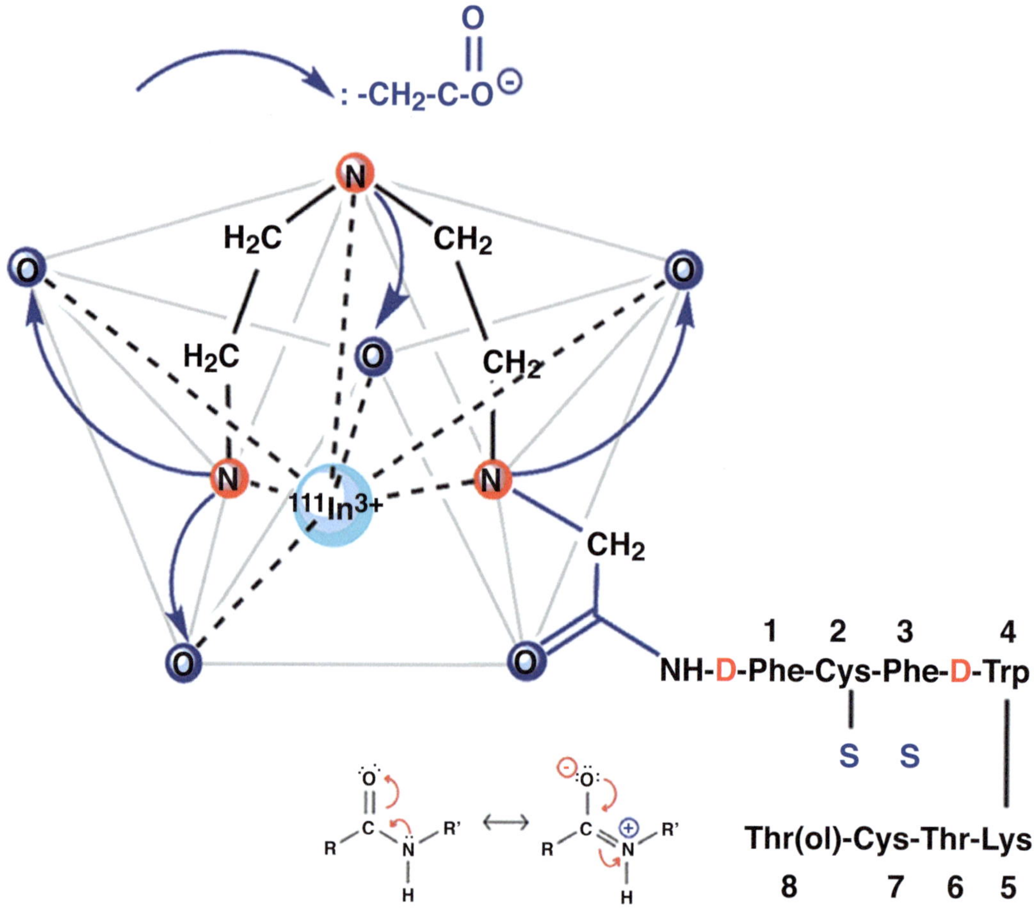

Fig. 4.14 The established distorted square antiprism geometry of the $^{111}In^{3+}$ ion with the DTPA moiety (coordination number: 7) in the [^{111}In-DTPA⁰-D-Phe¹]-Octreotide molecule. The Indium atom in the above structure has been drawn off-centered to facilitate the visualization. The eighth coordination position of the $^{111}In^{3+}$ ion may interact, although weakly, with the carbonyl oxygen of the amide bond (the resonance structures of the amide bond are shown below the DTPA moiety) [74, 75]

1. An appropriate aliquot of the Indium In-111 Chloride Sterile Solution vial was aseptically removed using the needle provided only (to avoid unwanted ions that tend to leach from the needles, as Al^{3+}, Cd^{2+}, etc., in the strongly acidic solution) and a shielded, sterile syringe.
2. The Indium In-111 Chloride Sterile Solution was injected into the Octreoscan™ Reaction Vial.
3. The Octreoscan™ Reaction Vial was swirled gently until the lyophilized pellet was completely dissolved.
4. The [^{111}In-DTPA⁰-D-Phe¹]-Octreotide solution was incubated at or below 25 °C for a minimum of 30 min. Note: A 30 min incubation time is required. Shorter incubation periods were avoided, as they could result in inadequate labeling.

5. Using proper shielding, the vial contents were visually inspected. The solution should be clear, colorless, and free of particulate matter. If not, the solution should not be used. It should be disposed in a safe and approved manner.

6. The [^{111}In-DTPA^0-D-Phe^1]-Octreotide pooled solution was assayed using a suitably calibrated ionization chamber.

7. The labeling yield of the pooled reconstituted vials was checked before administration to the patient, according to the instructions given below. If the radiochemical purity was less than 90%, the product was not used.

8. The reaction vial containing the pooled [^{111}In-DTPA^0-D-Phe^1]-Octreotide solution was stored at or below 25 °C (77 °F) until use and it was used within 2 h after the complexation reaction.

9. The pooled preparation can be diluted to a maximum volume of 10 mL with 0.9% Sodium Chloride Injection, USP immediately prior to injection, if desired. The sample should be drawn up into a shielded, sterile syringe and then administered to the patient.

4.6.4 Determination of the [^{111}In-DTPA^0-D-Phe^1]-Octreotide Labeling Yield [72]

4.6.4.1 Required Materials

1. Waters Sep-Pak™ C18 Cartridge, Part No. 51910
2. Methanol, 15 mL (Caution: toxic and flammable)
3. Distilled water, 20 mL
4. Disposable syringes:
   2–10-mL, no needle required
   2–5-mL, no needle required
   1–1-mL, with needle
5. Three disposable culture tubes or vials, minimum 10-mL capacity
6. Ion chamber

4.6.4.2 Preparation of the Sep-Pak™ Cartridge

1. The Sep-Pak™ cartridge was rinsed with 10 mL methanol as follows: a 10-mL syringe is filled with 10 mL methanol, the syringe was attached to the longer end of the Sep-Pak™ cartridge and the methanol was pushed through the cartridge. The eluate was discarded in a safe and approved manner.

2. Similarly, The Sep-Pak™ cartridge was also rinsed with 10 mL water. Caution was exercised, as the cartridge must kept wet, with no air bubbles trapped. If an air bubble was present, the cartridge was rinsed with additional 5 mL of water and the eluate was discarded.

4.6.4.3 Sample Analysis

1. An aliquot (0.05–0.1 mL) of the [^{111}In-DTPA^0-D-Phe^1]-Octreotide solution was withdrawn from the reaction vial, by using a 1-mL syringe. The preparation was applied to the Sep-Pak™ cartridge through the longer end of the cartridge.

2. Using a disposable 5-mL syringe, slowly (in dropwise manner) 5 mL water was pushed through the longer end of the cartridge and the eluate was collected in a counting vial. This eluate was labeled as Fraction 1.

3. Similarly, the cartridge was eluted with 5 mL methanol slowly, so that the elution occurred in a dropwise manner. This fraction was also collected in another counting vial and was labeled as Fraction 2. Two 5-mL portions of air were pushed through the longer end of the cartridge and the eluate was collected with Fraction 2.

4. The Sep-Pak™ cartridge was placed in a third vial for the assay.

4.6.4.4 Assay

1. The activity of Fraction 1 was assayed in a suitably calibrated ionization chamber. This fraction contains the hydrophilic impurities (e.g., unbound indium In-111).

2. The activity of Fraction 2 was also assayed. This fraction contained the [^{111}In-DTPA^0-D-Phe^1]-Octreotide.

3. Finally, the activity of the Sep-Pak™ cartridge was also assayed. This component contains the remaining non-elutable impurities.

4. All the materials used in the preparation, the sample analysis, and the assay were

subsequently disposed of in a safe and approved manner.

4.6.4.5 Calculations

1. Percent of [^{111}In-DTPA^0-D-Phe^1]-Octreotide = (Fraction 2 Activity/Total Activity) × 100%

   Where Total Activity = Fraction 1 + Fraction 2 + activity remaining in Sep-Pak™

   If this value was less than 90%, the preparation was not used and it was discarded in a safe and approved manner.

2. Percent of hydrophilic impurities = (Fraction 1 Activity/Total Activity) × 100%

3. Percent of non-elutable impurities = (Activity remaining in Sep-Pak™ cartridge/Total Activity) × 100%

4.6.5 Precautions

4.6.5.1 General

1. Therapy with octreotide acetate can elicit severe hypoglycemia in patients with insulinomas. Since [^{111}In-DTPA^0-D-Phe^1]-Octreotide is an octreotide analog, an intravenous line is recommended in any patient suspected of having an insulinoma. An intravenous solution containing glucose should be administered just before and during administration of [^{111}In-DTPA^0-D-Phe^1]-Octreotide.

2. Since [^{111}In-DTPA^0-D-Phe^1]-Octreotide is eliminated primarily by renal excretion, use in patients with impaired renal function should be carefully considered.

3. To help reduce the radiation dose to the thyroid, kidneys, bladder, and other target organs, patients should be well hydrated before the administration of [^{111}In-DTPA^0-D-Phe^1]-Octreotide. An increased fluid intake and frequent voiding were encouraged for 1 day after administration of this drug. In addition, a mild laxative (e.g., bisacodyl or lactulose) was recommended to the patients before and after the administration of [^{111}In-DTPA^0-D-Phe^1]-Octreotide.

4. The prepared [^{111}In-DTPA^0-D-Phe^1]-Octreotide solution should always be tested for labeling yield prior to administration. The product had to be used within 6 h of preparation.

5. Components of the kit are sterile and nonpyrogenic. To maintain sterility, it is essential that directions are followed carefully. Aseptic technique must be used during the preparation and administration of [^{111}In-DTPA^0-D-Phe^1]-Octreotide.

6. Octreotide acetate and the natural somatostatin hormone have been associated with cholelithiasis, presumably by altering fat absorption and possibly by decreasing motility of the gallbladder. However, a single dose of [^{111}In-DTPA^0-D-Phe^1]-Octreotide is not expected to cause cholelithiasis [72].

4.6.6 Adverse Reactions

The [DTPA^0-D-Phe^1]-Octreotide is derived from Octreotide, which is used as a therapeutic agent to control symptoms from certain tumors. The following adverse effects have been observed in clinical trials at a frequency of less than 1% of 538 patients: dizziness, fever, flush, headache, hypotension, changes in liver enzymes, joint pain, nausea, sweating, and weakness. These adverse effects were transient. During clinical trials, there was one reported case of bradycardia and one case of decreased hematocrit and hemoglobin. The usual diagnostic dose of [^{111}In-DTPA^0-D-Phe^1]-Octreotide is approximately 5–20 times less than the Octreotide therapeutic dose, therefore it is considered subtherapeutic, but this not the case when the [^{111}In-DTPA^0-D-Phe^1]-Octreotide is used for tumor therapy. The following adverse reactions have been associated with diagnostic doses of octreotide (10 μg of the peptide) in 3–10% of patients: nausea, injection site pain, diarrhea, abdominal pain/discomfort, loose stools, and vomiting. Hypertension and hyper- and hypoglycemia have also been reported with the use of Octreotide. The above adverse effects were more likely to occur with the administration of the 40–50 μg peptide doses used in each tumor radiotherapy session [72].

4.6.7 Dosage and Administration

For radiotherapeutic applications, 4–5 vials of the diagnostic kit were used, with a total peptide amount of 40–50 µg with the total added radioactivity of ^{111}InCl$_3$ ranging between 110–160 mCi (4070–5920 MBq), depending on the patient's weight and dosimetric data. Before administration, the patient as adequately hydrated. After administration, the patient was encouraged to drink fluids liberally. Elimination of extra fluid intake will help reduce the radiation dose by flushing out unbound [^{111}In-DTPA^0-D-Phe^1]-Octreotide by glomerular filtration. It was also recommended that a mild laxative (e.g., bisacodyl or lactulose) be given to the patient starting the evening before the radioactive drug administration and it was continued for 48 h after the procedure. Ample fluid uptake was imperative during this period as a support both to renal elimination and the bowel-cleansing process.

The calculated intravenous dose of the [^{111}In-DTPA^0-D-Phe^1]-Octreotide preparation was confirmed by a suitably calibrated radioactivity ionization chamber immediately before administration. The [^{111}In-DTPA^0-D-Phe^1]-Octreotide preparation, as with all intravenously administered products, was inspected visually for particulate matter and discoloration prior to administration. Preparations containing particulate matter or discoloration were not administered and they were disposed of in a safe manner, in compliance with the regulations. Aseptic techniques and effective shielding were employed in withdrawing doses for administration to patients. Waterproof gloves were worn during the administration procedure. The [^{111}In-DTPA^0-D-Phe^1]-Octreotide was never administered mixed with TPN (TPN: Total Parenteral Nutrition) solutions or through the same intravenous line [71, 72].

4.7 Clinical Pharmacology of [¹¹¹In-DTPA⁰-D-Phe¹]-Octreotide

[DTPA^0-D-Phe^1]-Octreotide is a DTPA conjugate of Octreotide, which is a long-acting analog of the human hormone, SST. Therefore, its labeled derivative ([^{111}In-DTPA^0-D-Phe^1]-Octreotide) binds to SSTRs on cell surfaces throughout the body. Within an hour after the injection, most of the dose of [^{111}In-DTPA^0-D-Phe^1]-Octreotide distributes from plasma to extravascular body tissues and concentrates in tumors containing a high density of SSTRs. After background clearance, visualization of somatostatin receptor-rich tissue is achieved. In addition to somatostatin receptor-rich tumors, the normal pituitary gland, thyroid gland, liver, spleen, and urinary bladder are also visualized in most patients, as is the bowel, to a lesser extent. Excretion is almost exclusively via the kidneys.

The binding of the labeled ligand [^{111}In-DTPA^0-D-Phe^1]-Octreotide to its appropriate receptor (SSTR) is followed by the internalization of the formed ligand-receptor complex via a clathrin-coated invagination of the plasma membrane, a temperature-dependent process known as receptor-mediated endocytosis. This process constitutes the major internalization pathway. The resulting vesicles shed their clathrin coat and fuse with endosomes, whose acidic environment causes the dissociation of the [^{111}In-DTPA^0-D-Phe^1]-Octreotide-SSTR complex (see Fig. 4.14). The SSTR is then recycled on the cell surface and the labeled peptide is further metabolized to ^{111}In-DTPA-D-Phe. The polarity and charge of this metabolite are responsible for its trapping inside the cell, since the ^{111}In-DTPA-D-Phe is a negatively charged molecule and therefore it cannot passively pass through the hydrophobic lysosomal or cell membranes. Moreover, part of the In-111 label may dissociate from the DTPA moiety and it migrates towards the nucleus through the nuclear pores, where it gets attached via an unknown biochemical mechanism. The emitted Auger electrons of In-111 are thus capable of releasing their energy at close proximity to the cell nucleus with high radiobiological effects (RBEs). In case the I-125-labeled Octreotide ([^{125}I-Tyr^3]-Octreotide) analogue is used, such a trapping is not possible, since the various I-125-containing degradation products leave the cell quite fast. In this case, the I-125 decaying atoms do not have the chance to deposit their energy in the intracellular environment, despite the high Auger electron yield per decay of I-125 and the long half-life of this isotope, thus rendering the I-125-labeled Octreotide analogues unfit as PRRT agents (PRRT: Peptide receptor radiotherapy) [18, 25, 28, 76–80].

Besides the direct and indirect radiotoxic effects of the Auger-emitting In-111 label, after their transport inside the cells, the "bystander effect" further augments the PRRT efficacy. The "bystander effect" is mediated through the local release of cytokines and free radicals from the radiation-damaged cells, which thus induce the death in non-irradiated adjacent cells through this mechanism. The observed discrepancy between the estimated from microdosimetry and the actual radiotherapeutic effects has been partially attributed to the "bystander effect" [10, 81].

During the development phase of in vitro saturable peptide binding assays, such as receptor binding assays and radioimmunoassays, it became evident that the much needed maximization of the assay sensitivity required the highest signal-to-background noise (S/N) ratio possible. Therefore, by lowering the mass of the radioligand and/or maximizing its specific radioactivity led to the improvement in the S/N ratio [82, 83]. Octreotide belongs to the family of the regulatory peptides and consequently its respective receptors (SSTRs) are characterized by high affinity but of low capacity (therefore, they are easily saturable). In the administered labeled Octreoscan™ preparations, approximately 90% of the administered peptide is in its unlabeled form ([DTPA^0-D-Phe^1]-Octreotide), unavoidably decreasing the in vivo binding of its labeled form ([^{111}In-DTPA^0-D-Phe^1]-Octreotide), due to the anticipated competition between the labeled and the unlabeled ligands for the limited number of the same somatostatin receptor sites [84].

However, the anticipated maximum % uptake of the labeled ligand though, when the lowest possible dose of the highest specific radioactivity [^{111}In-DTPA^0-D-Phe^1]-Octreotide was administered, failed to materialize. What was in reality observed, when the % of the radioactivity uptake was plotted vs. the injected peptide mass, was a bell-shaped curve, suggesting that two opposite effects are operating in vivo. According to Breeman et al. [85], the negative effect, due to the

saturation of the receptor sites when increasing total peptide amounts are present (as mentioned previously, ≈90% of the administered ligand remains unlabeled), appears to be counterbalanced by the positive effect that the higher amount of the ligand has on the endocytosis rate of the ligand-receptor complex. Thus, in order to achieve the optimum sensitivity in the scintigraphic detection of somatostatin receptor-positive tissues (i.e. tumors) an optimum dose of total peptide ligand is essential (at least 10 μg) and this has been taken into consideration in the Octreoscan™ kit formulation. It should be kept in mind though, since all the regulatory peptide receptors get saturated very rapidly, that the range of the optimal % uptake versus the injected mass of the ligand is fairly narrow; for this reason, the highest possible specific activity of the labeled ligand is absolutely essential, especially for *Peptide Receptor Radionuclide Therapy* (*PRRT*) applications, along with clinical studies for optimization of the total mass of the ligand to be administered [86]. Later results by Lewis et al. though [87], in a tumor-bearing rat model with ^{64}Cu-TETA-Tyr^3-Octreotate, seem to contradict the above interpretation of the experimental data, since in this model at least, increasing amounts of the "cold" peptide (10–5000 ng of TETA-Tyr^3-Octreotate) along with a constant amount of radioactive peptide (5 μCi/0.2 MBq ^{64}Cu-TETA-Tyr^3-Octreotate) decreased the % radioactivity uptake of the various organs, as expected (competition between "cold" and radioactive peptide for a limited number of available receptors).

Comparing the specific activities of labeled DOTA- and DTPA-peptides with In-111, Y-90 and Lu-177, the highest specific activity of the ligand was obtained with [^{111}In-DTPA^0-D-Phe^1]-Octreotide (1.7 GBq•nmole^{-1}), while the specific activity of Lu-177 and Y-90 labeled DOTA-peptides did not exceed in practice the 0.5 GBq•nmole^{-1}. The lower specific activity of Lu-177 and Y-90 labeled DOTA-peptides is believed to be the result of competing ion contaminant levels and the low DOTA-complexation reaction rate. A constraint on the maximum specific activity to be kept always in mind in the preparation of various labeled peptides is the integrity of the labeled compound due to radiolysis, of more concern if α- and β-emitters are used, a fact that gives a definite additional advantage to the Auger-emitting labels [88, 89].

4.7.1 Pharmacokinetics

The injected [¹¹¹In-DTPA⁰-D-Phe¹]-Octreotide leaves the plasma rapidly with one-third of the injected radioactivity dose remaining in the blood pool at 10 min after administration. Plasma levels continue to decline so that by 20 h post injection, about 1% of the radioactive dose is found in the blood pool. The biological half-life of [¹¹¹In-DTPA⁰-D-Phe¹]-Octreotide is 6 h. Half of the injected dose is recoverable in urine within 6 h after injection, 85% is recovered in the first 24 h, and over 90% is recovered in urine by 2 days. Hepatobiliary excretion represents a minor route of elimination, and less than 2% of the injected dose is recovered in feces within 3 days after the [¹¹¹In-DTPA⁰-D-Phe¹]-Octreotide injection [72].

4.7.2 Metabolism

For several hours after the administration of [¹¹¹In-DTPA⁰-D-Phe¹]-Octreotide, plasma radioactivity is predominantly in its parent form. Ten percent of the radioactivity excreted is non-peptide-bound [72].

4.7.3 Pharmacodynamics

[¹¹¹In-DTPA⁰-D-Phe¹]-Octreotide binds to cell surface somatostatin receptors. In nonclinical pharmacologic studies, the hormonal effect of Octreoscan in vitro is one-tenth that of octreotide. Since diagnostic imaging doses of [¹¹¹In-DTPA⁰-D-Phe¹]-Octreotide are lower than the therapeutic doses of "cold" octreotide, the [¹¹¹In-DTPA⁰-D-Phe¹]-Octreotide does not exert clinically significant somatostatin-mediated effects if administered for imaging applications, but with the radiotherapeutic peptide doses, cau-

tion should be exercised and measures should be taken to avoid any complications. [¹¹¹In-DTPA⁰-D-Phe¹]-Octreotide is cleared from the body primarily by renal excretion but its elimination has not been studied in anephric patients or in those with poorly functioning kidneys. It is not known [¹¹¹In-DTPA⁰-D-Phe¹]-Octreotide can be removed by dialysis. Dosage adjustments in patients with decreased renal function have not been studied [25, 77].

Small peptides and protein fragments of appropriate charge and size (MW < 70 kDa) are initially filtered through the glomeruli and then get reabsorbed in the proximal tubules. The non-specific receptor system of megalin/cubulin (Fig. 4.15) contributes most to their reabsorption, through receptor-mediated endocytosis. Megalin and cubulin are multiligand, structurally dissimilar endocytic receptors (megalin is a transmembrane protein, while cubulin is not) located at the apical membrane of the proximal tubular cells and they operate in a synergistic fashion (Fig. 4.15). Studies in megalin-deficient mice revealed that the [¹¹¹In-DTPA⁰-D-Phe¹]-Octreotide renal uptake was only 15–30% of that in the control mice [28, 56, 89–91].

After lysosome processing of the endocytosed [¹¹¹In-DTPA⁰-D-Phe¹]-Octreotide, the trapped polar In-111 labeled degradation products in the proximal tubular cells burden the radiosensitive kidneys with unwanted radiation load (kidneys are the dose-limiting organs in PRRT). The renal uptake of [¹¹¹In-DTPA⁰-D-Phe¹]-Octreotide appears to be facilitated by the electrostatic interaction between the slightly positive net charge of the molecule at a pH range 5–7, which is the usual pH range of the glomerular filtrate and the negatively charged proximal tubular cell surface. In Fig. 4.16, the electrophoretic mobility data on cellulose acetate (CAE: Cellulose Acetate Electrophoresis) of three Octreotide-based peptides with different net charge and lipophilicity are shown [12, 38, 80, 89]. In a comparative study of the renal uptake and metabolism between [¹¹¹In-DTPA⁰-D-Phe¹]-Octreotide and the modified [¹¹¹In-DTPA⁰-Asp⁰-D-Phe¹]-Octreotide and [¹¹¹In-DTPA⁰-D-Phe⁻¹-Asp⁰-D-Phe¹]-Octreotide, it was concluded that the insertion of a negatively

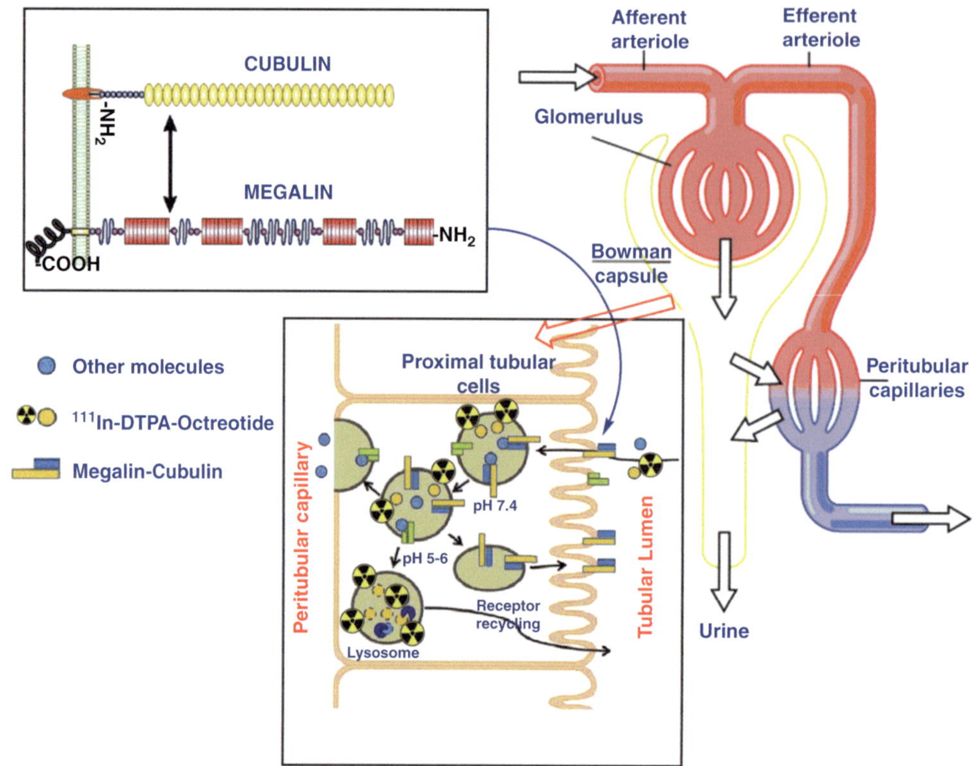

Fig. 4.15 Schematic depiction of the protein and peptide handling by the proximal tubular cells. The megalin/cubulin system located at the apex of the proximal tubular cells (nonselective system) mediates the reabsorption process for the [¹¹¹In-DTPA⁰-D-Phe¹]-Octreotide, along with other molecules (i.e. albumin, vitamins, aminoacids). The acidic environment of the lysosomes leads to the trapping of labeled hydrolysis products of the [¹¹¹In-DTPA⁰-D-Phe¹]-Octreotide molecule and contributes to the undesirable renal irradiation

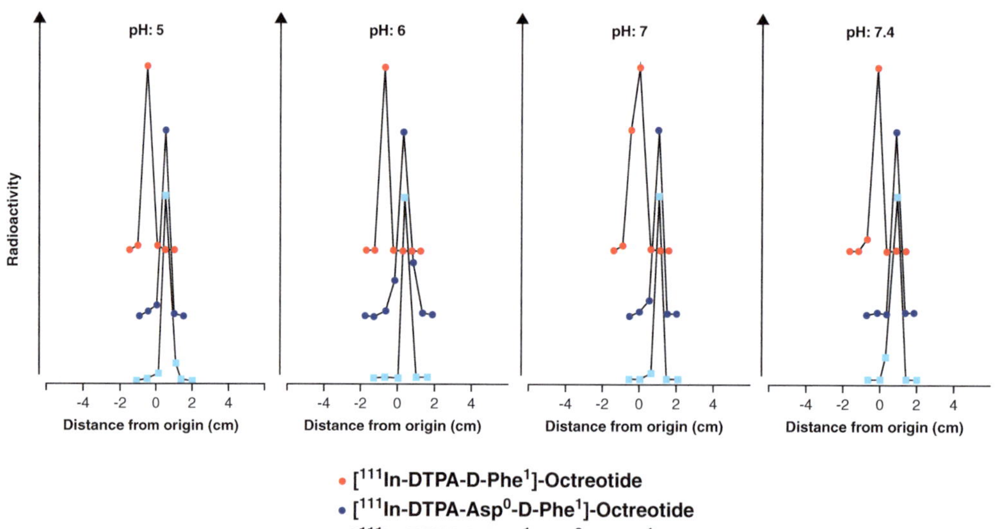

Fig. 4.16 The cellulose acetate electrophoresis (CAE) behavior of three structurally related peptides, at four different pH solutions, simulating urine and blood. The peptides differ in their net charge and lipophilicity [27, 89]

charged aspartic acid at the aminic end of the Octreotide molecule decreases its renal uptake due to the developing electrostatic repulsion, as it approaches the negatively charged proximal tubular cells. This result was further supported by the data of Akizawa et al. [27, 89].

4.8 Concluding Remarks

[^{111}In-DTPA^0-D-Phe^1]-Octreotide is a theragnostic radiopharmaceutical, which permits molecular imaging (SPECT or SPECT/CT) studies for acquisition of useful pre-therapy data (biodistribution, dosimetry, critical organ or tissue and the maximum tolerated dose), despite the limitations of In-111 as an Auger-emitting radionuclide. [^{111}In-DTPA^0-D-Phe^1]-Octreotide has been in use for more than two decades, mainly as an imaging agent and the experience that has been acquired formed the basis for the reevaluation of Auger emitters as radiotherapeutic agents. Indeed, extensive studies have proved that the small volume micrometastases of SSTR-expressing tumors can be successfully contained and possibly circulating tumor cells as well. Based on the findings of imaging results, dose ranging experiments, for higher dose-targeted molecular therapy and increased effectiveness, are thus allowed. All these factors lead to a tailored imaging and therapy approach to the same patient with [^{111}In-DTPA^0-D-Phe^1]-Octreotide as the modern personalized medicine approach dictates [80].

However, there is always ample room for improvement. Increasing the % uptake of the somatostatin analogue was an important step in this process, after the introduction of [DOTA^0-D-Phe^1-Tyr^3]-Octreotate (in which the C-terminal threoninol is replaced with threonine) by Kwekkeboom et al [88], which exhibited a nine-fold increased affinity for the SSTR$_2$ expressed by tumor cells compared with the affinity of [DOTA^0-D-Phe^1-Tyr^3]-Octreotide. The dimerization of the octreotide peptide ligand has been conclusively shown to increase the SSTR binding affinity with reduced background, opening the door to another possibility for improving the behavior of this class of ligands in the tumor radiotherapy set-ting [92]. Furthermore, experimental results with modifications in the incubation buffer used for the preparation of the In-111-labeled Octreotide analogue, which results in increased specific activity of the administered radiopharmaceutical and also the attachment of a nuclear localization sequence (NLS: Nuclear Localization Sequence) on the Octreotide molecule, are expected to augment the anti-tumor efficacy of these analogues, by maximizing the energy deposition of the Auger electrons in the region of the cell nucleus [3, 41, 93–97]. In addition, pharmacologic intervention for the sensitization of the replicating tumor cells, by interfering with the repair mechanisms of the DNA damage, is another clever strategy to increase therapeutic efficacy of the Auger-emitting radioligands. This approach has been attempted with Olaparib, a poly-[ADP-ribose]-polymerase 1 (PARP-1) inhibitor, which augments the cytotoxicity of the administered dose of the In-111-labeled preparation, by increasing the number of cytotoxic DSBs [98]. And lastly, the charge-modification of the NH$_2$-terminal-labeled somatostatin analogues, with the insertion of a negatively charged aspartic acid moiety therein, by facilitating its kidney excretion and reducing significantly the unwanted and deleterious kidney irradiation, allows the increase of the total administered Auger-emitter dose for higher therapeutic efficacy [27, 46].

References

1. Brazeau P, Vale W, Burgus R, et al. Hypothalamic polypeptide that inhibits the secretion of imunoreactive pituitary growth hormone. Science. 1973;179:77–9.
2. Weckbecker G, Lewis I, Albert R, et al. Opportunities in somatostatin research: biological, chemical and therapeutic aspects. Nat Rev Drug Discov. 2003;2:999–1017. https://doi.org/10.1038/nrd1255.
3. Bushberg JT, Seibert JA, Leid EM. The essential physics of medical imaging. 2nd ed. Philadelphia: Lippincott Williams & Wilkins; 2002.
4. De Lecea L, Criado JR, Prospero-Garcia O, et al. A cortical neuropeptide with neuronal depressant and sleep-modulating properties. Nature. 1996;381:242–5.
5. Gottero C, Prodam F, Destefanis S, et al. Cortistatin-17 and -14 exert the same endocrine activities

as somatostatin in humans. Growth Hormon IGF Res. 2004;14:382–7.

6. IUPAC-IUB Common Biochem Nomenclature. An one-letter notation for amino acid sequences. Tentative rules. Biochemistry. 1968;7:2703–5. https://doi.org/10.1021/bi00848a001.

7. Elliott DE. Somatostatin. 2001. https://epdf.tips/somatostatin9b1681210755ce0bffeb-5c27a17209b838154.html. Accessed 19 Oct 2018.

8. Bronstein-Sitton N. Somatostatin and the somatostatin receptors: versatile regulators of biological activity. 2018. https://www.alomone.com/article/somatostatin-somatostatin-receptors-versatile-regulators-biological-activity. Accessed 15 Oct 2018.

9. Barbieri F, Bajetto A, Pattarozzi A, et al. Peptide receptor targeting in cancer: the somatostatin paradigm. Int J Pept. 2013;2013:926295, 20 p. https://doi.org/10.1155/2013/926295.

10. Körner M, Reubi JC. Somatostatin. In: Kastin A, editor. Handbook of biologically active peptides. 1st ed. USA: Elsevier; 2006. p. 435–43.

11. Patel YC. Somatostatin and its receptor family. Front Neuroendocrinol. 1999;20:157–98.

12. Dalm DU, de Jong M. Comparing the use of radiolabeled SSTR agonists and an SSTR antagonist in breast cancer: does the model choice influence the outcome? EJNMMI Radiopharm Chem. 2017;2:11. https://doi.org/10.1186/s41181-017-0030-z.

13. Tulipano G, Schulz S. Novel insights in somatostatin receptor physiology. Eur J Endocrinol. 2007;156:S3–S11. https://doi.org/10.1530/eje.1.02354.

14. Reubi JC, Waser B, Mäcke H, et al. Highly increased ^{125}I-JR11 antagonist binding in vitro reveals novel indications for sst2 targeting in human cancers. J Nucl Med. 2017;58:300–6. https://doi.org/10.2967/jnumed.116.177733.

15. Hubalewska-Dydejczyk A, Signore A, de Jong M, Dierckx RA, Buscombe J, van de Wiele C, editors. Somatostatin analogues: from research to clinical practice. Hoboken: Wiley; 2015.

16. Günther T, Tulipano G, Dournaud P, et al. International Union of Basic and Clinical Pharmacology. CV. Somatostatin receptors: structure, function, ligands, and new nomenclature. Pharmacol Rev. 2018;70:763–835. https://doi.org/10.1124/pr.117.015388.

17. Patel RC, Kumar U, Lamb DC, et al. Ligand binding to somatostatin receptors induces receptor-specific oligomer formation in live cells. Proc Natl Acad Sci U S A. 2002;99:3294–9. https://doi.org/10.1073/pnas.042705099.

18. Reubi JC, Schonbrunn A. Illuminating somatostatin analog action at neuroendocrine tumor receptors. Trends Pharmacol Sci. 2013;34:676–88. https://doi.org/10.1016/j.tips.2013.10.001.

19. Reubi JC, Waser B, Schaer J-C, et al. Somatostatin receptor sst_1–sst_5 expression in normal and neoplastic human tissues using receptor autoradiography with subtype-selective ligands. Eur J Nucl Med. 2001;28:836–46. https://doi.org/10.1007/s002590100541.

20. Csaba Z, Peineau S, Dournaud P. Molecular mechanisms of somatostatin receptor trafficking. J Mol Endocrinol. 2012;48:R1–R12.

21. Fani M, Nicolas GP, Wild D. Somatostatin receptor antagonists for imaging and therapy. J Nucl Med. 2017;58:61S–6S. https://doi.org/10.2967/jnumed.116.186783.

22. Hofland LJ, Lamberts SWJ. The pathophysiological consequences of somatostatin receptor internalization and resistance. Endocr Rev. 2003;24:28–47. https://doi.org/10.1210/er.2000-0001.

23. Zhang X, Kim K-M. Multifactorial regulation of G protein-coupled receptor endocytosis. Biomol Ther. 2017;25:26–43.

24. Hanyaloglu AC, von Zastrow M. Regulation of GPCRs by endocytic membrane trafficking and its potential implications. Annu Rev Pharmacol Toxicol. 2008;48:537–68. https://doi.org/10.1146/annurev.pharmtox.48.113006.

25. Breeman WA, de Jong M, Kwekkeboom DJ, et al. Somatostatin receptor-mediated imaging and therapy: basic science, current knowledge, limitations and future perspectives. Eur J Nucl Med. 2001;28:1421–9. https://doi.org/10.1007/s002590100502.

26. Fani M, Braun F, Waser B, et al. Unexpected sensitivity of sst2 antagonists to N-terminal radiometal modifications. J Nucl Med. 2012;53:1481–9. https://doi.org/10.2967/jnumed.112.102764.

27. Oshima N, Akizawa H, Kawashima H, et al. Redesign of negatively charged ^{111}In-DTPA-octreotide derivative to reduce renal radioactivity. Nucl Med Biol. 2017;48:16–25.

28. Melis M, Krenning EP, Bernard BF, et al. Localisation and mechanism of renal retention of radiolabelled somatostatin analogues. Eur J Nucl Med Mol Imaging. 2005;32:1136–43. https://doi.org/10.1007/s00259-005-1793-0.

29. Fani M, Del Pozzo L, Abiraj K, et al. PET of somatostatin receptor-positive tumors using ^{64}Cu- and ^{68}Ga-somatostatin antagonists: the chelate makes the difference. J Nucl Med. 2011;52:1110–8. https://doi.org/10.2967/jnumed.111.087999.

30. Ginj M, Zhang H, Waser B, et al. Radiolabeled somatostatin receptor antagonists are preferable to agonists for in vivo peptide receptor targeting of tumors. Proc Natl Acad Sci U S A. 2006;103:16436–41. https://doi.org/10.1073/pnas.0607761103.

31. Kassis AI. Therapeutic radionuclides: biophysical and radiobiologic principles. Semin Nucl Med. 2008;38:358–66. https://doi.org/10.1053/j.semnuclmed.2008.05.002.

32. Kassis AI, Adelstein SJ. Considerations in the selection of radionuclides for cancer therapy. In: Welch MJ, Revanly CS, editors. Handbook of radiopharmaceuticals: Wiley; 2005. p. 767–93. https://doi.org/10.1002/0470846380.ch27.

33. Howel RW. Auger processes in the 21st century. Int J Radiat Biol. 2008;84:959–75. https://doi.org/10.1080/09553000802395527.

34. Duparc OH. Pierre Auger-Lise Meitner: comparative contributions to the Auger effect. Int J Mat Res (formerly Z Metallkd). 2009;100:1162–6. https://doi.org/10.3139/146.110163.

35. Feinendegen LE. Biological damage from the Auger effect, possible benefits. Radiat Environ Biophys. 1975;12:85–99.

36. Howell RW. Radiation spectra for Auger-electron emitting radionuclides: report No. 2 of AAPM Nuclear Medicine Task Group No. 6. Med Phys. 1992;19:1371–83. https://doi.org/10.1118/1.596927.

37. Lee BQ, Kibédi T, Stuchbery AE, et al. Atomic radiations in the decay of medical radioisotopes: a physics perspective. Comput Math Methods Med. 2012;2012:651475, 14 p. https://doi.org/10.1155/2012/651475.

38. McMillan DD, Maeda J, Bell JJ, et al. Validation of ^{64}Cu-ATSM damaging DNA via high-LET Auger electron emission. J Radiat Res. 2015;56:784–91. https://doi.org/10.1093/jrr/rrv042.

39. Cornelissen B, Vallis KA. Targeting the nucleus: an overview of Auger-electron radionuclide therapy. Curr Drug Discov Technol. 2010;7:263–79. https://doi.org/10.2174/157016310793360657.

40. Falzone N, Cornelissen B, Vallis KA. Auger emitting radiopharmaceuticals for cancer therapy. In: Gómez-Tejedor G, Fuss M, editors. Radiation damage in biomolecular systems. Biological and medical physics, biomedical engineering. Dordrecht: Springer; 2012.

41. Piroozfar B, Raisali G, Alirezapour B, et al. The effect of ^{111}In radionuclide distance and Auger electron energy on direct induction of DNA double strand breaks: a Monte Carlo study using Geant4-toolkit. Int J Radiat Biol. 2018;94(4):385–93. https://doi.org/10.1080/09553002.2018.1440329.

42. Bin Othman M, Mitry NR, Lewington VJ, et al. Re-assessing gallium-67 as a therapeutic radionuclide. Nucl Med Biol. 2017;46:12–8. https://doi.org/10.1016/j.nucmedbio.2016.10.008.

43. Thisgaard H. Accelerator based production of Auger-electron-emitting isotopes for radionuclide therapy. Dissertation, Risø National Laboratory for Sustainable Energy, Technical University of Denmark. 2008.

44. Thisgaard H, Jensen M. Sb-119: a potent Auger emitter for targeted radionuclide therapy. Med Phys. 2008;35:3839–46. https://doi.org/10.1118/1.2963993.

45. Stepanek J, Larsson B, Weinreich R. Auger-electron spectra of radionuclides for therapy and diagnostics. Acta Oncol. 1996;35:863–8. https://doi.org/10.3109/02841869609104038.

46. Fisher DR, Shen S, Meredith RF. MIRD dose estimate report No. 20: radiation absorbed-dose estimates for ^{111}In- and ^{90}Y-ibritumomab tiuxetan. J Nucl Med. 2009;50:644–52. https://doi.org/10.2967/jnumed.108.057331.

47. Lahiri S, Maiti M, Ghosh K. Production and separation of ^{111}In: an important radionuclide in life sciences: a mini review. J Radioanal Nucl Chem. 2012;297:309–18. https://doi.org/10.1007/s10967-012-2344-3.

48. Schlyer DJ. Production of radionuclides in accelerators. In: Welch MJ, Redvanly CS, editors. Handbook of radiopharmaceuticals: radiochemistry and applications. Hoboken: Wiley; 2003. p. 1–71.

49. Kocher DC. Radioactive decay data tables. DOE/TIC-11026, 115. 1981.

50. Tuck DG. Critical survey of stability constants of complexes of indium. Pure Appl Chem. 1983;55:1477–528.

51. Anderson CJ, Welch MJ. Radiometal-labeled agents (non-technetium) for diagnostic imaging. Chem Rev. 1999;99:2219–34. https://doi.org/10.1021/cr980451q.

52. Dilworth JR, Pascu SI. The radiopharmaceutical chemistry of gallium (III) and indium (III) for SPECT imaging. In: Long N, Wong W-T, editors. The chemistry of molecular imaging. 1st ed: Wiley; 2015. p. 165–76. https://doi.org/10.2967/jnumed.110.075101.

53. Harrison RC. Indium chemistry in radiopharmaceutical development. In: Cox PH, Mather SJ, Sampson CB, Lazarus CR, editors. Progress in radiopharmacy. Leiden: Martinus Nijhoff Publishers; 1986. p. 173–96.

54. Liu S. The role of coordination chemistry in the development of target-specific radiopharmaceuticals. Chem Soc Rev. 2004;33:445–61. https://doi.org/10.1039/b309961j.

55. Martell AE, Hancock RD. Factors governing the formation of complexes with unidentate ligands in aqueous solution. Some general considerations. In: Metal complexes in aqueous solutions. Springer US; 1996. p. 15–61.

56. Vegt E, de Jong M, Wetzels JFM, et al. Renal toxicity of radiolabeled peptides and antibody fragments: mechanisms, impact on radionuclide therapy, and strategies for prevention. J Nucl Med. 2010;51:1049–58. https://doi.org/10.2967/jnumed.110.075101.

57. Deferm C, Onghena B, Hoogerstraete V, et al. Speciation of indium (III) chloro complexes in the solvent extraction process from chloride aqueous solutions to ionic liquids. Dalton Trans. 2017;46:4412–21. https://doi.org/10.1039/c7dt00618g.

58. Ferri D. Complex formation equilibriums between indium (III) and chloride ions. Acta Chem Scand. 1972;26:733–46.

59. Harris WR, Chen Y, Wein K. Equilibrium constants for the binding of indium (III) to human serum transferrin. Inorg Chem. 1994;33:4991–8.

60. Yeh SM, Meares CF, Goodwin DA. Decomposition rates of radiopharmaceutical indium chelates in serum. J Radioanal Chem. 1979;53:327–36. https://doi.org/10.1007/bf02517931.

61. Layne WW, Hnatowich DJ, Doherty PW, et al. Evaluation of the viability of In-111-labeled DTPA coupled to fibrinogen. J Nucl Med. 1982;23:627–30.

62. Hsieh W-Y, Liu S. Synthesis, characterization, and structures of indium In(DTPA-BA$_2$) and

yttrium Y(DTPA-BA$_2$)(CH$_3$OH) complexes (BA benzylamine): models for [111]In- and ^{90}Y-labeled DTPA-biomolecule conjugates. Inorg Chem. 2004;43:6006–14.

63. Narita H, Tanaka M, Shiwaku H, et al. Structural properties of the inner coordination sphere of indium chloride complexes in organic and aqueous solutions. Dalton Trans. 2014;43:1630–5. https://doi.org/10.1039/c3dt52474d.

64. Sun Y, Motekaitis RJ, Martell AE, et al. N,N′-bis(2-mercaptoethyl)ethylenediamine-N,N′-diacetic acid; an effective ligand for indium(III). Inorgan Chim Acta. 1995;228:77–9. https://doi.org/10.1016/0020-1693(94)04392-9.

65. Ivanova VY, Chevela VV, Bezryadin SG. Complex formation of indium (III) with citric acid in aqueous solution. Russ Chem Bull. 2015;64:1842–9. https://doi.org/10.1007/s11172-015-1082-4.

66. Silva AMN, Kong X, Parkin MC, et al. Iron (III) citrate speciation in aqueous solution. Dalton Trans. 2009;0:8616–25. https://doi.org/10.1039/b910970f.

67. Thompson LCA, Pacer R. The solubility of indium hydroxide in acidic and basic media at 25°C. J Inorg Nucl Chem. 1963;25:1041–4. https://doi.org/10.1016/0022-1902(63)80039-1.

68. Maloney TJ, Camp AE Jr. Purification of indium 111. US Patent 6,162,648, 19 Dec 2000. 2000.

69. Brom M, Joosten L, Oyen WJG, et al. Improved labelling of DTPA- and DOTA conjugated peptides and antibodies with ^{111}In in HEPES and MES buffer. EJNMMI Res. 2012;2:4. https://doi.org/10.1186/2191-219X-2-4.

70. Balon HR, Brown TLY, Goldsmith SJ, et al. The SNM practice guideline for somatostatin receptor scintigraphy 2.0. J Nucl Med Technol. 2011;39:317–24.

71. Limouris GS, Chatziioannou A, Kontogeorgakos D, et al. Selective hepatic arterial infusion of In-111-DTPA-Phe[1]-octreotide in neuro-endocrine liver metastases. Eur J Nucl Med Mol Imaging. 2008;35:1827–37.

72. OctreoScan™ package insert, Petten, The Netherlands, Mallinckrodt Medical B.V. September 2017 (revision).

73. Bakker WH, Albert R, Bruns C, et al. [^{111}In-DTPA-D-Phe[1]]-octreotide, a potential radiopharmaceutical for imaging of somatostatin receptor-positive tumors: synthesis, radiolabeling and in vitro validation. Life Sci. 1991;49:1583–91. https://doi.org/10.1016/0024-3205(91)90052-d.

74. Maecke HR, Riesen A, Ritter W. The molecular structure of indium-DTPA. J Nucl Med. 1989;30:1235–1.

75. Siddons CJ. Metal ion complexing properties of amide donating ligands. Dissertation, University of North Carolina at Wilmington. 2004.

76. Bavelaar BM, Lee BQ, Gill MR, et al. Subcellular targeting of theranostic radionuclides. Front Pharmacol. 2018;9:996. https://doi.org/10.3389/fphar.2018.00996.

77. Capello A, Krenning EP, Wout AP, et al. Peptide receptor radionuclide therapy in vitro using [^{111}In-DTPA[0]]-octreotide. J Nucl Med. 2003;44:98–104.

78. Reubi JC. Peptide receptors as molecular targets for cancer diagnosis and therapy. Endocr Rev. 2003;24:389–427. https://doi.org/10.1210/er.2002-0007.

79. Reubi JC, Schär J-C, Waser B, et al. Affinity profiles for human somatostatin receptor subtypes SST$_1$–SST$_5$ of somatostatin radiotracers selected for scintigraphic and radiotherapeutic use. Eur J Nucl Med. 2000;27:273–82. https://doi.org/10.1007/s002590050034.

80. van Essen M, Sundin A, Krenning EP. Neuroendocrine tumours: the role of imaging for diagnosis and therapy. Nat Rev Endocrinol. 2014;10:102–14. https://doi.org/10.1038/nrendo.2013.246.

81. Mariani G, Bodei L, Adelstein SJ, et al. Emerging roles for radiometabolic therapy of tumors based on auger electron emission. J Nucl Med. 2000;41:1519–21.

82. Eckelman WC, Frank JA, Brechbiel M. Theory and practice of imaging saturable binding sites. Invest Radiol. 2002;37:101–6.

83. Gokce A, Nakamura RM, Tubis M, et al. Synthesis of indium-labeled antibody-chelate conjugates for radioassays. Int J Nucl Med Biol. 1982;9:85–95. https://doi.org/10.1016/0047-0740(82)90034-1.

84. Jonard P, Jamar F, Walrand S. Effect of peptide amount on biodistribution of Y-86-DOTA-Tyr[3]-octreotide (SMT487). J Nucl Med. 2000;41:260 p.

85. Breeman DWAP, Kwekkeboom DJ, Kooij PPM, et al. Effect of dose and specific activity on tissue, distribution of indium-111-pentetreotide in rats. J Nucl Med. 1995;36:623–7.

86. Wout AP, Breeman D, Kwekkeboom J, et al. Effect of dose and specific activity on tissue, distribution of indium-111-pentetreotide in rats. J Nucl Med. 1995;36:623–7.

87. Lewis JS, Lewis MR, Cutler PD, et al. Radiotherapy and dosimetry of ^{64}Cu-TETA-Tyr[3]-octreotate in a somatostatin receptor-positive, tumor-bearing rat model. Clin Cancer Res. 1999;11:3608–16. https://doi.org/10.1158/1078-0432.CCR-04-1084.

88. Kwekkeboom J, Bakker DH, Kooij WP, et al. [^{177}Lu-DOTA[0]-Tyr[3]]-octreotate: comparison with [^{111}In-DTPA[0]]-octreotide in patients. Eur J Nucl Med. 2001;28:1319–25.

89. Akizawa H, Arano Y, Mifune M. Effect of molecular charges on renal uptake of ^{111}In-DTPA-conjugated peptides. Nucl Med Biol. 2001;28:761–8.

90. Christensen EI, Birn H. Megalin and cubilin: multifunctional endocytic receptors. Nat Rev Mol Cell Biol. 2002;3:258–67. https://doi.org/10.1038/nrm778.

91. De Jong M, Barone R, Krenning E, et al. Megalin is essential for renal proximal tubule reabsorption of [^{111}In-DTPA[0]]-Octreotide. J Nucl Med. 2005;46:1696–700.

92. Dong C, Zhao H, Yang S, et al. ^{99m}Tc-labeled dimeric octreotide peptide: a radiotracer with high tumor uptake for single-photon emission computed tomography imaging of somatostatin receptor subtype 2-positive tumors. Mol Pharm. 2013;10:2925–33. https://doi.org/10.1021/mp400040z.

93. Chen P, Wang J, Hope K, et al. Nuclear localizing sequences promote nuclear translocation and enhance the radiotoxicity of the anti-CD33 monoclonal antibody HuM195 labeled with ^{111}In in human myeloid leukemia cells. J Nucl Med. 2006;47:827–36.

94. Ginj M, Hinni K, Tschumi S, et al. Trifunctional somatostatin-based derivatives designed for targeted radiotherapy using Auger electron emitters. J Nucl Med. 2005;46:2097–103.

95. Hillyar C. Auger electron radionuclide therapy utilizing F3 peptide to target the nucleolus. Dissertation, Jesus College, University of Oxford. 2015.

96. Cornelissen B, Able S, Kersemans V, et al. Nanographene oxide-based radioimmunoconstructs for in vivo targeting and SPECT imaging of HER2-positive tumors. Biomaterials. 2013;34:1146–54. https://doi.org/10.1016/j.biomaterials.2012.10.054.

97. Kersemans V, Kersemans K, Cornelissen B. Cell penetrating peptides for in vivo molecular imaging applications. Curr Pharm Des. 2008;14:2415–27. https://doi.org/10.2174/138161208785777432.

98. Nayak TK, Atcher RW, Prossnitz ER, et al. Enhancement of somatostatin-receptor-targeted ^{177}Lu-[DOTA^0-Tyr^3]-octreotide therapy by gemcitabine pretreatment-mediated receptor uptake, up-regulation and cell cycle modulation. Nucl Med Biol. 2008;35:673–8. https://doi.org/10.1016/j.nucmedbio.2008.05.003.

Regulations and Requirements of Scientific Centers Performing Radiopeptide Therapies

5

Maria I. Paphiti

5.1 Introduction

Radiopeptide Therapy or Peptide Receptor Radionuclide Therapy (PRRT) is a multidisciplinary and technically demanding procedure, and many emerging centers underestimate the expertise required to perform safe and successful treatment with radionuclides or "byproduct material" such as with ^{111}In-Octreotide. First and foremost, a multidisciplinary treatment protocol should be well established for the patient treatment. This includes the structured interaction between diagnostic imaging, nuclear medicine, requirements and provisions for radiation safety, multidisciplinary care team, and surgical oncology nursing staff, release and follow-up procedures.

5.1.1 Multidisciplinary Approach

Scientific centers performing radiopeptide infusions should be ideally characterized by a multidisciplinary approach to the design, delivery, and reappraisal of primary or metastatic neuroendocrine tumor treatment, or by referral from a multidisciplinary team consisting of specialists such as surgeon, pathologist, oncologist, (inter-ventional) radiologist, nuclear medicine physician, radiotherapist, and gastroenterologist [Appendix, Table 5.4 Multidisciplinary board (Limouris et al. 2008)] [1]. The primary purpose of this board is to study and decide the treatment plan; setting up priorities for each therapy step also includes several subcategories and alternative therapeutic modalities according to disease progression.

5.1.2 Radiopeptide Infusion Team

Once the eligibility criteria (Hicks et al. 2017) [2] are completed, then the PRRT protocol could be preceded. Complete clinical history as well as patient's consent should be obtained. At least 24 h prior the diagnostic angiography and the radiopeptide infusion procedure, patients' written consent should be documented. According to the recommendations by the radiopeptide therapy consortium (RPTC) [1] the team performing radiopeptide infusions should include staff having experience in the following:

1. Care for the overall medical treatment of the cancer patient
2. Perform vascular catheterization
3. Perform and interpret radiologic scans
4. Assume the responsibility of the delivery of the ^{111}In-Octreotide and be the authorized user
5. Establish radiation safety

M. I. Paphiti (✉)
National Health System, Athens, Greece

© Springer Nature Switzerland AG 2021
G. S. Limouris (ed.), *Liver Intra-arterial PRRT with ^{111}In-Octreotide*,
https://doi.org/10.1007/978-3-030-70773-6_5

While the interventional radiologist is particularly responsible for the angiography procedure, further care for the treated patients is usually assumed by the referring clinician or another designated number of the multidisciplinary board.

Prior to the radiopeptide Infusion, the technical complexity, any potential consequences or difficulties, and possible risks during the therapy procedure should be explained analytically to the patient in a dedicated counseling interview.

Once the radiopeptide infusion has been completed, each case should be reviewed again by the multidisciplinary team to inform the team members with respect to subsequent treatment decisions. On discharge of the patient, recommendations and information leaflet on further hydration, nutrition, medication, radiation safety instructions, follow-up visits, and contact details in case of post procedural side effects should all be given in hand.

5.2 Legal Regulations of Scientific Centers Performing Radiopeptide Therapies

5.2.1 Licensing

Radioactive material for diagnosis or therapy should only be used and stored at medical institutions that have the license and the appropriate designed facilities. The administration of therapeutic doses of radionuclides must be under the responsibility of a physician who is licensed under national regulations to administer radioactive materials to humans. Medical physicists are also subject to licensing since they are responsible for the radiation protection and safety use of radionuclides. Of course, the licensing requirements for the nuclear therapy ward may vary from country to country and may even include a minimum design and construction requirements, the necessary facilities, and the equipment as well **(IAEA, Nuclear medicine resources manual, 2006)** [3].

Considering, however, the case of radiopeptide infusions a special license is needed additionally in most European Countries from the appropriate national authorities or professional bodies since such infusions are regarded as a "clinical trial" and moreover this license is individualized for each patient defining the number of therapy cycles and the quantity of administered radionuclide.

For the case of intra-arterial administration procedure, which is performed within the radiology catheterization room and not in the nuclear medicine department, a specific authorization is additionally requested in order to satisfy all the radiation protection requirements and avoid any contamination hazard. (Appendix, Table 5.5: Hospital requirements for initiating radiopeptide therapies).

5.2.2 Appropriate Facilities and Equipment

The instrumentation in nuclear medicine could be classified into four main sections:

(a) Single photon imaging equipment (including SPECT, SPECT/CT) and dual photon imaging equipment (combining the various approaches to PET such as PET/CT, PET/MRI)
(b) Some nonimaging instruments such as isotope dose calibrator, portable contamination monitor (acoustic dose rate meter), and survey radiation detectors for survey of photons and beta radiation
(c) Phantoms: ^{57}Co sheet for uniformity tests, resolution bar, and SPECT for quality control measurements.
(d) Tools for handling and storing radioactive materials. Radio wash liquids for decontamination procedures.

Reliability of imaging instrumentation is critical to the practice of nuclear medicine and even more they are extremely sensitive to environmental conditions and consequently strict control of temperature and humidity is a must, as well as a continuous and stable power supply by the help of UPS unit. Regular assessment is required to confirm the equipment's performance and quality control protocols must be organized according the NEMA standards to ensure stable practice.

In the case of interventional nuclear medicine additional care must be taken in the angiography room, in order to exclude the problem of contamination. Several factors should be cared of such as e.g. the following:

- Controllable access to angiography room
- Floors impervious to liquids
- Special care for the angiography unit so as case of contamination could be avoided (pedals should be draped with plastic covers placed as a precautionary measure)
- Staff should have passive personnel dosimeters as well as active personnel dosimeters for direct reading during the isotope administration.
- Protective clothing (e.g. appropriate lab gown) is necessary to prevent the transfer of contamination hazard. Overshoes, caps, masks and thick gloves for protection of external beta radiation hazard must be in hand.
- The delivery catheter and all other contamination material that are potentially radioactive should be disposed according the radiation protection regulations.

5.3 Quality Control and Documentation of Radionuclides Applied

5.3.1 Introduction

All radiopharmaceuticals administered to patients should be checked and recorded down carefully before the administration procedure in order to ensure the correct amount of activity, the quality and efficacy of the product so as safety is under warranty in all subjects. Since testing is not possible in order to cover all the required control testing procedures, it is good to develop at least a quick quality control protocol

and documentation of the product. This chapter outlines the necessary steps and techniques that should be considered.

5.3.2 Documentation

Documentation is required in order to set out all the necessary standards and requirements into which radiopharmacy operates. Four areas to take care are the following:

(a) Storage conditions: Once the product has been introduced to the hospital, special storage conditions are required to be satisfied, such as the suitable temperature, so as the product remains stable up to the administration time.

(b) Full records and receipts of all the administered radionuclides relating to the activity, calibration, and expiration time must be carefully double checked.

(c) Definition of the standards to which the radiopharmacy operates: control checks of dose calibrators and safety cabinets.

(d) Records of disposal material: Disposal materials should be checked and disposed according the national legislation.

5.3.2.1 Radionuclide Activity

It is necessary to ensure that the correct activity is administered to the patient and thus requirement of measurement is needed by the help of dose calibrator. For this case, special care should be considered in the measurement of activity before and after dispensing the radiopharmaceutical keeping the same measurement conditions in order to have a more reliable measurement.

5.3.2.2 Radiochemical Purity

The radiochemical purity is defined as the proportion of the total radioactivity of the nuclide concerned present in the stated chemical form. For most radiopharmaceuticals the radiochemical purity will be expected to be greater than 95%, in order to proceed for administration.

For radiopharmaceuticals purchased in their final form, such as ^{111}In, manufacturers will normally declare the radiochemical purity, and the radiopharmacy need not perform any further determinations.

However, for the case of radiopharmaceuticals prepared "in-house," either totally from original materials or purchased kits, radiochemical purity should be established prior to the administration, in order to check the suitability of the final product. Low radiochemical purities may lead to an unintended biodistribution of the radiopharmaceutical. For diagnostic cases, this may lead to a false diagnostic result but for therapeutic radiopharmaceuticals it can produce significant dosimetry problems.

A range of techniques are available for such determinations, but it is preferable to choose a technique which is simple, fast, and reliable to catch the timing of administration.

The simplest and most widely used technique is that of planar chromatography, which employs suitable stationary material (e.g. porous paper or thin layers of silica gel) and readily available mobile phases (e.g. saline, acetone, and butanone). **IAEA-TECDOCs 649 and 805** [4, 5].

5.3.2.3 Disposal of Radioactive Waste

Radioactive waste from nuclear medicine procedures could be hazardous and a good management is needed in order to ensure that the radiation exposure to an individual (general public, radiation worker, patient) and the environment does not exceed the prescribed safe dose limits (Table 5.1).

When disposing of waste, attention should be paid to the following points:

– Once the surface dose rate in any individual bag of waste is below of 5 mGy/h or $\leq 5\,\mu$ Sv/h **(European Directive 2011/70 EURATOM, 19-7-2011)** [6] it can be disposed of. (Check with the local regulatory authority).
– Radioactive waste could be disposed according **(European Directive 2013/59 EURATOM, 5-12-2013)** [7] whenever the radioactive concentration (KBq/Kgr) reaches a certain amount for each different radionuclide, e.g. for the case of In-111 it is 100 KBq/Kgr.
– Always disposable gloves should be worn and caution exercised when handling sharp items such as syringes.
– Before disposure, any labels and radiation symbols should be removed.
– Waste should be placed in a locally appropriate waste disposal container, such as a biological waste bag; two bags is always advisable to minimize the risk of spillage

Table 5.1 Recommended dose limits in planned exposure situations

Type of limit	Occupational	Public
Effective dose[a]	20 mSv/year, averaged over defined periods of 5 years[e]	1 mSv/year[f]
Annual equivalent dose in:		
Lens of the eye[b]	**20 mSv**	**15 mSv**
Skin[c,d]	500 mSv	50 mSv
Hands and feet	500 mSv	–
Effective dose to the foetus[g]	1 mSv	1 mSv

[a]Limits on effective dose are for the sum of the relevant effective doses from external exposure in the specified time period and the committed effective dose from intakes of radionuclides in the same period. For adults, the committed effective dose is computed for a 50-year period after intake, whereas for children it is computed for the period up to age 70 years

[b]**This limit is a 2011 ICRP recommendation** [9]

[c]The limitation on effective dose provides sufficient protection for the skin against stochastic effects

[d]Averaged over 1 cm^2 area of skin regardless of the area exposed

[e]With the further provision that the effective dose should not exceed 50 mSv in any single year. Additional restrictions apply to the occupational exposure of pregnant women

[f]In special circumstances, a higher value of effective dose could be allowed in a single year, provided that the average over 5 years does not exceed 1 mSv per year

[g]The dose to pregnant women is limited up to 1 mSv/year, based on which the fetus is regarded as a member of the public

5.4 Release of the Patient

5.4.1 Radiation Safety Issues, General Principles

When the patient is hospitalized following radionuclide therapy, the people at risk of exposure may include hospital staff who may be radiation workers (occupational exposure) or not. Of course, radiation workers are effectively trained with radiation and they know how to work in order to avoid contamination and minimized the radiation hazard by the help of suitable facilities. But concerning the public at large, a significant problem may be arising once the patient has been released. According to the current radiation protection regulations (ICRP and IAEA) no dose limits for patients have been established, but for staff and members of the public, dose constraints have been provided and accepted by law in most of the European countries. Examples of the dose limits according the **ICRP 103, European Directive 2013/59/05-12-2013, EURATOM** [8] are presented in Table 5.1: Recommended dose limits in planned exposure situations.

5.4.2 Discharge Limits (ICRP Recommendations)

Patients may be discharged from hospital or clinic following radionuclide therapy treatment when an estimate of the effective dose to any member of the general public should not exceed 1 millisievert (mSv) in a year. This dose limit applies to adults and children, including the unborn child as well as to persons who may contact the patient, for example, through work, travel, social, or domestic activities. Adult family members or persons who care for the patient are not necessarily subject to the 1 mSv dose limit for members of the public. The effective dose for those persons helping the patient or living with them should not exceed the dose constraint of 5 mSv.

Mind that recommendations regarding release of patients after therapy with unsealed radionuclides many vary widely around the world.

Hospitalization or release, in-patient or out-patient, has been based on one or more of the following reasons:

(a) A requirement for regulatory compliance, based on the following:
- Dose limits or constraints from the ICRP, international, or national bodies as prescribed in the previous paragraph.
- The residual activity in the patient.
- The dose rate at a specified distance from the patient.

(b) Isolation of the patient to reduce dose to the public and family.

(c) Issues associated with the patient:
- A medical condition that requires hospitalization.
- A mental condition that might reduce compliance.
- Their home circumstances.

5.4.2.1 Guidance Based on Retained Activity

Many countries and regulatory authorities use an approach to patient release after radionuclide therapy based on the activity retained in the patient. This can be in addition to the dose limit/constraint approach described by ICRP, but in some cases, retained activity could be used in parallel (**IAEA, Safety reports series No 63**) [10]. Limits for retained activity are not provided for all the therapeutic radionuclides; most of the recommendations, are relating with I-131 therapies (**European Commission: Radiation Protection 97, 1998**) [11] since it is the oldest formality for therapy in nuclear medicine.

Retained activity could be applied only for photon emitting radionuclides and for the measurements a basic radiation detector is needed. The following points should be considered:

1. Define a fixed distance from a standing patient which is distinguish marked for dose rate measurement such as 1 m.
2. Immediately after the administration and before any excretion, measurement of dose rate from the patient at this fixed distance should be done.

3. More future measurements post administration could be obtained at this distance and the retained activity at any time of measurement is estimated from:

$$A_\mathrm{R} = \frac{A_0 D}{D_0}$$

where,

A_R is the retained activity at the time of measurement

A_0 is the administered activity

D_0 is the dose rate immediately after administration and

D is the dose rate at the time of measurement.

In general, for practical purposes, it is convenient to relate the activity remaining in the patient at the time of discharge to exposure of the public and family.

Table 5.2: Activities (MBq) for release of patients depending on the external doses to other people (mSv effective dose) has been provided by US **NRC, 1997** [12] and such data is especially useful indeed.

Table 5.2 Activities (MBq) for release of patients depending on the external doses to other people (mSv effective dose)

Radionuclide	Half life	MBq for 5 mSv	MBq for 1 mSv
Cr-51	28 days	4800	960
Cu-64	13 h	8400	1700
Cu-67	61 h	14,000	2900
Ga-67	78 h	8700	1700
I-123	13 h	6000	1200
I-125	60 days	250	50
I-131	8 days	1200	240
In-111	67 h	2400	470
P-32	14.29 days	a	a
Re-186	90 h	28,000	5700
Re-188	17 h	29,000	5800
Sm-153	47 h	26,000	5200
Sn-117m	13.61 days	1100	210
Sr-89	50.5 days	a	a
Tc-99m	6 h	28,000	5600
Tl-201	74 h	16,000	3100
Y-90	64 h	a	a

aNo value given because of minimal exposures of the public

Table 5.3 Activities and dose rates below which patient release is authorized

Radionuclide	Activity (GBq)	Dose rate at 1 m (mSv/h)
Ga-67	8.7	0.18
I-123	6.0	0.26
I-131	1.2	0.07
In-111	2.4	0.2
P-32	a	a
Re-186	28	0.15
Re-188	29	0.20
Sm-153	5–26	0.06–0.3
Sr-89	a	
Tc-99m	28	0.58
Tl-201	16	0.19
Y-90	a	

aNo value given because of minimal exposures of the public

From the same document, Table 5.3 tabulates activities and dose rates below which patient release is authorized.

5.4.2.2 Specific Instructions at Releasing the Radioactive Patient

At discharge, an official detailed report is given to the patient's referring clinician reporting all the relevant information regarding the administrating dose of the isotope, the date of delivery, and contact restrictions for the meta-infusion days.

Additional recommendations and instructions for the patient or legal guardian shall be written, provided with a view to the restriction of doses to persons in contact with the patient as far as reasonably achievable, and information on the risks of ionizing radiation. The IAEA gives example information/leaflet in Safety Reports Series No. 63 [9].

Some of the specific instructions are concerning the spread of contamination, minimization of exposure to family members, cessation of breast-feeding, and conception after therapy. The amount of time that each precaution should be implemented should be determined according to the retained activity in patients prior to discharge and on the estimation of the dose that is mighty to be received by carers and comforters or members of the public. For example, patients travelling after radionuclide therapy with a private automobile rarely present a hazard if the patient is keeping the 1 m distance from the other passengers and the travel time is short but, for longer times and traveling by public transport, special instructions are necessary.

In conclusion specific radiation protection consultations for the patient and the family members should be well organized, taking care of all the possibilities and situations by the medical physicist or by the radiation protection officer to avoid any hazard and risk.

Appendix

Table 5.4 Multidisciplinary board

Multidisciplinary team approach to reviewing liver cancer patients
Interventional radiologist
Hepatic surgeon
Medical oncologist
Nuclear medicine physician
Pain physician or anesthetist
Gastroenterologist/hepatologist
Radiation physicist
Dedicated clinical (surgical) oncology nursing staff
Desirable
One site consultant medical physicist
Radiologists

Table 5.5 Hospital requirements for initiating radiopeptide therapies

Country	^{111}In-Octreotide License	Specific authority to use radioisotopes within angiography suite
Austria	+	+
Belgium	+	+
Denmark	+	+
Finland	+	−
France	+	+
Germany	+	+
Greece	+	+
Ireland	+	+
Italy	+	+
Poland	+	+
Portugal	+	−
Scotland	+	−
Slovenia	+	+
Spain	+	−
Sweden	+	−
Switzerland	+	−
The Netherlands	+	+
Turkey	+	−
UK	+	+

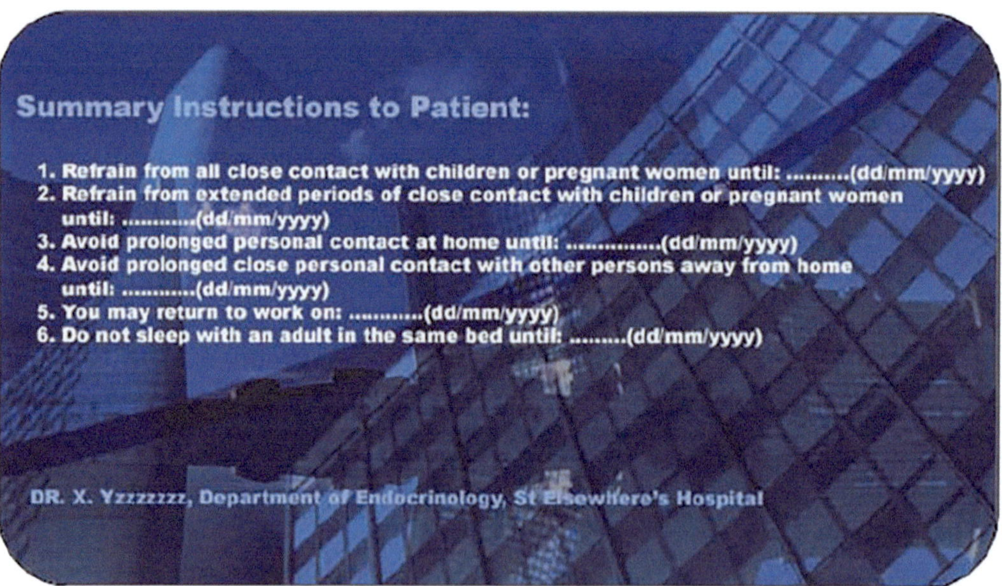

IAEA: Examples of information/leaflet in Safety Reports Series No. 63

References

1. Limouris GS, Chatziioannou A, Kontogeorgakos D, et al. Selective hepatic arterial infusion of In-111-DTPA-Phe1-octreotide in neuroendocrine liver metastases. Eur J Nucl Med Mol Imaging. 2008;35(10):1827–37.
2. Hicks RJ, Kwekkeboom DJ, Krenning E, et al. ENETS Consensus guidelines for the standards of care in neuroendocrine neoplasia: peptide receptor radionuclide therapy with radiolabeled somatostatin analogues. Neuroendocrinology. 2017;105(3):293–309.
3. IAEA. Nuclear medicine resources manual. 2006.
4. IAEA-TECDOCs 649.
5. IAEA-TECDOCs 805.
6. European Directive 2011/70 EURATOM, 19-7-2011.
7. European Directive 2013/59 EURATOM, 5-12-2013.
8. ICRP publication 103 (The 2007 recommendations of the international commission on radiological protection).
9. ICRP 2011 annual report.
10. IAEA, Safety report series No 63 "Release of patients after radionuclide therapy".
11. European Commission. Radiation protection following iodine-131 therapy (exposures due to out-patients or discharged in-patients), radiation protection 97. Luxembourg: European Commission; 1998.
12. Nuclear Regulatory Commission. Release of patients administered radioactive materials, regulatory guide no. 8.39. Washington, DC: US Govt Printing Office; 1997.

Georgios S. Limouris

6.1 Introduction

The treatment of liver neuroendocrine metastases continues to be a major doctor's dilemma because a majority of the patients suffer from extensive unresectable disease. Apart from surgical resection which is the treatment of choice, *systemic therapy, hepatic artery (chemo) embolisation and radiofrequency ablation* have been claimed to have proven clinically beneficial. Patients with the objective of *surgery* with a curative intention are few because of the wide incidence of the disease [1, 2] and because this procedure is not allowed in many cases. In fact, in a majority of them, only an excision procedure is carried out, while complete resection is opted for less than 10% of the patients [3]. In *systemic therapy,* the use of intravenous chemotherapy does not lead to the best expected results. This is due to diverse variables that include type of chemotherapy, stage of disease, progression and toxicity [4, 5]. From the panel of local ablation techniques *(chemo) embolisation* [6, 7] and *percutaneous radiofrequency ablation* [8], two minimally invasive procedures are usually done in an interventional radiology department. For both these procedures, it is necessary that the number of liver lesions are limited, no more than 3, a crite-

rion that should not be ignored as in a majority of the neuroendocrine liver metastases cases, these are more.

In 1993, Eric Krenning employed ^{111}In-Octreotide (Octreoscan, Mallinckrodt, Petten, the Netherlands) for therapeutic purposes in the treatment of NETs [9, 10] via intravenous infusions, exploiting the Auger and Internal Conversion Electron emission of Indium-111 [10, 11]. This treatment modality is aimed at destroying the tumor tissue with the help of the high linear energy transfer delivered from these electrons [12]. However, a disadvantage of this procedure was the increased retention of the radiolabel in the kidneys and spleen, considered as the critical organs [13, 14]. That study aimed to assess and evaluate the usefulness of the procedure in long term in non-resectable liver metastases caused by NETs.

To maximise the linear energy transfer onto the tumor, achieve a larger lesion, destroy and, in parallel, reducing the delivered dose to the critical organs (kidneys and spleen), we decided to modify, in our institution, the way of ^{111}In-Octreotide administration by applying radioactivity as close as possible to the malignancy after selective catheterisation of the hepatic artery [15, 16]. To the best of our knowledge, this is the first time that this approach has been adopted on a routine basis. However, while some cases could not be treated intra-arterially either because the patient refused to be catheterised or

G. S. Limouris (✉)
Nuclear Medicine, Medical School, National and Kapodistrian University of Athens, Athens, Greece
e-mail: glimouris@med.uoa.gr

G. S. Limouris (ed.), *Liver Intra-arterial PRRT with ^{111}In-Octreotide*,
https://doi.org/10.1007/978-3-030-70773-6_6

the anatomic variants of the arterial net inhibited the intra-arterial approach. PRRT was performed intravenously in only 10 cases, while 86 treated intra-arterially.

According to Hirmas et al. [17], in the gastrointestinal system, particularly, the most common, malignant NETs arise from the midgut. For such patients presenting with metastatic disease, Yao et al. and Modlin et al. have reported a 5-year survival rate of less than 50% [18, 19]. NET classification was introduced by the European Neuroendocrine Tumor Society (ENETS) in 2006 and 2007 [20, 21], without taking into account the Ki-67 index. However, the ENETS, the American Joint Committee on Cancer (AJCC) and the WHO classification (2010) included the Ki-67 labelling cutoff of <3% to define low-grade (G1), 3–20% for intermediate-grade (G2) and >20% for high-grade (G3) NETs (Table 6.1) [20, 21].

To stratify the best possible NET treatment strategy, a multidisciplinary approach for their management is required that can ensure a consistent and optimal level of care (Table 6.2). If NETs are resectable, the surgery consists of the treatment of choice.

In the case of unresectable disease, in tandem treatments, including obligatory somatostatin analogue therapy with Octreotide or Lanreotide,

Table 6.1 NETs 2010-WHO classification for digestive system NETs

Differentiation	Grade	Mitoses per 10 HPFs	Ki-67 index
Well-differentiated	Low-Grade (G1)	<2	<3%
Well-differentiated	Intermediate-Grade (G2)	2–20	3–20%
Poorly differentiated	High-Grade (G3)	>20	>20%

HPFs high power fields

Table 6.2 Multidisciplinary team's approach to review NET patients

Nuclear medicine physician	Hepatic surgeon
Interventional radiologist	Medical oncologist
Radiation physicist	Pathologist
Colorectal surgeon	Anesthesiologist
Gastroenterologist	Dedicated nursing staff

PRRT, Everolimus (mTOR inhibitor) or Sunitinib (tyrosine kinase inhibitor) [22].

The purpose of this study was to study, evaluate and report on PRRT carried out by using ^{111}In-Octreotide, intravenously implemented, high dose treatment as a treatment option for unresectable, multiple and small-in-size (up to 20 mm in their major diameter) liver metastases.

6.1.1 Patients

Ten patients (4 women, 6 men; age range: 49–76 years, median age 64, 5 years) with unresectable neuroendocrine liver metastases, confirmed by biopsy, were administered 4070–5920 MBq (110–160 mCi) per session intravenously (Table 6.3) after centesis of the dorsal vein hand system or the antecubital vein. Repetitions did not exceed the nine sessions, and the treatment intervals were of 5–8 weeks. The study was approved by the Institutional Committee on Human Investigation and Ethics of the "Aretaieion" University Hospital. Informed consent was signed by each of the patients participating in this study.

Liver metastases originating from mediastinum ($n = 1$) lungs ($n = 4$), head of pancreas ($n = 2$), sigmoid ($n = 1$) and small intestine ($n = 2$).

According to the RECIST criteria [23, 24], the disease was not measurable in two of the patients because the lesions were diffused within the liver parenchyma. The eligibility criterion for PRRT was the unresectable nature of the liver metastases that had shown resistance to systemic chemotherapy as could be seen in contrast with the help of a material-enhanced computed tomography (CT) scan and/or a magnetic resonance imaging (MRI) image. Besides the confirmed biopsy (Fig. 6.1) from the primaries, no additional histologic proof was obtained in the treated liver lesion because of the risk of possible biopsy complications (i.e. haemorrhage, metastatic spread). Contra-indications of PRRNT were a Karnofsky index of <40, pleural or abdominal effusions, renal impairment (serum creatinine

Table 6.3 Patients' characteristics and PRRT results using ^{111}In-Octreotide intravenously

Patient/gender	Age (in years)	No. of sessions/cumul. activ. (GBq)	CR	PR	SD	PD	PFS	OS
1. ANT.ANS./M	57	1/5.92	–	–	–	+	7	11
2. KAT.ALH./F[a]	70	5/29.60	–	–	–	+	3	6
3. MAN.NIK./M	53	4/23.32	–	–	–	+	10	19
4. SOT.STA./F	76	9/53.28	–	–	+	–	26	32
5. ROU.KON./M	68	4/23.68	–	–	–	+	9	19
6. MPO.NIK./M	60	3/17.20	–	–	+	–	12	17
7. THE.KYR./F	49	2/10.92	–	–	+	–	17	35
8. MPA.XRI./M	65	3/17.40	–	–	–	+	5	11
9. MAL.VAS./F	64	2/11.84	–	–	–	+	4	11
10. GAZ.NIK./M[a]	70	6/35.52	–	–	–	+	8	18

[a]Non-measurable disease; *CR* complete response; *PR* partial response; *SD* stable disease; *PD* progressive disease; *PFS* progression-free survival; *OS* overall survival

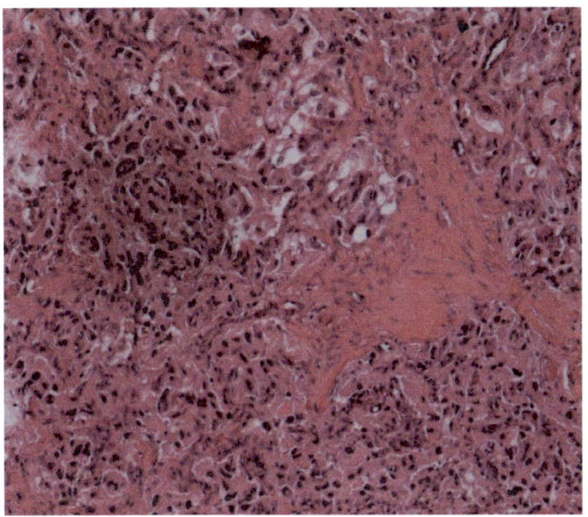

Fig. 6.1 Histological section of a well-differentiated mammary NET (Haematoxylin-Eosin ×10)

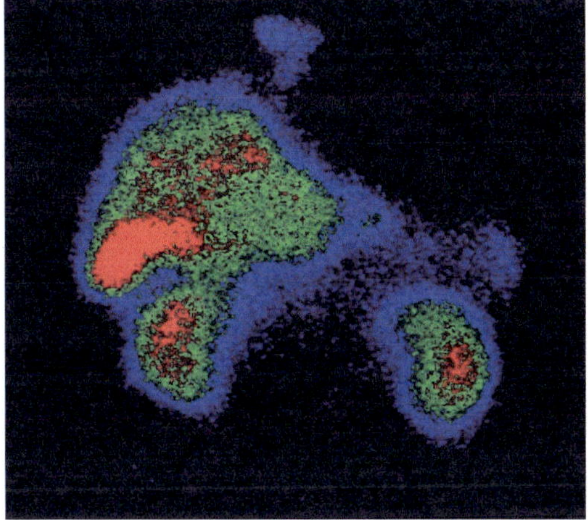

Fig. 6.2 A 'grade IV' OctreoScan visual score

>1, 7 mg/dL), serum haemoglobin ≤9.0 g/dL, total white blood cell (WBC) count ≤2 × 10^9/L, platelet count ≤75 × 10^9/L and serum creatinine concentration ≤1.7 mg/dL. All ten patients had undergone complete surgical resection of primary cancer.

The assumption for the patients to be treated with ^{111}In-Octreotide was that the intense degree of the radionuclide tumor uptake on the diagnostic OctreoScan scintigraphy to be as high as the half uptake in the normal parenchyma of the spleen and left kidney (visual score 4) before the therapy (Fig. 6.2).

6.1.2 Preliminary Results

In the sub-group of 17 GEP–NET-patients that were intra-arterially infused [25], CR was seen in 1 (6%), PR in 8 (47%), SD in 3 (18%) and PD in 5 (29%). ^{111}In-Octreotide was obtained from Mallinckrodt (Petten, Holland) and prepared 'in-house' as described previously [25]. Before the infusion of the radiopharmaceutical, Ondansetron (8 mg) was administered intravenously. To reduce the radiation dose to the kidneys, intravenous infusion of amino acids (2.5% arginine and 2.5% lysine in 1 L 0.9% NaCl) was started 30 min before the administration of the radiopharmaceutical and lasted for 4 h. Additionally, to reduce myelotoxicity, 75 mg of DTPA in trip-trop diluted in about 200 mL normal saline water was also infused 30 min before the initialisation of the radiopeptide therapy, also lasting for about 4 h. Patients were treated up to a cumulative intended dose from 160 mCi (5.92 GBq) to 1440 mCi (53.28 GBq) ^{111}In-Octreotide. Routine haematology, liver and kidney function tests were performed after three therapy cycles during follow-up. A CT or MRI scan was performed before and at the end of the entire therapeutic scheme. Thereafter, every case was seen as an outpatient.

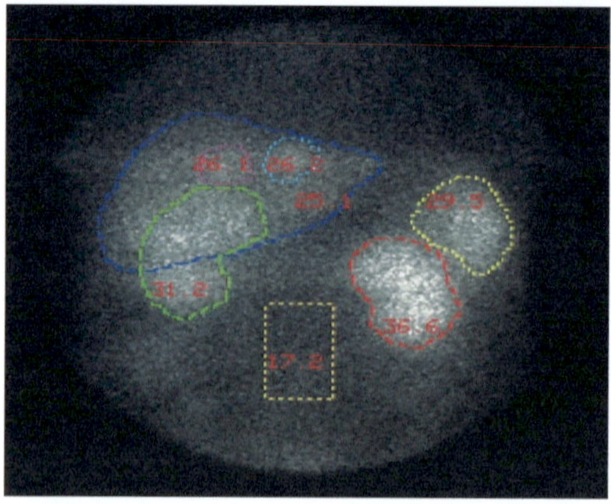

Fig. 6.3 Delineation of organs and creation of Region of Interest (ROIs) on planar Octreoscan for quantitative dosimetry

6.1.3 Equipment and Procedure

The infusions were conducted at the Nuclear Medicine Department of the "Aretaieion" University Hospital. The size and location of the neuroendocrine nodules were assessed using the Couinaud nomenclature [26, 27] based on consensus between the two observers who compared the images obtained with each of the radiologic techniques.

6.1.4 Intravenous Infusion

[111]In-Octreotide solution was administered via a three-cock catheter; the radionuclide infusion lasted for 20–30 min to avoid side effects, i.e. hypotony, nausea or vomiting. The time interval between consecutive sessions was 7–8 weeks. However, in cases with long-lasting post-treatment, subacute, haematologic toxicity, the intended interval was postponed to 9–10 weeks. The radioactive material was injected by the nuclear physician, covered by a 0.787-inch-thick lead shield (barrel). At the end of the procedure, a 10 mL saline flush was given to deplete any radioactivity that remained in the three-cock catheter wall. Just after the end of the infusion, a stop-cock heparinised catheter was ante-cubitally inserted to drain blood samples 2 h, 4 h, 8 h and 24 h post-catheterisation for dosimetric calculations. For the same reasons, 24 h urine was collected. No pain, except some discomfort during or after the infusion, headache and nausea was noticed. Patients remained obligatory for 24 h in a single bedroom with its own toilet dedicated for hot (radionuclide treated) patients. At the time of the patient discharge behaviour, instructions were given to constrain the doses received by the members of the public and the close family taking into account the dose rate (mSv/h) at 1 m distance from the patient's body.

Planar and SPECT scans were performed for all therapy cycles to calculate tumor and critical organ doses, followed by quantitative dosimetry (Fig. 6.3). Accordingly, absorbed doses delivered to liver metastases, kidneys and red marrow were calculated using OLINDA 1.1 program, and the response assessment was classified, based on RECIST criteria. Response to salvage PRRT was assessed by CT/MRI scans performed before, during and after the end of the treatment, and monthly ultrasound images were studied for liver follow-up measurements. Toxicity (WHO criteria) was measured using blood and urine tests of renal, hepatic and bone marrow functions. PFS analysis was performed with the help of the Kaplan-Meier survival plot.

6.1.5   Blood Sampling

Blood sampling was performed 24 h after the administration. The absorbed dose to the blood was mainly caused by beta radiation originating from activity in the blood. The activity in the blood is determined in a well counter from aliquots of non-heparinised blood samples. Whole blood samples (about 2 mL) were collected at 2, 4, 8 and 24 h post-infusion. The first sample was drawn from the contra-lateral arm within 10 min.

6.2 ^{111}In-Octreotide Treatment Results

6.2.1   Liver Metastatic Load

None of the 10 treated patients resulted in either CR or PR. (Table 6.3): Three out of the ten cases resulted in disease stabilisation, whereas the other seven did not respond at all and died within approximately one and a half years after the end of the therapeutic scheme due to disease aggravation (Table 6.3). The 12-month PFS and OS ratio was 3/10 (30.0%) and 6/10 (60.0%), respectively; the median PFS in months was 8.5 and for OS 17.5 (Fig. 6.4).

A Grade II to III erythro-, leuko- and thrombocytopenia occurred in all PD cases. Dosimetric calculations (Table 6.4) were found as follows:

(a) Liver Tumor 11.2 mGy/MBq, (b) Liver 0.40 mGy/MBq, (c) Kidneys 0.51 mGy/MBq, (d) Spleen 1.56 mGy/MBq, (e) bone marrow 0.022 mGy/MBq.

6.2.2   Follow-Up

Patients were in close contact with our institution as it was recommended to them that they perform bi- to tri-monthly ultrasonography of the upper and lower abdomen and undergo specific laboratory examinations that were performed for WBC

Table 6.4 Tumor-absorbed dose comparison between i.v. and i.a. administration of ^{111}In-DTPA^{0}-Octreotide

	Intra-arterial infusion	Intravenous infusion
Liver dose	0.14 (mGy/MBq)	0.40 (mGy/MBq)
Kidney dose	0.41 (mGy/MBq)	0.51 (mGy/MBq)
Tumor dose	15.20 (mGy/MBq)	11.20 (mGy/MBq)
Spleen dose	1.40 (mGy/MBq)	1.56 (mGy/MBq)
Bone marrow dose	0.0035 (mGy/MBq)	0.022 (mGy/MBq)
Tumor/liver dose ratio	108.57[a]	28.00
Tumor/ kidney dose ratio	37.07	21.96

[a]The average absorbed dose per session to a tumor for a spherical mass of 10 gr was estimated to be 10.8 mGy/MBq, depending on the tumor's histotype

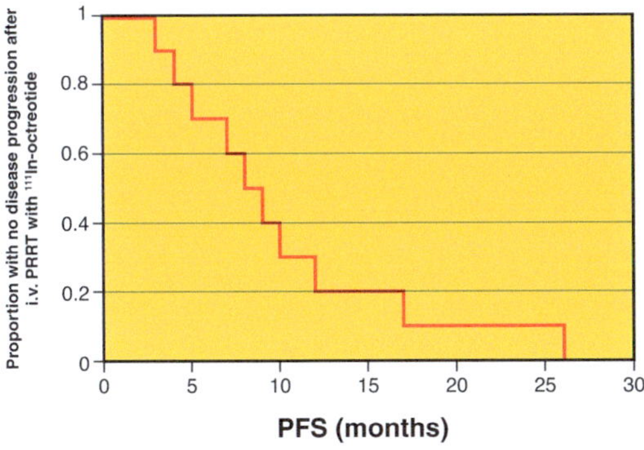

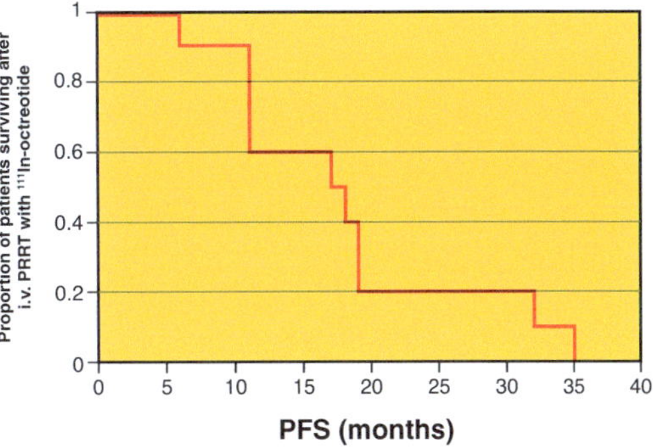

Fig. 6.4 Kaplan-Meier curves for progression-free (left) and overall survival (OS) (right) of ten NETs, intravenously treated with ^{111}In-Octreotide

and RBC counts, platelet counts, haemoglobin, creatinine and Cr-A levels. CT and/or MRI scans were also performed before the initialisation of the therapy and every 6 months thereafter. All laboratory values were compared with the previous ones as well as with ultrasonography, CT and MRI scan images that were obtained before the initialisation of the treatment to assess any changes in tumor consistency and size. As detailed archives are kept for every case, patients were requested to present at the nuclear medicine division at least thrice every year for the evaluation of the response to the procedures that were done based on RECIST guidelines, whereby the disease was classified into two categories, i.e. (a) measurable and (b) non-measurable. In the first category, the nodules had to be distinguished in terms of their diameters that are easily measurable, whereas the second category was that of diffused malignancy. Diameter measurements were performed by using the longest cross-sectional diameter on U/S scans and finally confirmed by CT and/or MRI scan images.

6.3   Discussion

Combating the liver metastatic disease continues to be a major dilemma for the scientists concerned (oncologists, nuclear physicians, gastroenterologists and surgeons) including invasive, minimally invasive and non-invasive therapeutic schemes. A combination of the aforementioned techniques might be the treatment of choice after a thorough evaluation of the malignancy as a whole (generally) and in appropriate hierarchy of the treating methodologies in particular after taking into account the multidisciplinarity of the specialities involved. From the non-invasive therapeutic schemes, Everolimus or Sunitinib and chemotherapeutics aimed to improve possible liver nodule receptibility by trying to ablate, as efficiently as possible, the aggressiveness of the cancerous cell(s). Even though chemotherapy is used and continues to be the treatment of choice to confront the progression of the malignancy, its toxicity limits its application. Surgical liver nodule excision, on the other hand, is regarded as the

treatment of preference despite the fear of a further metastatic spread post-surgery. In cases that are eligible for surgery, a 5-year survival rate of 21–44% has been achieved [28]. Given that the neuroendocrine disease spread is highly variable, depending on a plethora of factors, such as the site of the tumor, its origin, tumor functionality or non-functionality, differentiation, receptor homogeneity, mitotic indexes and size that tremendously impact therapy response, an in tandem treatment of PRRT with Octreotide or Lanreotide, Everolimus, and less often with Sunitinib and Streptozotocin, prolongs progression-free survival, overall survival and quality of life among the patients. PRRT combined with other anticancer therapies have appeared to be safe, but, to date, only phase-II clinical trials have been reported in this regard, leaving numerous possible options for further research [28, 29]. Based on worldwide reports, infusing radiopeptide therapies in combination with different therapeutic modalities have proved to be more effective in the manipulation of the neuroendocrine character of these tumors [30]. Tandem schemes with ^{111}In-Octreotide are not recommended as ^{111}Indium's Auger and Internal Conversion Electron emission is not considered as an appropriate candidate for PRRT armamentarium due to electrons' extremely short path length of 2–500 nm.

As it can be derived, in the therapeutic cycle for each patient the response is strongly dependent on the classification category of the neuroendocrine disease. A diffused, non-measurable disease consists of the first main factor of resistance to an efficient response. Practically, the disease has no hope for improvement unless a tiny tumor degeneration degree, whereas the tumor size is, surprisingly, a secondary factor of resistance to an objective response. It should not be ignored that the main drawback of ^{111}In emission is its extremely short range, incapable to destroy a larger cell number than as might be achieved by the use of ^{90}Y or ^{177}Lu, both being addressed approximately to a 250 and 50 cell population, respectively [31]. On the other hand, this short emission does not aggravate the disease apart from some side effects such as transient diarrhoea.

As the majority of the patients do not favour systemic schemes or surgery as well, the PRRT population with the final therapeutic results 'partial response' is not permitted to be abandoned without any further care and treatment. The best solution could be to convince them to shift towards a surgical excision in case the eligibility criteria allow it or to a radiofrequency ablation procedure. Additionally, the simplicity of the radionuclide intra-hepatic infusion allows it to be considered as a preparative procedure for a furthermore potent therapeutic solution. U/S is requested as a follow-up obligatory exam every quarter to evaluate the disease's behaviour and to permit shifting to a more invasive therapeutic modality.

To our knowledge, the advantages of this methodology are that it is: (a) minimally invasive, performed after centesis of the femoral artery and insertion of an appropriate endovascular catheter up to proper hepatic, right or left hepatic artery depending on the vaso-anatomical status of the patient; (b) a super-selective methodology that is systematic and has a targeted character. As it is obvious that much closer to the lesion the radioactivity is delivered such that its uptake by the cellular receptors is higher and hence it has a more destructive effect on the tumor; (c) a simple infusion and not an embolisation. Practically, there are no side effects either during or after the procedure; (d) independent of using a specific tracer to transport the radioactive material to the target as radiolabelled Octreotide is by its nature receptor-trapped and specific.

A drawback of this study however was that it lacked a control group. So, a comparison in terms of the survival advantage with the radionuclide perfusion managed group was not possible.

On the other hand, as the majority of the treated patients had discontinued or finished with chemotherapeutic schemes, the results of the radioactive infusions (tumor shrinkage or consistency changes) could be attributed to the contribution of the radioactive effect (Auger and Internal Conversion electron emission).

We studied the PRRT outcome with ^{111}In-Octreotide, intravenously administrated, in 10 patients suffering from NETs with primaries of different origin. Comparing the international references as a whole, of several expert reports on PRRT (Table 6.5) using ^{111}In-Octreotide an objective response (CR + PR) was observed in 20/139 (14.4%) of the treated cases, whereas the outcome of our tiny cohort is higher, giving an objective response rate of 30%. In 1994, in his first ^{111}In-Octreotide study Eric Krenning [9], including only one patient, reported an ORR of 100.0%, after a cumulative activity of 20.3 GBq.

Table 6.5   Experts working with ^{111}In-Octreotide

Author	No of pts	Cumul. activ. (GBq)	CR	PR	SD	PD
Krenning et al. (1994), *ref. no 19, 20*	1	20.30	–	1 (100%)	–	–
Tiensuu Janson et al. (1999) ref. no 21	5	18.00	–	2 (40%)	3 (60%)	–
Caplin et al. (2000) *ref. no 22*	8	3.10–15.20	–	–	7 (87.5%)	1 (12.5%)[a]
Valkema *et al.* (2002)	26	4.7–160.00	–	2 (8%)	15 (58%)	9 (35%)
Anthony et al. (2002)	26	6.7–46.60	–	2 (8%)	21 (81%)	3 (11%)
Buscombe *et al.* (2003)	12	3.1–36.60	–	2 (17%)	7 (58%)	3 (25%)
Nguyen et al. (2004) *ref. no 23*	15	21.00	–	–	13 (87%)	2 (13%)
Delpassand *et al.* (2008)	29	35.3–37.30	–	2 (7%)	16 (55%)	11 (38%)
Limouris et al. (2008)[b]	17	13.0–77.00	1 (6%)	8 (47%)	3 (18%)	5 (29%)
Limouris GS (this study)	10	5.92–53.28	–	–	3 (30%)	7 (70%)

[a]Unrelated to the tumor cause
[b]Exclusively intra-arterially

In a ^{111}In-Octreotide study by Tiensuu Janson et al. [32] in a cohort of 5 NETs a 100% control disease (CR, PR or SD) was also reported after a cumulative activity of 18 GBq. In 2000, Caplin et al. [33] in a cohort of 8 NETs, treated with ^{111}In-Octreotide of a dosage ranging from 3.10 to 15.20 GBq achieved an SD in 7 (87.5%) patients whereas the remaining one died due to reasons unrelated to the disease. In 2002, Valkema et al. [34] in a study of 26 NETs treated with ^{111}In-Octreotide 2 (8%) patients had PR, 15 (58%) SD and 9 (35%) PD, after a cumulative activity ranging from 4.7 to 160 GBq. The same year, Anthony et al. [35] in 26 NET patients reported a PR in 2 (8%), a SD in 21 (81%) and PD in 3 (11%) after a cumulative activity of ^{111}In-Octreotide ranging from 6.7 to 46.6 GBq. Buscombe et al. in 2003 [36], in a study of 12 NET patients treated cases implementing ^{111}In-Octreotide reported a PR in 2 (17%), an SD in 7 (58%) and a PD in 3 (25%) after a cumulative activity ranging from 3.1 to 36.6 GBq. In a study by Nguyen et al. in 2004 [37] on 15 NETs, treated with ^{111}In-Octreotide after a cumulative activity of 21 GBq, an SD was reached in 13 (87%), whereas the rest 2(13%) patients showed PD. In a study of 29 NET patients, Delpassand et al. [38] reported PR in 2 (7%), SD in 16 (55%) and PD in 11 (38%) patients after a cumulative activity ranging from 35.3 to 37.30 GBq. Finally, in preliminary data of a prospective study of 17 NET patients from our Institution, in 2008, treated with ^{111}In-Octreotide intra-arterially, after catheterisation of the hepatic artery we achieved a CR IN 1 (6%), a PR in 8 (47%), an SD in 3 (18%) and a PD in 5 (29%), after a cumulative activity ranging from 13 to 77 GBq.

6.4   Conclusion

[111]In-Octreotide was infused in repeated high doses ranging from 4.070 GBq (110 mCi) to 5.920GBq (160 mCi) with a time interval of 6–8 weeks between sessions. This treatment was well-tolerated in all the patients without any marked side effects or complications being observed subsequently. According to the RECIST criteria, a disease control could be achieved in only 3 out of 10 patients. In the other 7 patients, disease progression was recorded, and all of them died approximately 4–7 months after the end of the therapeutic scheme. Radiopeptide intravenous infusions with high activity of ^{111}In-Octreotide even well-tolerated in all patients were disappointing and are not suggested as a therapeutic treatment option in patients with neuroendocrine disease.

References

1. Que FG, Nagorney DM, Batts KP, et al. Hepatic resection for metastatic neuroendocrine carcinomas. Am J Surg. 1995;169:36–43.
2. McEntee GP, Nagorney DM, Kvols LK, et al. Cytoreductive hepatic surgery for neuroendocrine tumors. Surgery. 1990;108:1091–996.
3. Padhani A, Ollivier L, Ihse I, Persson B, et al. Neuroendocrine metastases of the liver. World J Surg. 1995;19:76–82.
4. Neary PC, Redmond PH, Houghton T, et al. Carcinoid disease: review of the literature. Dis Colon Rectum. 1997;40:349–62.
5. Diaco DS, Hajarizadeh H, Mueller CR, et al. Treatment of metastatic carcinoid tumors using multimodality therapy of octreotide acetate, intra-arterial chemotherapy, and hepatic arterial chemoembolization. Am J Surg. 1995;169:523–8.
6. Brown KT, Koh BY, Brody LA, et al. Particle embolization of hepatic neuroendocrine metastases for control of pain and hormonal symptoms. J Vasc Interv Radiol. 1999;10:397–403.
7. Diculescu M, Atanasiu C, Arbanas T, et al. Chemoembolization in the treatment of metastatic ileocolic carcinoid. Rom J Gastroenterol. 2002;11:141–7.
8. O'Toole D, Maire F, Ruszniewski P. Ablative therapies for liver metastases of digestive neuroendocrine tumors. Endocr Relat Cancer. 2003;10:463–8.
9. Krenning EP, Kooij PPM, Bakker WH, et al. Radiotherapy with a radiolabeled somatostatin analogue, [111In-DTPA-D.Phe1]—octreotide; a case history. Ann N Y Acad Sci. 1994;733:496–506.
10. Krenning EP, Kwekkeboom DJ, Bakker WH, et al. Somatostatin receptor scintigraphy with [111In-DTPA-d-Phe1] and [123I-Tyr3]-octreotide: the Rotterdam experience with more than 1000 patients. Eur J Nucl Med. 1993;20:716–31.
11. Adelstein SJ. The Auger process: a therapeutic promise? AJR. 1993;160:707–13.
12. Krenning EP, de Jong M, Kooij PP, et al. Radiolabelled somatostatin analogues for peptide receptor

scintigraphy and radionuclide therapy. Ann Oncol. 1999;10(Suppl 2):S23–9.

13. Wiseman GA, Kvols LK. The radiolabelled MIBG and Somatostatin analogues. Semin Nucl Medicine XXV. 1995;3:272–8.

14. De Jong M, Bakker WH, Krenning EP, et al. Yttrium-90 and Indium-111 labeling, receptor binding and biodistribution of [DOTA, D-Phe^1, Tyr^3]-octreotide; a promising somatostatin analogue for radionuclide therapy. Eur J Nucl Med. 1997;24:368–71.

15. Limouris GS, Lyra M, Skarlos D, et al. Electron therapy with In-111 pentetreotide in hepatocellular carcinoma. In: Bergmann H, Köhn H, Sinzinger H, editors. Radioactive isotopes in clinical medicine and research XXIII. Birkhäuser, Basel: Advances in Pharmacological Sciences; 1999.

16. Limouris GS, Voliotopoulos V, Dimitropoulos N, et al. Auger-electron therapeutic effectiveness in neuroendocrine and non-tumors using indium-111 labeled pentetreotide. Nucl Med Commun. 2000;21(6):590. [abstr]

17. Hirmas N, Jadaan R, Al-Ibraheem A. Peptide receptor radionuclide therapy and the treatment of gastroentero-pancreatic neuroendocrine tumors: current findings and future perspectives. Nucl Med Mol Imaging. 2018;52(3):190–9.

18. Yao JC, Hassan M, Phan A. One hundred years after "carcinoid": epidemiology of and prognostic factors for neuroendocrine tumors in 35,825 cases in the United States. J Clin Oncol. 2008;26:3063–72.

19. Modlin IM, Lye KD, Kidd M. A 5-decade analysis of 13,715 carcinoid tumors. Cancer. 2003;97:934–59.

20. Rindi G, Klöppel G, Alhman H. TNM staging of foregut (neuro) endocrine tumors: a consensus proposal including a grading system. Virchows Arch. 2006;449:395–401.

21. Rindi G, Klöppel G, Couvelard A, et al. TNM staging of midgut and hindgut (neuro) endocrine tumors: a consensus proposal including a grading system. Virchows Arch. 2007;451:757–62.

22. Frilling A, Clift AK. Therapeutic strategies for neuroendocrine liver metastases. Cancer. 2015;121:1172–86.

23. Therasse P, Arbuck SG, Eisenhauer EA, et al. New guidelines to evaluate the response to treatment in solid tumors. European Organization for Research and Treatment of Cancer, National Cancer Institute of the United States, National Cancer Institute of Canada. J Natl Cancer Inst. 2000;92:205–16.

24. Padhani AR, Ollivier L. The RECIST criteria: implications for diagnostic radiologists. Br J Radiol. 2001;74(887):983–6.

25. Limouris GS, Chatziioannou A, Kontogeorgakos D, et al. Selective hepatic arterial infusion of In-111-DTPA-Phe1-octreotide in neuroendocrine liver metastases. Eur J Nucl Med Mol Imaging. 2008;35:1827–37.

26. Lafortune M, Mardore F, Patriquin H, et al. Segmental anatomy of the liver; a US approach to the Couinaud nomenclature. Radiology. 1991;181:443–8.

27. Couinaud C. Le Foie. Etudes anatomiques et chirurgicales. Paris: Masson & Cie; 1957.

28. Mazzaferro V, Pulvirenti A, Coppa J. Neuroendocrine tumors metastatic to the liver: how to select patients for liver transplantation? J Hepatol. 2007;47(4):460–46.

29. Bison SM, Konijnenberg MW, Melis M. Peptide receptor radionuclide therapy using radiolabeled somatostatin analogs: focus on future developments. Clin Transl Imaging. 2014;2(1):55–66.

30. Cidon EU. New therapeutic approaches to metastatic gastroenteropancreatic neuroendocrine tumors: a glimpse into the future. World J Gastrointest Oncol. 2017;9(1):4–20.

31. Senekowitsch-Schmidtke R, Huber R, Seidl C. Alpha-emitting radionuclides for therapy in oncology. In: Limouris GS, Biersack H-J, Shukla SK, editors. Radionuclide therapy for oncology, current status and future aspects. Athens: Mediterra; 2003. p. 135–40.

32. Tiensuu Janson E, Eriksson B, Oberg K. Treatment with high dose [(111) In-DTPA-D-PHE1]-octreotide in patients with neuroendocrine tumors–evaluation of therapeutic and toxic effects. Acta Oncol. 1999;38(3):373–7.

33. Caplin ME, Miclcarek W, Buscombe JR, et al. Toxicity of high-activity In-111 octreotide therapy in patients with disseminated neuroendocrine tumours. Nucl Med Commun. 2000;21:97–102.

34. Valkema R, De Jong M, Bakker WH, et al. Phase I study of peptide receptor radionuclide therapy with [In-DTPA] octreotide: the Rotterdam experience. Semin Nucl Med. 2002;32(2):110–22.

35. Anthony LB, Woltering EA, Espanan GD, et al. Indium-111-pentetreotide prolongs survival in gastroenteropancreatic malignancies. Semin Nucl Med. 2002;32:123–32.

36. Buscombe JR, Caplin ME, Hilson AJW. Long-term efficacy of high-activity ^{111}In-pente-treotide therapy in patients with disseminated neuroendocrine tumors. J Nucl Med. 2003;44(1):1–6.

37. Nguyen C, Faraggi M, Giraudet A-L. Long-term efficacy of radionuclide therapy in patients with disseminated neuroendocrine tumors uncontrolled by conventional therapy. J Nucl Med. 2004;45:1660–8.

38. Delpassand ES, Sims-Mourtada J, Saso H, et al. Safety and efficacy of radionuclide therapy with high-activity In-111 pentetreotide in patients with progressive neuroendocrine tumors. Cancer Biother Radiopharm. 2008;23:292–300.

Intra-arterial Radiopeptide Infusions with High Activity of ^{111}In-Octreotide: From "Aretaieion Protocol" to the Temporal Intra-arterial Port Installation

7

Georgios S. Limouris

7.1 Introduction

Contemporary aspects of neuroendocrine tumors (NETs) emerge on tissues containing cells derived from the neural crest, the neuroectoderm, and the embryonic endoderm [1]. Although these tumors can occur everywhere in the human body, the majority of them appear along the axis of the gastrointestinal tract, particularly lungs, mediastinum, stomach, intestine, pancreas (Fig. 7.1), including gastrinomas, insulinomas, VIPomas, glucagonomas, PPomas, somatostatinomas, and carcinoids [1]. Catecholamine-secreting neoplasms such as pheochromocytomas, paragangliomas, the myeloid carcinoma of the thyroid gland, the primary neuroendocrine carcinoma of the skin [also known as Merkel-cell carcinoma (Fig. 7.2)], tumors of the pituitary and parathyroid gland and broncho-pulmonary neoplasms belong to the family of non-gastroenteropancreatic neuroendocrine tumors (non-GEP-NETs). Non-GEP-NETs can occur in the frame of hereditary neoplastic syndromes. These include multiple endocrine neoplasms type 1 and 2 (MEN1 and MEN2), von Hippel Lindau disease (VHL), type 1 neuro-fibrosis (NF1), and Carney syndrome [1–5]. However, the majority, of non-GEP-NETs appear as nonhereditary (sporadic) single tumors.

Neuroendocrine tumors are rather rare neoplasms with an incidence today of about 6/100,000 [6]. They are categorized in functional and non-functional, the latter often presenting as a large solid bleeding mass. The functional NETs take up precursors of biologically active amines to produce active ones after subsequent intracellular decarboxylation and to store them in secretory vesicles. As a result, these **A**mine **P**recursor **U**ptake and **D**ecarboxylation cells, enabled to develop distinct clinical syndromes, i.e. flushing, skin rush, diarrhea, and hypoglycemia (the so-called carcinoid syndrome), are named APUD according to AGE Pearse, in 1969 [7], (Fig. 7.3) [8]. About one-half

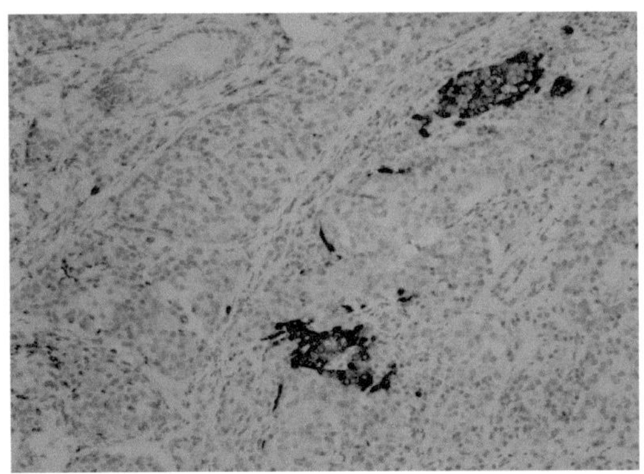

Fig. 7.1 Histological section of a well-differentiated pancreatic NET; positive immunore-action to somatostatin (Immunostain ×10)

G. S. Limouris (✉)
Nuclear Medicine, Medical School, National and Kapodistrian University of Athens, Athens, Greece
e-mail: glimouris@med.uoa.gr

© Springer Nature Switzerland AG 2021
G. S. Limouris (ed.), *Liver Intra-arterial PRRT with ^{111}In-Octreotide*,
https://doi.org/10.1007/978-3-030-70773-6_7

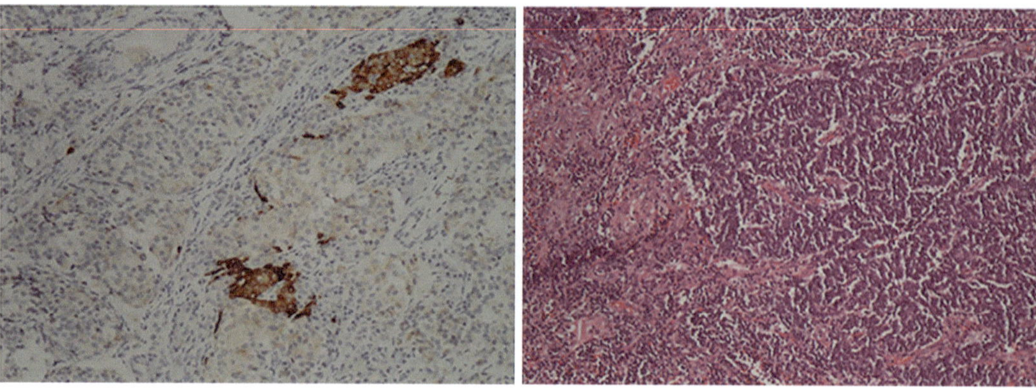

Fig. 7.2 Histological section of a Merkel cell carcinoma of the skin, metastatic to lymph node (Hematoxylin + Eosin ×10)

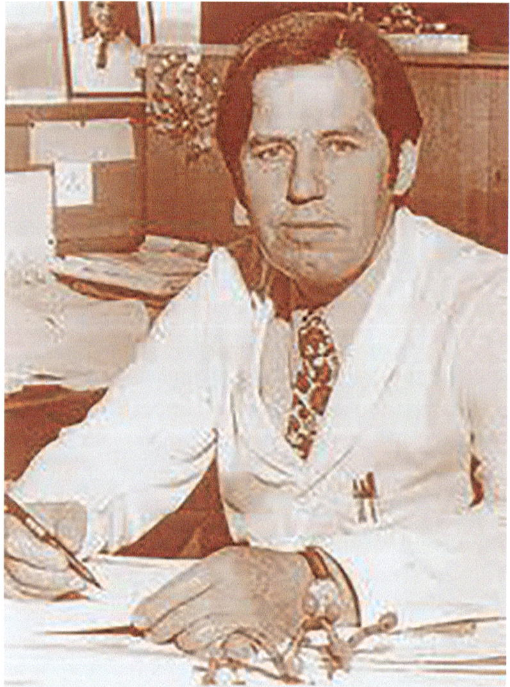

Fig. 7.3 Anthony Guy Everson Pearse 1906–2003 [8, 7]

of all NETs are described as nonfunctional, meaning that the patients do not have hormone-related symptoms. Both functional and nonfunctional have the unique feature of several somatostatin peptide receptor over-expressions.

7.2 The Therapeutic Approach of NENs

7.2.1 NETs' Treatment Background

Albeit the worldwide research, it is worth to note that over the last 30 years, no significant improvement in the survival of patients with NETs in the general population could be observed. For this reason, to promote the optimum care provided to these neoplasms, a better understanding of their biology might be needed, with emphasis on molecular genetics and the improvement of experimental models. Furthermore, at clinical practice level, it is important to develop more reliable serological markers as well as methods to allow for accurate tumor detection for even smaller lesions.

Treatment for neuroendocrine tumors depends upon the location of the tumor, whether the cancer has given metastases, spread to other areas of the body i.e. liver, bone, lymph nodes, and if the tumor is secreting hormones, responsible for symptoms. Treatment modalities against primary or metastatic neuroendocrine tumors can be categorized as: (a) invasive, i.e. *surgical resection*, (b) minimally invasive or ablative or locoregional, i.e. selective trans-arterial (chemo) *embolization* [TA (C) E], radiofrequency *ablation* [RFA], laser-induced thermotherapy [LITT], selective internal radiotherapy [SIRT], and (c) systemic standard therapy.

7.2.2 NETs and Curative Surgery (In This Volume, Chaps. 18 and 19)

Curative surgery should be considered whenever possible even in the presence of metastatic disease, including localized metastatic disease to the liver, if considered potentially resectable and the patient can tolerate the surgery. Surgical resection is the treatment of choice for NETs. Specifically, GEP-NET patients should be considered potential candidates for curative surgery. Curative resection of the primary tumor and locoregional lymph node metastases improves outcomes in these patients, resulting in excellent 5- and 10-year survivals of 100% in stage 1 and stage 2 patients, and still favorable outcomes in stage 3 disease with 5- and 10-year survivals of more than 95% and 80%, respectively [9–14].

7.2.3 NETs and Minimally Invasive Modalities

The choice of the ablative or loco-regional procedures or minimally invasive modalities [15], i.e. radiofrequency ablation (RFA) [16–18] laser-induced thermotherapy (LITT) [19, 20] selective hepatic trans-arterial embolization (TAE) [21–24], trans-arterial chemo-embolization (TACE) [25, 26] and selective internal radiotherapy (SIRT) [27–31], depends on the local expertise, number and size of lesions, and location of liver involvement (in this volume, Chaps. 20 and 21).

7.2.4 NETs and Systemic Standard Treatment [32–35]

The use of *somatostatin analogs*, i.e. octreotide [36] pasireotide [37, 38] and lanreotide [39], is a standard therapy in functioning NETs of any size to confrontate flushing and diarrhea, being the cornerstone treatment for patients with advanced NETs. *Interferon alpha* [40] may also be considered for symptom control in some patients and is usually used as second-line therapy due to its less-favorable toxic profile. *Everolimus* [34, 35], registered for treatment of pancreatic NETs worldwide, inhibits *mammalian target of rapamycin* (mTOR), a serine–threonine kinase that stimulates cell growth, proliferation, and angiogenesis. *Sunitinib* [33] *and Pazopanib* [41, 42] are potent and selective multitargeted receptor tyrosine kinase inhibitors that block tumor growth and inhibit angiogenesis. They have been approved for renal cell carcinoma and soft tissue sarcoma by numerous regulatory administrations worldwide. Chemotherapy [32], on the other hand, with doxorubicin, streptozocin, fluorouracil, chlorozotocin [43, 44], or in combination shows equivocal and mediocre results.

Though surgery consists the only curative option for NETs, there is a lack of precision-consensus between their management and guidelines regarding optimal treatment approaches in the unresectable and/or metastatic setting. Consequently, on account of the limited availability of high-level clinical evidence, a multidisciplinary approach [15] for the management of NETs is a first-class strategy to ensure a consistent and optimal level of care (Table 7.1).

Table 7.1 Multidisciplinary team approach for neuroendocrine neoplasms

Nuclear medicine physician	Tumor surgeon
Interventional radiologist	Radiation physicist
Medical oncologist	Pathologist
Gastroenterologist	Dedicated nursing staff

Table 7.2 Classification of neuroendocrine neoplasms of the gastroenteropancreatic system (WHO 2017)

Grade	Differentiation	Ki-67%	Mitotic index (hpf)
G1	Well-differentiated NET	<3	**<2/10**
G2	Well-differentiated NET	3–20	2–20/10
G3	Well-differentiated NET or Poorly differentiated NET or NEC small and large cell type	>20	>20/10
≠	MiNEN*	≠	≠

NEN Neuroendocrine neoplasm (also called NET = neuroendocrine tumor), *NEC* neuroendo-crine carcinoma, *HPF* high power field, ≠ A mixed neoplasm with components of a nonendocrine carcinoma (mostly ductal adenocarcinoma or acinar cell carcinoma) combined with a neuroendocrine neoplasm. Usually both components are high-grade malignant carcinomas (G3), but occasionally one of the two or both components may belong to the G1/G2 category. Therefore, the components should be individually graded, using the respective grading systems for each
*Mixed neuroendocrine/non-neuroendocrine neoplasm

Recently, the new classification guidelines [45] for GEP-NETs (4th edition) and the World Health Organization (WHO) from 2017 [46] are enriched adding the proliferation Ki-67 and Mitotic Indexes[1] to the differentiation criteria (Table 7.2). Accordingly, well-differentiated tumors are grade 1 (Ki-67 <3% and MI <2/10 high power field (HPF)), grade 2 (Ki-67 3–20% and MI 2–20/10 HPF), and grade 3 (Ki-67 >20% and MI >20/10 HPF). There is a subdivision of tumors with a Ki-67 >20% and an MI >20/10 HPF into well-differentiated grade 3 NET and

---

[1] **Ki-67** is a *nuclear antigen* expressed in proliferating cells and is expressed during the GI, S, G2, and M phases of the cell cycle. Cells are then stained with a Ki-67 *antibody*, and the number of stained nuclei is then expressed as a percentage of total tumor cells. The name is derived from the city of origin (Kiel, Germany) and the "67" number of the original clone in the 96-well plate.

The **Mitotic Index**, expressed *as the number of cells per microscopic field* is determined by counting the number of cells undergoing mitosis through a light microscope on hematoxylin and eosin (H and E) stained sections. Usually the number of mitotic figures is expressed as the total number in a defined number of high-power fields, i.e., 10 mitoses in 10 high power fields. Since the field of vision area can considerably vary between different microscopes, the exact area of the high-power fields should be defined in order to compare results from different studies.

poorly differentiated neuroendocrine carcinoma (NEC), the latter being categorized into small cell and large cell carcinomas.

7.2.5 NETs and the Intra-arterial Peptide Receptor Radionuclide Therapy (PRRT) Concept; A Brief Introduction

In our Institution, PRRT was performed from 1997 up to 2012 using n.c.a. ^{111}In-Octreotide, routinely in high activities (12 cycles of 4070–5920 MBq (110–160 mCi) per session, per patient, intra-arterially) and thenceforth replaced by non-carrier added (n.c.a.) ^{177}Lu-DOTA-TATE (6 cycles of 7000 MBq (189 mCi) per session, per patient, intra-arterially, too), rather exclusively focused in cases with hepatic secondaries. A PRRT dosimetry-guided protocol was followed of a more personalized character for each case, based on patients' hematotoxicity, tumor behavior (RECIST 1.1.criteria), chromogranin-A serum levels and clinical (symptoms') profile, not exceeding the 2 Gy absorbed dose to bone marrow or the 23 Gy to the kidneys [47–52]. The PRRT therapeutic scheme was implemented in combination with octreotide-Long-Acting-Repeatable (30 mg per 20 days) or lanreotide (60 mg up to 120 mg per 20 days), as first-line therapy. As a final result, objective tumor response (CR + PR) was achieved in 47/86 (54.65%) patients, disease control (CR, PR or SD) in 70/86 (81.39%) with a 32 and 46.5 months median progression-free survival and overall survival, respectively. We describe the outcome of the n.c.a. ^{111}In-Octreotide treatment in 86 patients of various NET histotypes, where approximately more than 800 infusions were intra-arterially implemented after catheterization of the hepatic artery, a novelty unique worldwide in humans.

7.3 Patients and Methods

A total of 86 patients were treated with n.c.a. ^{111}In-Octreotide from April 1997 to February 2012 in our Institution. Patients were Greek citizens with NETs treated according to a standard protocol called "Aretaieion Protocol" [15, 53], devoted to the name of the University Hospital of the Nuclear Section in which it was developed.

Selective hepatic angiography was conducted with a digital angiographic unit (Optimus, Phillips, the Netherlands). A 5.0-F valved sheath (Introducer II-long sheath; Terumo; Tokyo, Japan) was inserted into the femoral artery with the patient under local anesthesia, which was induced by injecting 10 mL of 2% lidocaine subcutaneously (Xylocaine; Astra, Sweden). After obtaining arterial access, a diagnostic visceral arteriogram was performed to delineate the arterial supply to the tumor, determine the presence of variant arterial anatomy, and confirm portal vein patency, even though portal vein thrombosis does not necessarily constitute a contra-indication to perform trans-catheter arterial radionuclide infusion. Celiac and superior mesenteric arteriography was performed with a Cobra II 5.0-F catheter (Glidecath; Terumo, Japan), which was advanced into the proper hepatic artery by using a 0.035-inch gliding guide wire (Guide Wire M; Terumo, Japan). The catheter was then selectively inserted into the right or left hepatic or proper hepatic artery, dependent on the tumor intra-hepatic location. In seldom cases, when a very super-selective catheterization was necessary, a 2.8-F micro-catheter (Terumo, Japan) was coaxially used. The size and location of the neuroendocrine nodules was assessed using the Couinaud nomenclature [55] according to which the liver is divided into eight independent segments; each of which has its own vascular inflow, outflow, and biliary drainage (Fig. 7.4). Tumor size and location was evaluated

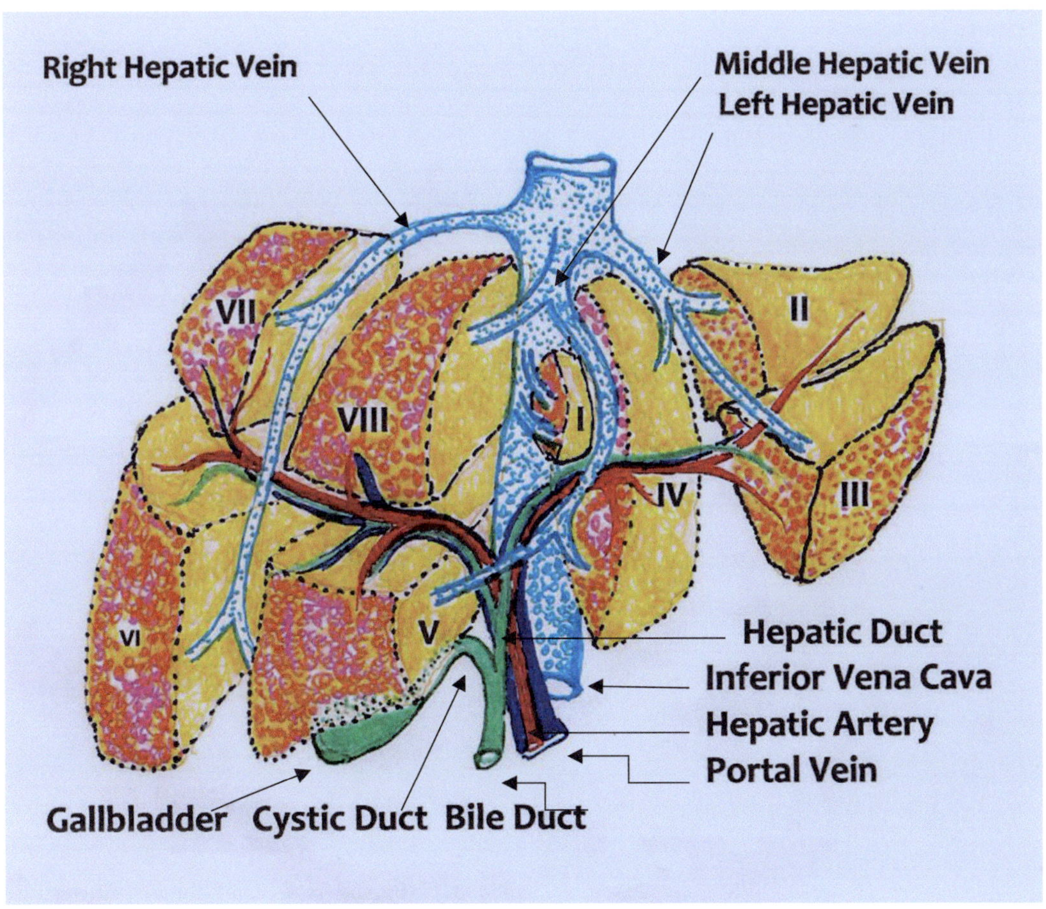

Fig. 7.4 Segmental anatomy of the liver, according to Couinaud nomenclature [54] nomenclature

by means of a consensus between two observers who compared the images obtained. Having safely positioned the catheter within the nearest artery to the tumor, intra-hepatic radionuclide infusion followed.

Angiogenesis is a key event in neoplasm progression and therefore a promising target in cancer treatment. SST-2 receptors, over-expressed in the endothelium of neuroendocrine character neo-plasmatic disease and used as the target of radiolabeled somatostatin analogues, are proved to serve as powerful anti-angiogenic targets with consequently potent anti-tumor activity (Fig. 7.5).

For evaluation, only patients who received at least in total 330 mCi (12.210 GBq) ^{111}In-Octreotide were included. The analysis of treatment efficacy comprises NET types, categorized into (Figs. 7.6 and 7.7), foregut, other foregut, midgut, hindgut,

and NETs of unknown origin. Other foregut NETs comprised two NETs of the brain (one meningioma and one oligodendroglioma), one of the stomach, one of the mesothorax, and three hepatocellular carcinomas with neuroendocrine characteristics. Assumption for PRRT with ^{111}In-Octreotide was a visual score 3–4 on OctreoScan scintigraphy prior to PRRT[2].

---

[2]Uptake on the OctreoScan was scored on planar images using a four-point scale; [grade 1: activity (uptake) equal to that in the normal liver, grade 2: activity (uptake) greater than that in the normal liver but less than that in the left kidney and spleen, grade 3: activity (uptake) equal to that in the left kidney, grade 4: activity (uptake) at least equal to the half of the sum of the activities in spleen and left kidney]. Purpose of this four-point scale is to assess candidacy for peptide receptor radionuclide therapy (PRRT), with a score mandatorily greater than 2, i.e., 3 and 4.

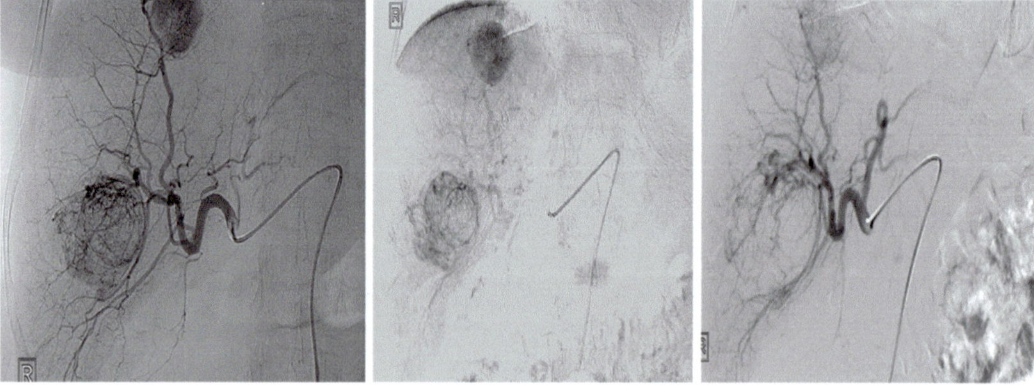

Fig. 7.5 Serial angiography of a patient with multiple hepatic metastases due to neuroendocrine tumor obviously shows the neo-vessel being destroyed after combined ^{111}In/^{177}Lu-radiopeptide treatment

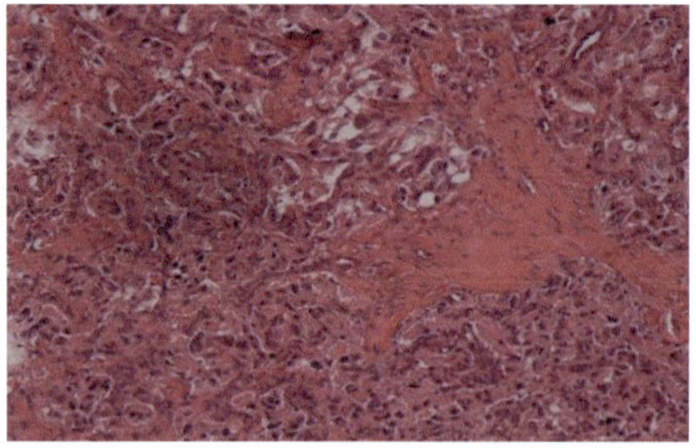

Fig. 7.6 Histological section of a well differentiated mammary NET (Hematoxylin + Eosin ×10)

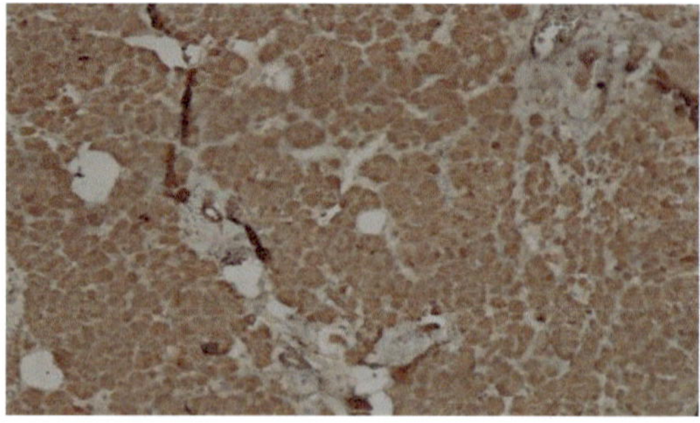

Fig. 7.7 Histological section of a well-differentiated pancreatic NET, showing extensive immunoreactions to Chromogranin (Immunostain ×10)

Other inclusion criteria were serum hemoglobin ≥ 9.7 g/dL, total white blood cell (WBC) count $\geq 2 \times 10^9$/L, platelet count $\geq 75 \times 10^9$/L, serum creatinine concentration ≤ 1.7 mg/dL), and Karnofsky Index (KI) ≥ 40. Preliminary results in a subgroup of these patients with GEP-NETs were reported previously [15]. All patients gave written informed consent, which was approved by the medical ethical committee of our hospital. ^{111}In-Octreotide was obtained from Mallinckrodt (Petten, Holland) and prepared "in house" as already described [15]. Before the infusion of the radiopharmaceutical, Ondansetron 8 mg was injected intravenously. To reduce the radiation dose to the kidneys, intravenous infusion of amino acids (2.5% arginine and 2.5% lysine in 1 L 0.9% NaCl) was started 30 min before the administration of the radiopharmaceutical and lasted for 4 h. The radiopharmaceutical was co-administered intravenously over 30 min. In cases of longer subacute hematologic toxicity, the intended continuing interval between treatments was 9 and 10 weeks. Patients were treated up to a cumulative intended activity from 330 mCi (12.210 GBq) to 2560 mCi (94.720 GBq) ^{111}In-Octreotide except in one case with excised bronchopulmonary primary, infused once, who received a cumulative activity of only 185 mCi (5 GBq).

7.3.1   Follow-Up and In Vivo Measurements

Routine hematology, liver, and kidney function tests were performed per three therapy cycles. Tumor response was assessed trimonthly on U/S and as far on CT or MRI before and at least 6 months after the initialization of the treatment or at the end of the entire therapeutic scheme, according to the Response Evaluation Criteria in Solid Tumors 1.1 (RECIST 1.1) criteria [51]. Thereafter every case was seen as an outpatient for follow-up.

7.3.1.1   Posttreatment and Follow-Up Studies

The aforementioned radionuclide infusion procedure was repeated 4–6 weeks apart. Initially, before the commencement of the treatment CT and/or MRI scans and U/S imaging was performed, being considered as the baseline of the pre-therapy lesion status. U/S was repeated monthly, just before the beginning of each session and being the main tool of the follow-up estimation. A second CT or MRI scan was requested at the end of the entire therapy scheme. Routine measurement of complete blood count, liver and kidney function tests, Chromogranin-A (Cr-A), and hormone levels as previously described will be measured before each session and at follow-up visits.

CT images Non-enhanced as well as contrast-enhanced CT images (5 mm slice thickness, 7-mm collimation, 1.50 pitch, 120 kVp, 220–250 mAs) was performed with model PQ 6000 (PICKER International, Highland Heights, Ohio) and Hi-Speed Advantage (GE Medical Systems, Milwauckee Wis) Spiral scanners (Fig. 7.8).

MR tomoscans Magnetic resonance (MR) images were obtained by using a 1.5-T Magnetom Vision Unit (Siemens) and two pulse sequences: T2-weighted turbo spin echo (4200/83 or 165 [repetition time ms/echo time ms], 7-mm slice thickness, 128×256 matrix, 3-min imaging time) and T1-weighted gradient echo with a fast low-angle shot technique (174.9/4.1, 80° flip angle, 7-mm section thickness, 128×256 matrix, 22-s imaging time) (Fig. 7.9).

U/S tomoscans The U/S scan images were acquired in the sagittal, transverse, and intercostal planes by using ATL 3000-HDI (Advanced Technology Laboratories, Bothell, Wash) and AU 590 (Esaote Biomedica, Genoa, Italy) units and a convex 4–2 MHz probe (Fig. 7.10).

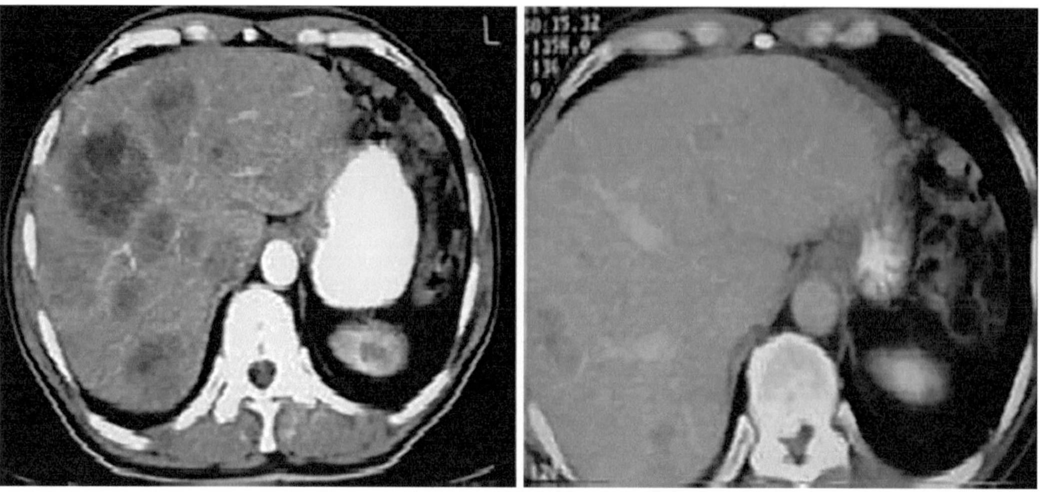

Fig. 7.8 Liver CT before [left] and after [right] the radiopeptide treatment completion

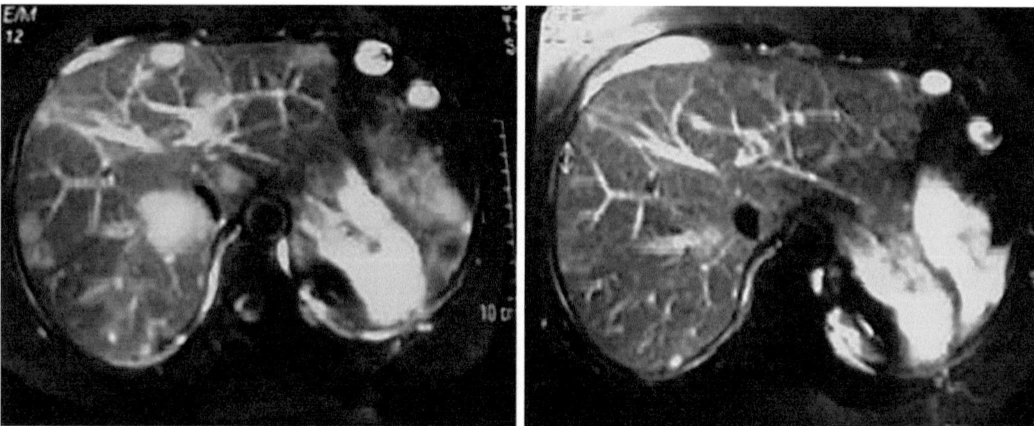

Fig. 7.9 Liver MRI before [left] and after [right] the radiopeptide treatment completion

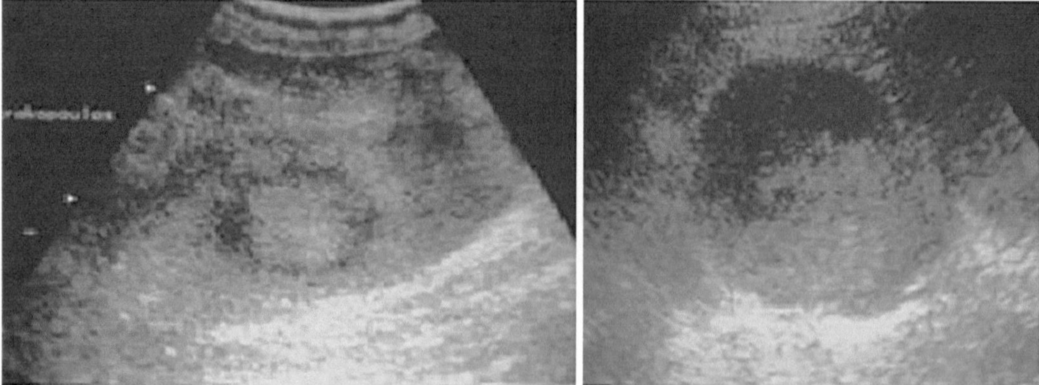

Fig. 7.10 Liver U/S [left] after the fourth and [right] the ninth session with ^{111}In-Octreotide completion

7.4 ^{111}In-Octreotide Treatment Evaluation

Baseline patient characteristics and response rates are presented in Table 7.3. All patients were under somatostatin analogues treatment. Best objective response rate (ORR) was defined as the proportion of patients achieving complete response (CR) and partial response (PR) at follow-up according to the RECIST 1.1 criteria. The ORR in the entire 86 patients was (47/86) 54.65%. SD was found in 23/86 (26.74%) of patients. PD as treatment outcome was observed in 16/86 (18.6%) of patients. For the entire group of 86 NET patients, the median OS was 46.5 months (95% CI, 11–120 months), whereas the median PFS was 32 months (95% CI, 0–110 months). The median OS ranged from 44 to 54 months with the longest OS in favor of the midgut cases. Exceptionally, the three cases of unknown origin reached a much longer OS of 61 months. Risk factors that might shorten/cut down/burden OS are bone morrow secondaries, nonmeasurable disease, and high Ki-67 index at baseline.

7.5 Discussion

According to Ertl et al. [56], Hofer and Hughes [57], Bradley et al. [58] and Feinendegen et al. [59] Auger electron emitters can be highly radio-toxic when they decay in the vicinity of DNA of the cell nucleus. After Howell et al. [60] and Rao et al. [61]some of them can be as radiotoxic as polonium-210 (^{210}Po) which emits 5.3 MeV alpha particles. Furthermore, reviews on the biological effects of Auger electron emitters published by Sastry and Rao in 1984 [62], Kassis in 2004 [63], Buchegger et al. in 2004 [64] and 2006 [65], and Nikjoo et al. in 2006 [66] consist of an excellent resource for a first-class detailed background and analysis on the field. The extreme radiotoxicity of Auger electron emitters prompted the aforementioned scientists to extensively investigate the radiobiological effects of Auger electrons and some others, among them our group (Figs. 7.11 and 7.12), to implement them routinely for thera-

peutic reasons in humans after the consent of the Ethical and Scientific Committee of our institution ("Aretaieion" University Hospital). Furthermore, we intended to prove their therapeutic efficacy to successfully confront mainly small (less than 20 mm) and micro-metastatic lesions, positive in somatostatin 2 (sst2) receptors. Worth mentioning is the support by the colleagues and leading scientists from the Interventional Radiology Clinic (Profs Vlahos Lambros and Chatzioannou Achilles), from the Oncology Unit (Prof Gennatas Konstantinos) from the II Surgery Clinic (Profs Voros Dionysios and Fragulidis Georgios), the Director of the Gastroenterological Clinic of National Health System Dr. Nikou Georgios of the "Laikon"

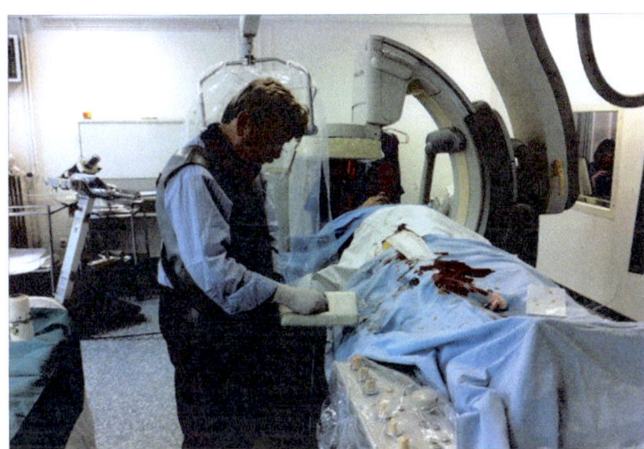

Fig. 7.11 National and Kapodistrian University of Athens-"Aretaieieon" Hospital Hemodynamic Theatre-I Department of Radiology: On the course of the intra-arterial procedure (GS Limouris)

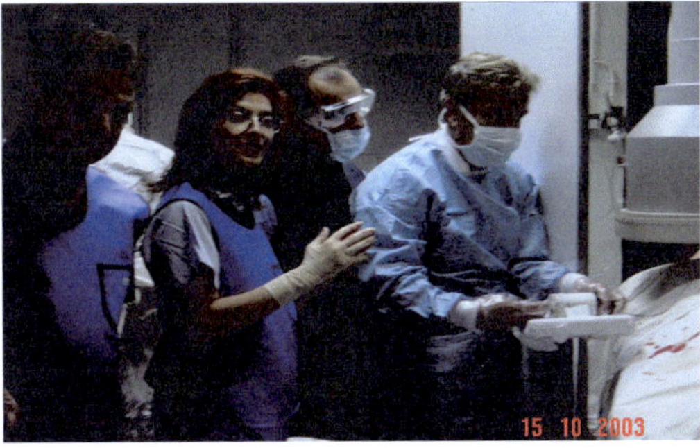

Fig. 7.12 National and Kapodistrian University of Athens—"Aretaieion" Hospital Hemodynamic Theatre-I Department of Radiology: On the course of the intra-arterial procedure (from left to right: V Skiadas, O Doryforou, A Chatziioannou, GS Limouris)

Table 7.3 Characteristics and response rates in patients treated with ^{111}In-Octreotide

Primary NET localization	No. of patients	Tumor histotype	CR (%)	PR (%)	SD (%)	PD (%)	Median PFS (months)	Median OS (months)
Foregut	39	smi, pancr, brpln	**2**	**16**	**12**	**9**	31	44
Non-PD	30	pancr, brlpn, hcc + neur, gastr, brain, hep hilus	2 (6.7)	16 (53.3)	12 (40.0)	0 (0.0)	42.5	50.6
PD	9	pancr, brlpn, mediast	0	0	0	9 (100)	3	17
Other foregut	7	hcc + neur, ming,dndrglio, gastr, mesent	**1** (14.3)	**2** (28.6)	**3** (42.8)	**1** (14.3)	31	38
Non-PD	6	Brain, gastr, hcc + neur	1	2	3	0	31	38
PD	1	hcc + neur, mediast	1 (16.7)	2 (**33.3**)	3 (50.0)	0 (0.0)	5	19
Midgut	27	mesent	**0**	**18**	**5**	**4**	36	54
Non-PD	23	smi, asc col, cecum, mesent	0 (0.0)	18 (72.3)	5 (21.7)	0 (0.0)	39	56
PD	4	smi	0	0	0	4 (100)	9	26.5
Hindgut	10	rect, colorect, prg	**0**	**5**	**3**	**2**	32.5	45
Non-PD	8	desc col, colorect, rect prg	0	5 (62.5)	3 (**37.5**)	0 (0.0)	37.5	51.0
PD	2	rect, desc col	0	0	0	2 (100)	6	**22**
Unknown	3	–	**0**	**3**	**0**	**0**	60	61
Functional	16	brlpn(2), gastr(1), jej(4), nisid(1), MEN I(1), desc col(2), uo(1), pancr(4),	0 (0.0)	7 (43.7)	5 (31.25)	4 (25.0)	23	34.5
Nonfunctional	70	pancr(22), brlpn(9), smi(11), jej(1), rect(1), hcc + neur(2), uo(2), desc col(3), gastr(1), rect prg(1), asc col(2), colorect(1), mesent (3), mening(1), dndrglio(1), liver hil(1), ile(5), sigm(2), cecum(1)	3	38	16	11	33.5	51
Total	86		**3**	**44**	**23**	**16**	32	46.5

General Hospital and the MD PhD radiologist Dr. Dimitropoulos Nikolaos who encouraged us (the specialized physicians, physicists, PhD candidates and me) at the Nuclear Medicine Section to infuse ^{111}In-Octreotide as first-line therapy since 1997 up to 2012, performing exclusively intra-arterially, more than 800 infusions; additionally, to continue thereafter with non-carrier added [177]Lutetium DOTA TATE (around 50 infusions).

This scientific effort has led to the establishment of the "Aretaieion Protocol" [15, 53], where appart from the intra-arterially radionuclide infusion technique, nephroprotection with amino-acids and bone-marrow prophylaxis with 75 mg DTPA were taken as *"sine qua non"*. Furthermore, the temporary implementation of a port-system for those patients who wanted to avoid the discomfort of the intra-arterial procedure (Chap. 8, in this volume), was a special achievement, during this period; it has to be taken into account that PRRT with ^{111}In-Octreotide necessitated 12 sessions for an expected successful therapeutic result as well as the introduction of the "sonoporation concept" (Chap. 9, in this volume).

The results of this study demonstrate that PRRT with ^{111}In-Octreotide is a potent therapeutic option for liver metastasized patients with advanced grade 1 to 2 and even grade 3 NENs, which are of less than 20 mm in size or of micro-metastases. This treatment has limited side effects and is undisputably safe.

Preliminary results in initial ^{111}In clinical studies and efficacy: Analyzing the results of the first and initially (with ^{111}In-Octreotide) treated cohort 1 of 17 (6%) in 2008 [15] (Table 7.1) patients achieved a complete response (CR), 8 of 17 (47%) showed partial response (PR) and 3 (18%) stable disease (SD), whereas in the remaining 5 (29%) patients the disease progressed, the therapy was discontinued and the patients died shortly thereafter. Consequently, 71% of the patients showed some radiological benefit (CR or PR or SD) from the treatment. Worldwide, only a limited number of authors reported until today on the efficacy of treatments in GEP-NET-patients using high doses of ^{111}In-Octreotide (Table 7.1). Our results in the CR/PR group (53%, 9/17) substantially differ compared to those of Valkema et al. (8%, 2/16 patients [67], of Buscombe et al. (17%, 2/12 patients) [68] of Anthony et al. (8%, 2/6 patients) [69] and of Delpassand et al. (7%, 2/29 patients) [70]. A similar diverge is obvious in the SD group 18% (3/17 pts) compared to the 58% (15/26 pts) of Valkema et al. [67], 58% (7/12 pts) of Buscombe et al. [68], 81% (21/26 pts) of Anthony et al. [69], and 55% (16/29 pts) of Delpassand et al. [70]. The superiority of our results compared to the aforementioned authors might be explained by the intra-arterial route of infusions, where the tumor mean absorbed dose per session was estimated to be markedly higher compared to i.v. application (Table 7.3); a finding also reported by other authors [71, 72]. Summarizing the results of previous studies, it might/can be concluded that the application of ^{111}In-Octreotide leads indisputably to disease stabilization (SD) in previously progressive tumors, clinical symptomatic improvement, and biochemical (Cr-A) decline. The

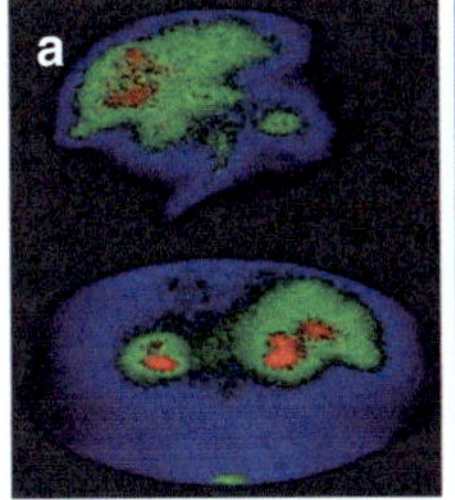
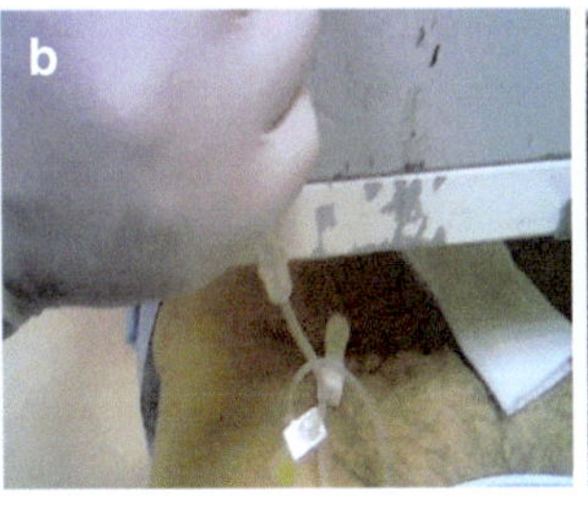
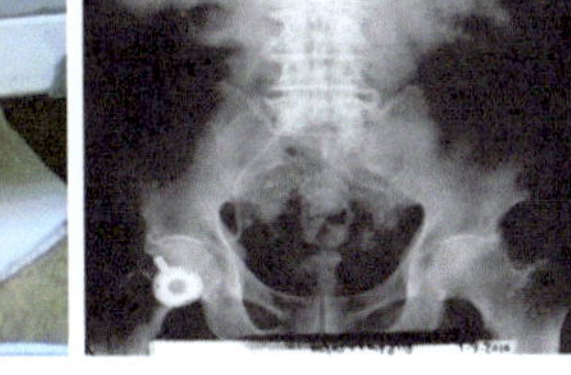
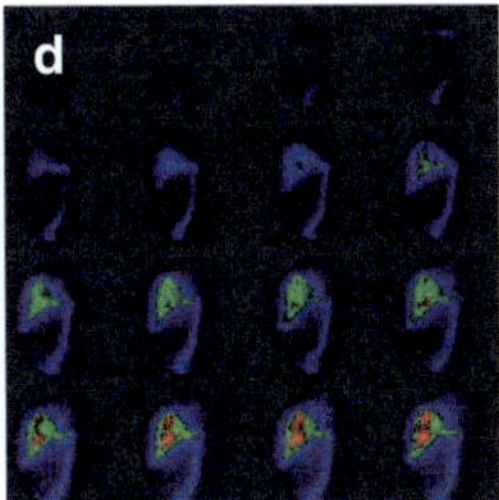

Fig. 7.13 (**a**) Radionuclide infusion through the drum-port system, temporarily implanted subcutaneously in the right iliac fossa area, (**b**) X-ray image (anterior view) of the patient's abdomen, (**c**) Dynamic (60 s, anterior view) scintimages obtained on the course of the infusion initialization and (**d**) static ones (anterior/posterior view) just after the end of the infusion (treatment) procedure

Table 7.4 Experts working with ^{111}In-Octreotide

Author	No of pts	cumul. activ. (GBq)	CR	PR	SD	PD
Krenning et al. (1994) [99]	1	20.3	–	1 (100%)	–	–
Caplin et al. (2000) [100]	8	3.10–15.200	–	–	7 (87.5%)	1 (12.5%)[a]
Tiensuu Janson et al. (1999) [101]	5	18.00	–	2 (40%)	3 (60%)	–
Nguyen et al. (2004) [102]	15	21.00	–	–	13 (87%)	2 (13%)
Valkema et al. (2002) [67]	26	4.7–160.0	–	2 (8%)	15 (58%)	9 (35%)
Anthony et al. (2002) [69]	26	6.7–46.6	–	2 (8%)	21 (81%)	3 (11%)
Buscombe et al. (2003) [68]	12	3.1–36.6	–	2 (17%)	7 (58%)	3 (25%)
Delpassand et al. (2008) [70]	29	35.3–37.3	–	2 (7%)	16 (55%)	11 (38%)[b]
Limouris et al. (2008) [15][c]	17	13.0–77.0	1 (6%)	8 (47%)	3 (18%)	5 (29%)

[a]Unrelated to the tumor cause
[b]Not clearly reported
[c]Exclusively intra-arterially

results of the clinical evaluation of the Auger electron emitter indium-111 conjugated to somatostatin analogues that target and exploit its receptor over-expression on neuroendocrine cells are encouraging, particularly as it was thereafter proven successful, for the eradication of small volume tumors [15] (Tables 7.4, 7.5 and 7.6).

7.5.1 The "Gnosti-Thera" Principle ["Gnosti-Thera" vs. "Thera-Nostics"]

In their Letter to the Editor [73] entitled: Why should we be concerned about a "g"? Frangos S and Buscombe JR aptly reported on the etymology of the term "Theranostics" (the concept from "diagnosis to therapy") which is uttered linguistically erroneously worldwide by the entire medical community.

The term "Theranostics," in addition to being an awkward title for a reputable international scientific journal, is repeated not only by colleagues noneducated in ancient Greek and Latin language but also strangely enough by native Greek- or Latin-originated scientists.

Additionally, the term "Theranostics" is also by definition wrong because therapy logically follows diagnosis and linguistically the appropriate approach is the synergy of these two words, where "diagnosis" precedes "therapy."

Table 7.5 Tumor-absorbed dose comparison between i.v. and i.a. administration of ^{111}In-Octreotide

Organ	Intra-arterial infusion	Intravenous infusion
Liver dose	0.14 (mGy/MBq)	0.40 (mGy/MBq)
Kidney dose	0.41 (mGy/MBq)	0.51 (mGy/MBq)
Tumor dose	15.20 (mGy/MBq)	11.20 (mGy/MBq)
Spleen dose	1.40 (mGy/MBq)	1.56 (mGy/MBq)
Bone marrow dose	0.0035 (mGy/MBq)	0.022 (mGy/MBq)
Tumor/liver dose ratio	108.57[a]	28.00
Tumor/kidney dose ratio	37.07	21.96

[a]The average absorbed dose per session to a tumor for a spherical mass of 10 g was estimated to be 10.8 mGy/MBq, depending on the histotype of the tumor

Furthermore, the second moiety (suffix) of the term "nostics" is leading inevitably towards the Greek word "νόστος" (nóstos) originated from the word "νέομαι" (néomai) meaning "repatriation" and furthermore nostalgy for return home (Sehnsucht nach etwas! in German); a linguistically erroneous word which alone does not express the precise meaning "from diagnosis to therapy".

Thus, the indisputable addition of "g" on the head of nostics, i.e., "gnostics" as it was aptly pointed out by the two colleagues, is a sine qua non, etymologically originated from the Greek word "know," "diagnosis" or the Latin word "cognosco," "diagnosis," and furthermore to reorder these two words (moieties) in their appropriate sequence.

According to the above exlanation, the proposed term "Gnosti-Thera," although not euphonic but etymologically correct, could be suggested for use in the place of "Thera-Nostics" or "Thera-Gnostics."

7.5.2 The Intra-arterial Infusion Concept

Intrahepatic radionuclide infusion after selective hepatic artery catheterization has proved to be simple to perform safe and effective therapeutic management of small ($\leq$20 mm) neuroendocrine hepatic secondaries, which are considered as inoperable. Compared to the other interventional techniques [74, 75] the methodology is almost invasive and short time lasting with negligible side effects. A relative drawback of the method is the slow tumor necrosis rate, requiring multiple treating sessions. Tumor melting areas shown on U/S scans are slowly growing, binding to each other and finally forming a large cavity, indicating necrosis. These tissue consistency changes can be easily followed up and evaluated by ultrasonography [76] (Fig. 7.13). The melting areas observed concern the neuroendocrine nodules, sparing the surrounding non-neuroendocrine healthy hepatic tissue. This is achieved due to the very short range of the Auger and Conversion electrons, the killing capability of which is limited up to 2–3 cells per decay [28]. Unfortunately, this very short range of the Auger and Conversion electrons consists a disadvantage of the procedure since multiple sessions are required for a potent tumor-cell destruction.

The radiopharmaceutical starts diffusing from the endpoint of the catheter into the branches of the hepatic artery towards the sinusoids of the neuroendocrine metastatic nodules following a pressure gradient that drains through rich vascular communications into the portal and/or hepatic veins [77, 78]. The radioactive distribution within and around the neuroendocrine nodules is related to the somatostatin receptor density of the cells as well as to the difference in vascularization between the neuroendocrine nodules and the surrounding normal hepatic parenchyma. The latter having a dual blood supply is mainly nourished by the hepatic artery [79], which provides about two-thirds of the blood flow, whereas the remaining one-third is provided by the portal vein [80, 81]. On the other hand, the increased somatostatin receptor-density acts like a magnet; the higher the receptor density of the tumor, the stronger the tracer gradient towards the receptors and hence the accumulation of the radiopharmaceutical.

Another parameter that gravely anticipates the large melting of the tumor and consequently the efficacy of the technique is the tumor shape and size. Neuroendocrine nodules of large volume of infiltrations spread into the hepatic parenchyma (Fig. 7.14) have shown poor response from the

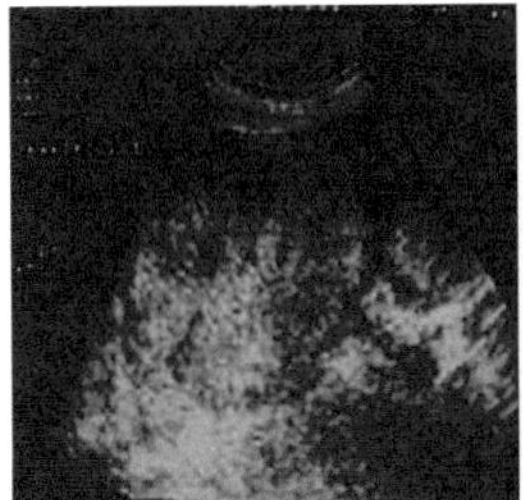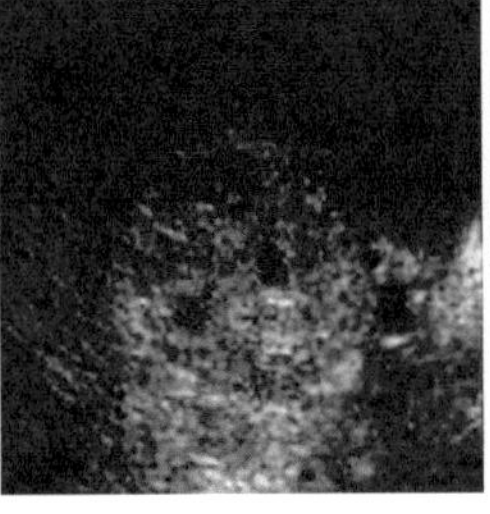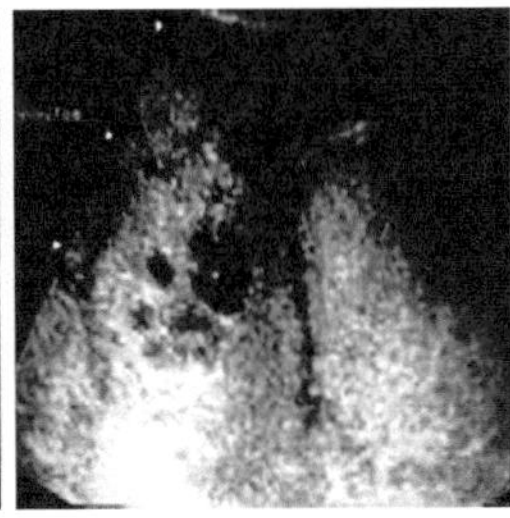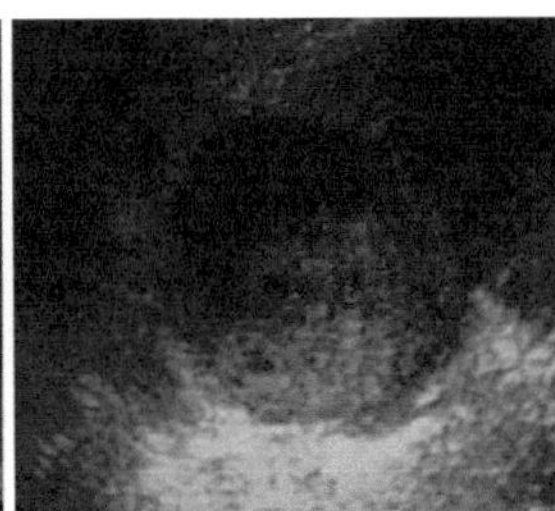

Fig. 7.14 Ultrasonographic evaluation of liver nodule before (5) and after (6) 5 sessions of octreotide treatment. Cystic degeneration of the nodule center and peripheral rim edema, as response to the therapeutic scheme. Cavity-type cystic degeneration of liver nodule in ultrasonographic examination. Swiss-cheese microcystic degeneration of liver nodule in ultrasonographic examination. Peripheral rim edema of liver nodule as first sign of tumor regression in U/S examination (Limouris et al. [76])

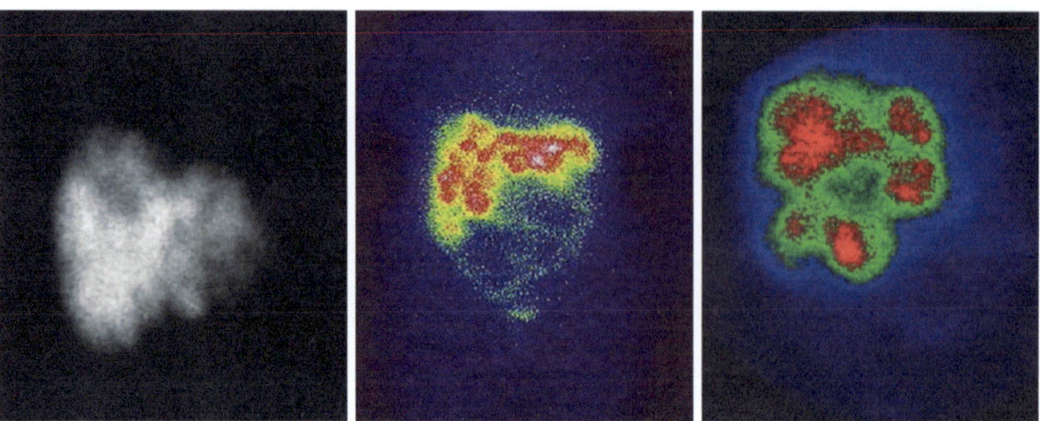

Fig. 7.15 Neuroendocrine secondaries of excised pancreatic NETs of large volume of infiltrations spread into the hepatic parenchyma (anterior view)

beginning of the treatment, because the indium-111 Auger and Conversion Electron ranges are insufficient to kill large tumor cell populations and essentially inhibit the progressive tumor growth (Fig. 7.15) [82].

The proliferation marker Ki-67 (this volume, Chap. 24) was almost routinely used for the grading of NETs [45, 83, 84]. A sample of 14 NEN patients out of the 86 treated with ^{111}In-Octreotide is tabulated in Table 7.6, related to their diameter.

7.5.3 Co-infusion of DTPA During Peptide Receptor Radionuclide Therapy with ^{111}In-Octreotide Reduces the Ionic Indium Contaminants

The Concept: In Peptide Receptor Radionuclide Therapy (PRRT) ^{111}In-Octreotide according to the manufacturer contains ~0.1% trivalent free ions of ^{111}In ($T_{ph1/2}$ = 2.83 days) and ^{114}In ($T_{p1/2}$ = 49.5 days). However since the mean patient activity per session usually ranges from 4070 MBq (110 mCi) to 7030 MBq (190 mCi) the amount of free ^{111}In^{3+} and ^{114}In^{+3} might provoke undesirable radiological burden to the patient, i.e., the often observed post-infusion myelotoxicity. According to pharmacokinetics, Indium trivalent (+3) ions accumulate in bone, liver, and spleen [85], bound to transferrin, a 80 kDa iron binding protein [86], inducing unwanted irradiation, particularly in bone marrow. Furthermore the trivalent indium anions mimic calcium bivalent ones accumulated in bone tissue where they participate in the hydroxyl-apatite formation. The tandem i.v. co-infusion of 75 mg of DTPA, diluted in 200–250 mL normal saline, 30 min before the commencement of the PRRT session in trip-trop infusion, continuing on the course of the procedure and lasting 4 h thereafter, competes with transferrin, forms trivalent DTPA complexes, by rerouting the ionic (free) indium fraction to renal clearance, and thus, effectively reducing blood pool activity and particularly bone marrow burden (Fig. 7.16).

Materials and Methods: Eighteen patients with neuroendocrine disease, age range 26–72 years, were treated with ^{111}In-Octreotide after selective hepatic artery catheterization. Nine out of them received a DTPA (Bristol-Myers Squibb) co-infusion in a dosage of 75 mg in 200 mL NaCl solution, in drip drop infusion, 30 min before the initialization of the session, lasting for about 4 h. Quantification of whole body scintigrams (30 min, 24 and 4 h p.i.) was performed [*MIRD Pamphlet No. 16 (J Nucl Med 1999, 40: 37S–61S)*]. Urinary and blood samples were collected during the patients' hospitalization and measured in a well-type scintilla-

Table 7.6 Ki-67 index vs tumor diameter in post-treated patients with ^{111}In-Octreotide

Patient's name	No. of foci	ø ≤ 2 cm	ø > 2 cm up to 4 cm	ø > 4 cm	Posttreatment foci/response	Ki-67
1. GAG.KON	5	–	–	4.8, 4.2, 6.8, 4.1	5/PD	>20%
2. XAT. VAS	2	–	–	4.1, 7.2	2/PD	>20%
3. SIM. PAN	3	–	–	4.6, 5.0, 5.2	3/PD	>20%
4. MPO.NAN	2	–	–	5.4, 6.3	2/PD	>20%
5. DRO.IOA	3	–	–	4.2, 5.0, 5.2	3/SD	>2–<20%
6. POL.IOA	3	–	2.8, 3.4, 3.2	–	3/SD	>2–<20%
7. TSO.GRI	5	0.8, 1.2, 1.1, 1.6, 1.9	–	–	1/PR	<2%
8. THER/KYR	4	0.8, 1.6, 1.9, 1.0	–	–	4/SD	>20%
9. BISTH. THEO	6	1.8, 1.1, 1.4, 0.8, 1.0, 1.6	–	–	6/SD	>20%
10. SOTH. STAV	5	1.4, 1.8, 1.6, 08, 1.2	–	–	5/SD	>20%
11. XRI.PAN	5	0.9, 1.2, 1.4, 1.8, 1.0	–	–	3/PR	<2%
12. BAT.ALE	5	–	2.0, 2.1, 3.1, 2.8, 3.5	–	2/PR	<2%
13. KAL. ANN	5	1.2, 0.8, 1.5, 1.8, 1.0	–	–	1/PR	<2%
14. POUT. AR	6	–	2.4, 2.0, 2.8, 3.0, 3.4, 3.8	–	3/PR	<2%

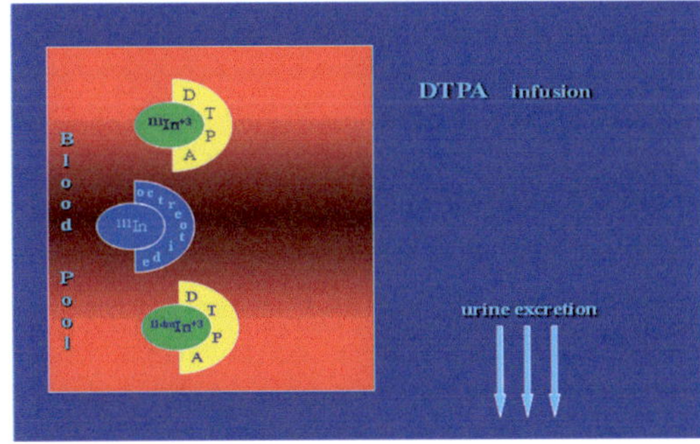

Fig. 7.16 Co-infusion of DTPA during peptide receptor radionuclide therapy with ^{111}In-Octreotide

tion counter. Exposure rate at 1 m patient's distance was recorded by means of an ionization chamber (Fig. 7.17).

Exposure rate measurements at 1 m distance from the patient were accomplished by means of an ionization chamber. The dose was estimated according to the MIRD schema [*MIRD Pamphlet No. 5 (revised J Nucl Med 1978)*].

Results: The activity and exposure rate half lives (h) in blood were 2.2 ± 0.4 and 1.2 ± 0.5 (rapid phase) without and with DTPA, respectively ($p < 0.05$) and for the slow phase 14 ± 8 and 12 ± 5 ($p > 0.05$). For the whole body the rapid phase for ^{111}In was 11 ± 3 and 8.1 ± 2 ($p < 0.001$) without DTPA and with DTPA respectively. For the whole body slow phase was 33 ± 12 and 33 ± 11 ($p > 0.05$) (Table 7.7).

Conclusion: DTPA co-infusions in PRRTs accelerate ^{111}In clearance, leading to the optimization of radiation protection of the clinical staff, the members of the family, and the public (97/43 EURATOM Directive); also, they significantly reduce the patients' radiobiological burden, contributing to the optimization of the treatment. Consequently it is strongly recommended in every PRRT [87].

Side effects of PRRT originated in general from bone marrow and kidneys. Co-infusion of lysine and arginine starting just before therapy

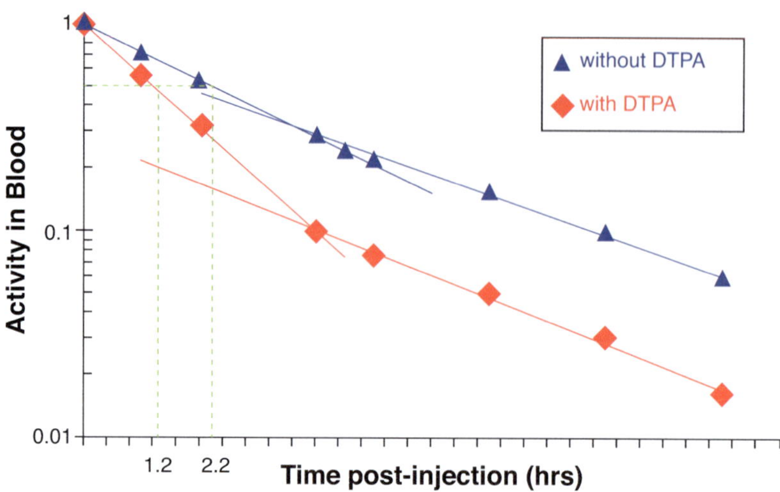

Fig. 7.17 Blood pool activity with and without DTPA co-infusion

Table 7.7 Activity and expose rate half life (h)

	Without DTPA	With DTPA	Difference
Blood (rapid)	2.2 ± 0.4	1.2 ± 0.5	$p < 0.05$
Blood (slow)	14 ± 8.0	12 ± 5.0	$p > 0.05$
Whole body	11 ± 3.0	7.8 ± 1.1	$p < 0.001$

lowers the radiation dose to the kidneys in patients treated with ^{90}Y or ^{177}Lu peptides, whereas for PRRT using ^{111}In-peptide intra-arterially it is practically not the case based on investigations performed by Kwekkeboom et al. (2001) and de Jong et al. (2004). Both authors proved that the pathlength of ^{111}In particularly can reach and affects the inner cortical zone of them and accordingly the kidney cannot by virtue be considered as a dose-limiting organ [88]. In his study, De Jong et al. [89] reported that ^{111}In-Octreotide distribution in the human kidney was investigated using SPECT scanning before and ex vivo kidney-autoradiography after surgery and indium's-111 radioactivity was localized predominantly in the inner zone of the renal cortex. Furthermore in the cortex, radioactivity is not distributed homogeneously, forming a striped pattern. These findings show that the average dose calculations using the MIRD scheme, assuming homogeneous renal radioactivity distribution, are virtually inadequate to accurately and precisely estimate the radiation dose to various parts of the kidney after PRRT.

On the course of the infusion, no pain was noticed, except for some abdominal discomfort in almost all patients, fatigue, headache, a temporary chest and head rush in 15 and blood pressure drop (from 140 to 9 mmHg)) in 21, as well as nausea, vomit, and diarrhoea on the first day p.i. All side effects disappeared shortly thereafter without any specific medical intervention. WHO toxicity grade I anemia occurred in 5 and grade I leuko-cytopenia and thrombocytopenia in 3. Severe (grade III and IV), mostly reversible, acute bone marrow toxicity was observed in 8/86 (10.5%) patients as a persistent hematological dysfunction. In 2/88 hairy cell leukemia was diagnosed and died shortly. Serum creatinine, transaminases, and alkaline phosphatase did not change in the entire group. Regarding the hormone levels, there were no abnormal values throughout the study for the whole group of patients. In contrast, a clear decrease in serum Cr-A was observed in SD and more obvious in partial and complete responders (Fig. 7.18), whereas in patients with progressive disease, a marked increase could be noticed.

Renal impairment and myelodysplasia (MDS)
We have observed renal impairment in six patients during follow-up after this therapy, not related to PRRT, as according to their medical history, all six candidates for therapy presented with impaired serum creatinine ranging from >1.2 mg% up to 2.0 mg% [90–94]. Acute leukemia and MDS are severe complications related to PRRT and occurred

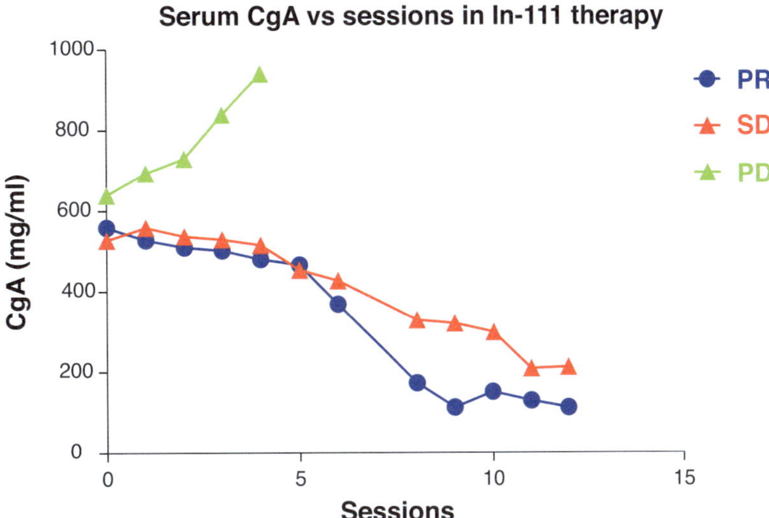

Fig. 7.18 Serum chromogranin-A levels during ^{111}In-Octreotide therapy in patients with PR, SD, and PD [1]

on average at 28 months after the first cycle with ^{177}Lu-DOTATATE for MDS, and after a median of 55 months for acute leukemia. Although none of our patients treated with ^{111}In-Octreotide were diagnosed with acute leukemia or MDS prior chemotherapy, recent reports suggest that there might be a higher risk of MDS or acute leukemia after alkylating chemotherapy [90–94].

Hormone-related side-effects or hormonal crises after PRRT with ^{111}In-Octreotide were not observed. However, when treating patients with functional neuroendocrine tumors, these hormone-related side effects should be taken into serious concern.

In the last two decades, many european authors have extensively reported on PRRT using [^{90}Y-DOTA[0],Tyr[3]]-Octreotide [90, 95–98]. Because of its higher energy, as compared with Indium-111, serious side effects have been noticed, e.g., transient grade 3 to 4 hematologic toxicity in 12.8% of patients and permanent grade 4 to 5 renal toxicity in 9.2% [90].

In 2008, we reported on 17 GEP-NET patients who were treated with n.c.a. ^{111}In-Octreotide [15]. In contrast to the former report, in this 86-patient cohort, the follow-up was much longer and the results are more representative in regard to the Auger electron efficacy in a multivariability of GEP-NET subtypes.

In this randomized study, the patients were all treated strictly according to the inclusion criteria, whereas an insistent active follow-up for many years makes the results by virtue noteworthy. Large tumor load or functional disease was dramatically slowed down, because PRRT was the best available treatment option at that time point. However, analysis of the patients with PD at baseline demonstrated only small differences in PFS and OS compared with all other NEN patients.

7.6 Conclusion

Considering the favorable high linear energy transfer of indium-111 Auger electron emission, it can be anticipated that the majority of diagnostically positive OctreoScans in small (less than 20 mm) neuroendocrine liver nodules, seems to be a first class candidates for this kind of treatment. The results so far are promising for the local control of such a histotype of malignancies. On the other hand, the relatively satisfactory long (>7 years) follow-up period of these patients encourages for a reliable estimation of the successful responders. The intra-arterial catheterization technique highly optimizes the received dose to the tumor, reducing consequently the burden of the critical organs. The tumoricidal effectiveness of PRRT with indium-111 Auger electron emission is judged by the overall survival and survival rate of these patients.

References

1. Barakat MT, Meeran K, Bloom SR. Neuroendocrine tumors. Endocr Relat Cancer. 2004;11:1–18.
2. Leotlela PD, Jauch A, Holtgrave-Grez H, et al. Genetics of neuroendocrine tumors and carcinoid tumors. Endocr Relat Cancer. 2003;10:437–50.
3. Thakker RV. Multiple endocrine neoplasia. Syndromes of the twentieth century. J Clin Endocrinol Metab. 1998;83(8):2617–20.
4. Thakker RV. Multiple endocrine neoplasia type 1. In: De Groot LJ, Jameson JL, editors. Endocrinology. 5th ed. Philadelphia: Elsevier Saunders Publs; 2006. p. 3509–31.
5. Gagel RF. Multiple endocrine neoplasia type 2. In: De Groot LJ, Jameson JL, editors. Endocrinology. 5th ed. Philadelphia: Elsevier Saunders Publs; 2006. p. 3533–50.
6. Lawrence B, Gustafsson BI, Chan A, et al. The epidemiology of gastro-entero-pancreatic neuroendocrine tumors. Endocrinol Metab Clin North Am. 2011;40:1–18.
7. Pearse AG. The cytochemistry and ultrastructure of polypeptide hormone-producing cells of the APUD series and the embryologic, physiologic and pathologic implications of the concept. J Histochem Cytochem. 1969;17:303–13.
8. Radu I. In memoriam of Professor A. G. E. Pearse (1916–2003). Roman J Morphol Embryol. 2005;46(3):257.
9. Chan MY, Ma KW, Chan A. Surgical management of neuroendocrine tumor-associated liver metastases: a review. Gland Surg. 2018;7(1):28–35.
10. Musunuru S, Chen H, Rajpal S, et al. Metastatic neuroendocrine hepatic tumors: resection improves survival. Arch Surg. 2006;141(10):1000–4.
11. Reddy SK, Clary BM. Neuroendocrine liver metastases. Surg Clin N Am. 2010;90(4):853–61.
12. Mayo SC, de Jong MC, Pulitano C, et al. Surgical management of hepatic neuroendocrine tumor metastasis: results from an international multi-institutional analysis. Ann Surg Oncol. 2010;17(12):3129–36.
13. Clary B. Treatment of isolated neuroendocrine liver metastases. J Gastrointest Surg. 2006;10(3):332–4.
14. Glazer ES, Tseng JF, Al-Refaie W, et al. Long-term survival after surgical management of neuroendocrine hepatic metastases. HPB. 2010;12(6):427–33.
15. Limouris GS, Chatziioannou A, Kontogeorgakos D, et al. Selective hepatic arterial infusion of In-111-DTPA-Phe1-octreotide in neuroendocrine liver metastases. Eur J Nucl Med Mol Imaging. 2008;35:1827–37.
16. O'Toole D, Maire F, Ruszniewski P. Ablative therapies for liver metastases of digestive neuroendocrine tumors. Endocr Relat Cancer. 2003;10:463–8.
17. Gillams A, Cassoni A, Conway G, et al. Radiofrequency ablation of neuro-endocrine liver metastases; the Middlesex experience. Abdom Imaging. 2005;30:435–41.
18. Eriksson J, Stålberg P, Nilsson A, et al. Surgery and radiofrequency ablation for treatment of liver metastases from midgut and foregut carcinoids and endocrine pancreatic tumors. World J Surg. 2008;32:930–8.
19. Tombesi P, Di Vece F, Sartori S. Laser ablation for hepatic metastases from neuroendocrine tumors. Am J Roentgenol. 2015;204:W732. https://doi.org/10.2214/AJR.14.14242.
20. Pacella CM, Nasoni S, Grimaldi F, et al. Laser ablation with or without chemoembolization for unresectable neuroendocrine liver metastases: a pilot study. Int J Endocr Oncol. 2016;3:97–107.
21. Brown KT, Koh BY, Brody LA, et al. Particle embolization of hepatic neuroendocrine metastases for control of pain and hormonal symptoms. J Vasc Interv Radiol. 1999;10:397–403.
22. Kanabar R, Barriuso J, McNamara MG, et al. Liver embolization for patients with neuroendocrine neoplasms: systematic review. Neuroendocrinology. 2021;111(4):354–69. https://doi.org/10.1159/000507194.
23. Pericleous M, Caplin ME, Tsochatzis E, et al. Hepatic artery embolization in advanced neuroendocrine tumors: efficacy and long-term outcomes. Asia Pac J Clin Oncol. 2016;12(1):61–9.
24. Chen JX, Rose S, White SB, et al. Embolotherapy for neuroendocrine tumor liver metastases: prognostic factors for hepatic progression-free survival and overall survival. Cardiovasc Intervent Radiol. 2017;40(1):69–80.
25. Sun JH, Zhou TY, Zhang YL, et al. Efficacy of transcatheter arterial chemoembolization for liver metastases arising from pancreatic cancer. Oncotarget. 2017;8(24):39746–55.
26. Diculescu M, Atanasiu C, Arbanas T, et al. Chemoembolization in the treatment of metastatic ileocolic carcinoid. Rom J Gastroenterol. 2002;11:141–7.
27. King J, Quinn R, Glenn DM, et al. Radioembolization with selective internal radiation microspheres for neuroendocrine liver metastases. Cancer. 2008;113:921–9.
28. Kennedy AS, Dezarn WA, McNeillie P, et al. Radioembolization for unresectable neuroendocrine hepatic metastases using resin 90Y-microspheres: early results in 148 patients. Am J Clin Oncol. 2008;31:271–9.
29. Braat AJAT, Prince JF, van Rooij R, et al. Safety analysis of holmium-166 microsphere scout dose imaging during radioembolisation work-up: a cohort study. Eur Radiol. 2018;28(3):920–8.
30. Braat AJAT, Kwekkeboom DJ, Kam BLR, et al. Additional hepatic 166Ho-radioembolization in patients with neuroendocrine tumours treated with 177Lu-DOTATATE; a single center, interventional, non-randomized, non-comparative, open label, phase II study (HEPAR PLUS trial). BMC Gastroenterol. 2018;18(1):84. https://doi.org/10.1186/s12876-018-0817-8.

31. Braat AJAT, Kappadath SC, Ahmadzadehfar H, et al. Radioembolization with 90Y resin microspheres of neuroendocrine liver metastases: international multicenter study on efficacy and toxicity. Cardiovasc Intervent Radiol. 2019;42(3):413–25.

32. Eriksson B, Annibale B, Bajetta E, et al. ENETS consensus guidelines for the standards of care in neuroendocrine tumors: chemotherapy in patients with neuroendocrine tumors. Neuroendocrinology. 2009;90:214–9.

33. Raymond E, Dahan L, Raoul JL, et al. Sunitinib malate for the treatment of pancreatic neuroendocrine tumors. N Engl J Med. 2011;364:501–13.

34. Yao JC, Lombard-Bohas C, Baudin E, et al. Daily oral everolimus activity in patients with metastatic pancreatic neuroendocrine tumors after failure of cytotoxic chemotherapy: a phase II trial. J Clin Oncol. 2010;28:69–76.

35. Yao JC, Shah MH, Ito T, et al. Everolimus for advanced pancreatic neuroendocrine tumors. N Engl J Med. 2011;364:514–23.

36. Modlin IM, Pavel M, Kidd M, et al. Review article: somatostatin analogues in the treatment of gastroenteropancreatic neuroendocrine (carcinoid) tumors. Aliment Pharmacol Ther. 2010;31:169–88.

37. Vitale G, Dicitore A, Sciammarella C, et al. Pasireotide in the treatment of neuroendocrine tumors: a review of the literature. Endocr Relat Cancer. 2018;25(6):R351–64.

38. Wolin E, Jarzab B, Eriksson B, et al. Phase III study of pasireotide long-acting release in patients with metastatic neuroendocrine tumors and carcinoid symptoms refractory to available somatostatin analogues. Drug Des Devel Ther. 2015;9:5075–86.

39. Godara A, Siddiqui NS, Byrne MM, et al. The safety of lanreotide for neuroendocrine tumor. Expert Opin Drug Saf. 2019;18(1):1–10.

40. Öberg K. Interferon in the management of neuroendocrine GEP tumors. Digestion. 2000;62(Suppl 1):92–7.

41. Grande E, Capdevila J, Castellano D, et al. Pazopanib in pretreated advanced neuroendocrine tumors: a phase II, open-label trial of the Spanish Task Force Group for Neuroendocrine Tumors (GETNE). Ann Oncol. 2015;26(9):1987–93.

42. Ahn HK, Choi JY, Kim KM, et al. Phase II study of pazopanib mono-therapy in metastatic gastroenteropancreatic neuroendocrine tumours. Br J Cancer. 2013;109:1414–9.

43. Kouvaraki MA, Ajani JA, Hoff P, et al. Fluorouracil, doxorubicin, and streptozocin in the treatment of patients with locally advanced and metastatic pancreatic endocrine carcinomas. J Clin Oncol. 2004;22:4762–71.

44. Moertel CG, Lefkopoulos M, Lipsitz S, et al. Streptozocin-doxorubicin, streptozocin-fluorouracil or chlorozotocin in the treatment of advanced islet-cell carcinoma. N Engl J Med. 1992;326:519–23.

45. Bosman FT. World Health Organization, International Agency for Research on Cancer. WHO classification of tumours of the digestive system. 4th ed. Lyon: IARC Press; 2010.

46. Rindi G, Klimstra DS, Abedi-Ardekani B, et al. A common classification framework for neuroendocrine neoplasms: an International Agency for Research on Cancer (IARC) and World Health Organization (WHO) expert consensus proposal. Mod Pathol. 2018;31:1770–86.

47. Sandström M, Garske U, Granberg D, et al. Individualized dosimetry in patients undergoing therapy with (177) Lu-DOTA-D-Phe (1)-Tyr (3)-octreotate. Eur J Nucl Med Mol Imaging. 2010;37:212–25.

48. Sandström M, Garske-Román U, Granberg D, et al. Individualized dosimetry of kidney and bone marrow in patients undergoing 177Lu-DOTA-octreotate treatment. J Nucl Med. 2013;54:33–41.

49. Kontogeorgakos D, Dimitriou P, Limouris GS, et al. Patient-specific dosimetry calculations using mathematic models of different atomic sizes during therapy with In-111-DTPA-D-Phe1 Octreotide infusions after catheterization of the hepatic artery. J Nucl Med. 2006;47(9):1476–82.

50. Garske-Román U, Sandström M, Fröss Baron K, et al. Prospective observational study of ^{177}Lu-DOTA-octreotate therapy in 200 patients with advanced metastasized neuroendocrine tumors (NETs): feasibility and impact of a dosimetry-guided study protocol on outcome and toxicity. Eur J Nucl Med Mol Imaging. 2018;45:970–88.

51. Eisenhauer EA, Therasse P, Bogaerts J, et al. New response evaluation criteria in solid tumors: revised RECIST guideline (version 1.1). Eur J Cancer. 2009;45:228–47.

52. Pazdur R. Endpoints for assessing drug activity in clinical trials. Oncologist. 2008;13:19–21.

53. Limouris GS, Karfis I, Chatziioannou A, et al. Super-selective hepatic arterial infusions as established technique ('Aretaieion' protocol) of 177 Lu DOTA-TATE inoperable neuroendocrine liver metastases of gastro-entero-pancreatic tumors. Q J Nucl Med Mol Imaging. 2012;56:551–8.

54. Davoodabadi A, Abdourrahimkashi E, Khamehchian T, et al. Effects of right hepatic artery ligation. Trauma. 2018;23(3):e63240. https://doi.org/10.5812/traumamon.63240.

55. Couinaud C. Le foie; études anatomiques et chirurgicales. Paris: Masson; 1957.

56. Ertl HH, Feinendegen LE, Heiniger HJ. Iodine-125, a tracer in cell biology: physical properties and biological aspects. Phys Med Biol. 1970;15:447–56.

57. Hofer KG, Hughes WL. Radiotoxicity of intranuclear tritium, iodine-125 and iodine-131. Radiat Res. 1971;47:94–109.

58. Bradley EW, Chan PC, Adelstein SJ. The radiotoxicity of iodin-125 in mammalian cells. I. Effects on the survival curve of radioiodine incorporated into DNA. Radiat Res. 1975;64:555–63.

59. Feinendegen LE. Biological damage from the Auger effect, possible benefits. Radiat Environ Biophys. 1975;12:85–99.

60. Howell RW, Narra VR, Rao DV, et al. Radiobiological effects of intracellular polonium-210 alpha emissions: a comparison with Auger-emitters. Radiat Prot Dosim. 1990;31:325–8.

61. Rao DV, Narra VR, Govelitz GF, et al. In vivo effects of 5.3 MeV alpha particles from Po-210 in mouse testes: comparison with internal Auger emitters. Radiat Prot Dosim. 1990;31:329–32.

62. Sastry KSR, Rao DV. Dosimetry of low energy electrons. In: Rao DV, Chandra R, Graham M, editors. . New York: American Institute of Physics; 1984. p. 169–208.

63. Kassis AI. The amazing world of Auger electrons. Int J Radiat Biol. 2004;80:789–803.

64. Buchegger F, Adamer F, Schaffland AO, et al. Highly efficient DNA incorporation of intratumourally injected [125I] iododeoxyuridine under thymidine synthesis blocking in human glioblastoma xenografts. Int J Cancer. 2004;110:145–9.

65. Buchegger F, Perillo-Adamer F, Dupertuis YM, et al. Auger radiation targeted into DNA: a therapy perspective. Eur J Nucl Med Mol Imaging. 2006;33:1352–63.

66. Nikjoo H, Girard P, Charlton DE, et al. Auger electrons—a nanoprobe for structural, molecular and cellular processes. Radiat Prot Dosim. 2006;122:72–9.

67. Valkema R, De Jong M, Bakker WH, et al. Phase I study of peptide receptor radionuclide therapy with [111In-DTPA°]Octreotide: the Rotterdam experience. Semin Nucl Med. 2002;32(2):110–22.

68. Buscombe JR, Caplin ME, Hilson JW. Long-term efficacy of high-activity 111In-pentetreotide therapy in patients with disseminated neuroendocrine tumors. J Nucl Med. 2003;44:1–6.

69. Anthony LB, Woltering EA, Espanan GD, et al. Indium-111-pentetreotide prolongs survival in gastroenteropancreatic malignancies. Semin Nucl Med. 2002;32(2):123–32.

70. Delpassand ES, Samarghandi A, Zamanian S. Peptide receptor radionuclide therapy with ^{177}Lu-DOTATATE for patients with Somatostatin receptor–expressing neuroendocrine tumors: the first US phase 2 experience. Pancreas. 2014;43(4):518–25. Lippincott Williams & Wilkins.

71. Pool SE, Kam B, Breeman WAP. Increasing intrahepatic tumour uptake of 111In-DTPA-octreotide by loco regional administration. Eur J Nucl Med Mol Imaging. 2009;36:S427.

72. Kratochwil C, Giesel FL, López-Benítez R, et al. Intraindividual comparison of selective arterial versus venous 68Ga-DOTATOC PET/CT in patients with gastroenteropancreatic neuro-endocrine tumors. Clin Cancer Res. 2010;16(10):2899–905.

73. Frangos S, Buscombe JR. Why should we be concerned about a "g"? Eur J Nucl Med Mol Imaging. 2019;46:519. https://doi.org/10.1007/s00259-018-4204-z.

74. Kress O, Wagner HJ, Wied M, et al. Transarterial chemoembolization of advanced liver metastases of neuroendocrine tumours; a retrospective single-center analysis. Digestion. 2003;68:94–101.

75. Dodd GD, Soulen MC, Kane RA, et al. Minimally invasive treatment of malignant hepatic tumours; at the threshold of major breakthrough. Radiographics. 2000;20:9–27.

76. Limouris GS, Dimitropoulos N, Kontogeorgakos D, et al. Evaluation of the therapeutic response to In-111-DTPA octreotide-based targeted therapy in liver metastatic neuroendocrine tumors according to CT/MRI/US findings. Cancer Biother Radiopharm. 2005;20(2):215–7.

77. Ueda K, Matsui O, Kawamori Y, et al. Hypervascular hepatocellular carcinoma; evaluation of the hemodynamics with dynamic CT during hepatic arteriography. Radiobiology. 1998;206:161–6.

78. Kanazawa S, Yasui K, Doke T, et al. Hepatic arteriography in patients with hepatocellular carcinoma: change in findings caused by balloon occlusion of tumor-draining hepatic veins. AJR Am J Roentgenol. 1995;165:1415–9.

79. Lautt WW, Greenway CV. Conceptual review of the hepatic vascular bed. Hepatology. 1987;7:952–63.

80. Breedis C, Young G. The blood supply of neoplasms in the liver. Am J Pathol. 1954;30:969–85.

81. Goseki N, Nokasa T, Endo M, et al. Nourishment of hepatocellular carcinoma through the portal blood flow with and without transcatheter arterial embolization. Cancer. 1995;76:736–42.

82. Krenning EP, de Jong M, Kooij PP, et al. Radiolabelled somatostatin analogue(s) for peptide receptor scintigraphy and radionuclide therapy. Ann Oncol. 1999;10(Suppl 2):S23–9.

83. Rindi G, Klöppel G, Alhman H, et al. TNM staging of foregut neuroendocrine tumors: a consensus proposal including a grading system. Virchows Arch. 2006;449:395–401.

84. Rindi G, Klöppel G, Couvelard A, et al. TNM staging of midgut and hindgut (neuro) endocrine tumors: a consensus proposal including a grading system. Virchows Arch. 2007;451:757–62.

85. Jandl JH, Katz JH. The plasma-to-cell cycle of transferrin. J Clin Invest. 1963;42(3):314.

86. Ka Luk C. Study of the nature of the metal-binding sites and estimate of the distance between the metal-binding sites in transferrin using trivalent lanthanide ions as fluorescent probes. Biochemistry. 1971;10(15):2838–43.

87. Limouris GS, Lamprakos L, Kontogeorgakos D, et al. Co-infusion of DTPA during peptide receptor radionuclide therapy with In-111 DTPA Octreotide reduces the ionic indium-111/114m contaminants. Eur J Nucl Med. 2006;33(Suppl 2):775. [abstract].

88. Kwekkeboom DJ, Bakker WH, Kooij PP, et al. [177Lu-DOTAOTyr3]Octreotate: comparison with [111In-DTPAo]octreotide in patients. Eur J Nucl Med. 2001;28(9):1319–25.

89. de Jong M, Valkema R, van Gameren A, et al. Inhomogeneous localization of radioactivity in the human kidney after injection of (111In-DTPA) octreotide. Nucl Med. 2004;45:1168–71.

90. Imhof A, Brunner P, Marincek N, et al. Response, survival, and long-term toxicity after therapy with the radiolabeled somatostatin analogue [90Y-DOTA]-TOC in metastasized neuroendocrine cancers. J Clin Oncol. 2011;29:2416–23.

91. Bodei L, Kidd M, Paganelli G, et al. Long-term tolerability of PRRT in 807 patients with neuroendocrine tumours: the value and limitations of clinical factors. Eur J Nucl Med Mol Imaging. 2015; 42:5–19.

92. Kesavan M, Claringbold PG, Turner JH. Hematological toxicity of combined 177Lu-octreotate radiopeptide chemotherapy of gastroentero-pancreatic neuroendocrine tumors in long-term follow-up. Neuroendocrinology. 2014;99:108–17.

93. Kwekkeboom DJ, de Herder WW, Kam BL, et al. Treatment with the radiolabeled somatostatin analog [177 Lu-DOTA 0,Tyr3]octreotate: toxicity, efficacy, and survival. J Clin Oncol. 2008;26: 2124–30.

94. Sabet A, Khalaf F, Yong-Hing CJ, et al. Can peptide receptor radionuclide therapy be safely applied in florid bone metastases? A pilot analysis of late stage osseous involvement. Nuklearmedizin. 2014;53:54–9.

95. Forrer F, Waldherr C, Maecke HR. Targeted radionuclide therapy with 90Y-DOTATOC in patients with neuroendocrine tumors. Anticancer Res. 2006;26:703–7.

96. Bushnell DL, O'Dorisio TM, O'Dorisio MS, et al. 90Y-edotreotide for metastatic carcinoid refractory to octreotide. J Clin Oncol. 2010;28(1):652–9.

97. Waldherr C, Pless M, Maecke HR, et al. The clinical value of [90Y-DOTA]-D-Phe1-Tyr3-octreotide (90Y-DOTATOC) in the treatment of neuroendocrine tumours: a clinical phase II study. Ann Oncol. 2001;12:941–5.

98. Valkema R, Pauwels S, Kvols L, et al. Survival and response after peptide receptor radionuclide therapy with [90Y-DOTA0,Tyr3]octreotide in patients with advanced gastroenteropancreatic neuroendocrine tumors. Semin Nucl Med. 2006;36(2):147–56.

99. Krenning EP, Kooij PPM, Bakker WH, et al. Radiotherapy with a radiolabeled somatostatin analogue, [In-DTPA-d-Phe]-octreotide. Annals of the New York Academy of Sciences. 1994;733(1 Molecular and):496–506.

100. Caplin ME, Mielcarek W, Buscombe JR, et al. Toxicity of high-activity 111In-octreotide therapy in patients with disseminated neuroendocrine tumors. Nuclear Medicine Communications. 2000;21(1):97–102.

101. Tiensuu Janson E, Eriksson B, Öberg K, et al. Treatment with high dose [111In-DTPA-D-PHE1]-octreotide in patients with neuroendocrine tumors. Evaluation of therapeutic and toxic effects. Acta Oncologica (Stockholm). 1999;38(3):373–77.

102. Nguyen C, Faraggi M, Anne-Laure Giraudet A-L, et al. Long-term efficacy of radionuclide therapy in patients with disseminated neuroendocrine tumors uncontrolled by conventional therapy. Journal of Nuclear Medicine. 2004;45(10)1660–68.

Ioannis L. Karfis

8.1 Introduction

Of the five somatostatin receptor subtypes discovered and coded, subtype-2 (SSTR2) is the most frequently overexpressed in the majority of neuroendocrine tumors (Table 8.1).

The ^{111}In-labeled somatostatin peptide analogue $DTPA^0$-Octreotide binds with high affinity to SSTR2 subtype. [111]In emits (a) gamma-photons of three 23 keV, 171 keV, and 245 keV energy photons used for imaging and (b) Auger and Internal Conversion electrons for therapeutic purposes, respectively. The ^{111}In-peptide complex after i.v. or i.a. administration penetrates into the cell by an endocytosis mechanism called internalization and fuses with the lysosomes where it is hydrolyzed. The radiolabeled fragment of the complex remains trapped in the lysosomes, with the receptor emerging on the surface of the cell membrane (like a recycling model) to recruit a new labeled peptide, and so on. The radioactive metabolite burdens the space around it with radiation originated from Auger and Internal Conversion electrons, not exceeding 20–25µm (from the point of its permanent installation, i.e.

Table 8.1 SSTRs overexpression in NENs

Neuroendocrine tumors	Somatostatin subtypes	expression
GH pituitary adenoma	SSTR2, SSTR5	++
Nonfunctioning pituitary adenoma	SSTR2, SSTR3	+
Carcinoid	SSTR, SSTR2, SSTR5	++
Gastrinoma	SSTR2	++
Insulinoma	SSTR1	+
Glucagonoma	SSTR2	++
Somatostatinoma	SSTR2	++
Peraganglioma	SSTR2	++
Pheochromocytoma	SSTR2	++
Myeloid thyroid cancer	SSTR3, SSTR5	+

the lysosomes). Looking thoroughly the histologic sample of a tumor of neuroendocrine character (Fig. 8.1), it is obvious that the double strand of DNA lies within the radius of action of the above electrons.

Hepatic radionuclide intra-arterial infusion (routinely using ^{111}In in the present study) is a pioneering treatment in Nuclear Medicine in patients with unresectable neuroendocrine hepatic metastases. However, in interventional radiology, repeated transhepatic infusions of chemotherapeutic agents by a transdermally implanted drum-catheter system is a process often used for the confrontation of unresectable liver tumors [2–9].

I. L. Karfis (✉)
Nuclear Medicine Department, Institute Jules Bordet, Bruxelles, Belgium
e-mail: ioannis.karfis@bordet.be

© Springer Nature Switzerland AG 2021
G. S. Limouris (ed.), *Liver Intra-arterial PRRT with ^{111}In-Octreotide*,
https://doi.org/10.1007/978-3-030-70773-6_8

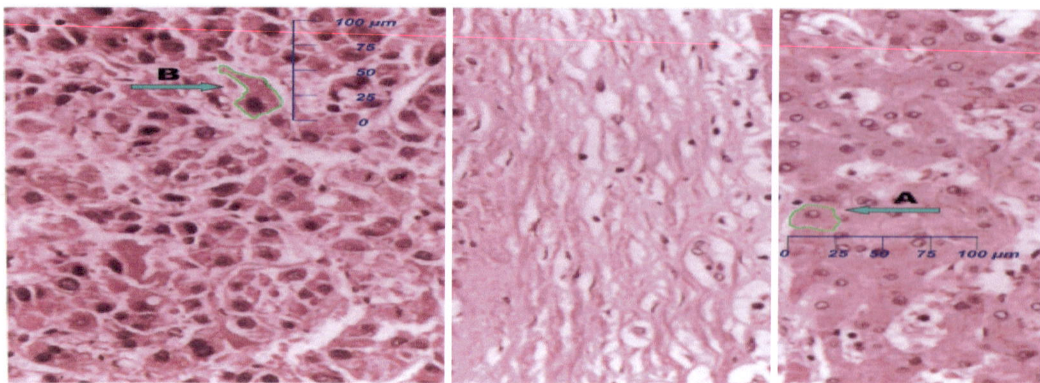

Fig. 8.1 On a histological sample of normal (**a**) and tumor liver cells (**b**) two micrometers (*in blue*) are superimposed. Cellular membrane is delineated *in green* (arrow). Nuclei of normal cells A and tumor cells B are well distinguished. Comparing cell dimensions and distances between cell surface and nuclei obviously can be elicited that DNA lies within the micrometer range of In-111 emissions (adapted and modified from Limouris et al. [1])

8.2 Installation of the Drum-Port System

8.2.1 Technical Details

The procedure was performed transarterially for all patients involved. Before insertion of the catheter, patients underwent CT-angiography to map the arterial network. The catheter was placed under local anesthesia immediately after angiography. Its distal end was positioned free in the proper hepatic artery without any distal fixation device.

A small reservoir "drum" (Figs. 8.2 and 8.3; Pakumed medical products, gmbh, Germany) was implanted in the lower right quadrant of the abdomen and specifically in the area of the right lumbar cavity, after subcutaneous sealing and fixing with a special inert suture thread. After this procedure, the proximal portion of the catheter is embedded in a subcutaneous tunnel with its proximal end attached to the drum, embedded in the subcutaneous space. Angiography was followed through the drum–catheter system to confirm its correct positioning and mounting. The subcutaneous tissue was rinsed with antibiotic solution, antiseptically sutured (skin was closed with liga-

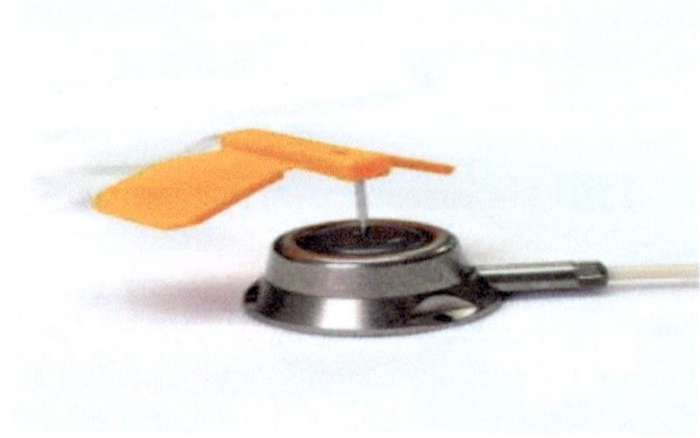

Fig. 8.2 A small reservoir "drum" made from titan and the "gripper needle" (in orange). [Courtesy of PakuMed]

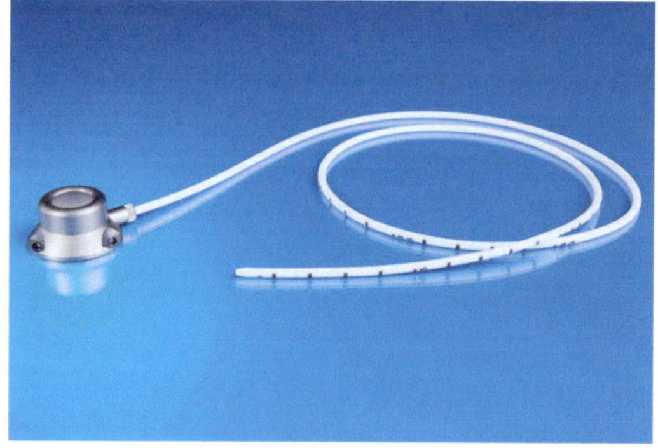

Fig. 8.3 A small reservoir "drum" made from titan, the "gripper needle" and the attached port (in white). [Courtesy of PakuMed]

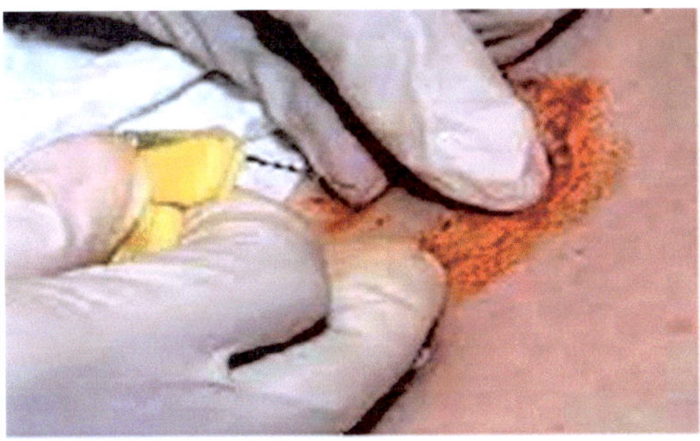

Fig. 8.4 After local antisepsis the port is stabilized with the forefinger and thumb of one hand and with the other the angular needle is vertically inserted in the center of the drum. [Courtesy of PakuMed]

ments), and after each administration of the radionuclide application, 2000 IU of heparin was administered through the drum to avoid systemic thrombosis. The needle used in the port has special angular features. Its introduction is painless. After local antisepsis, the port is stabilized between the forefinger and the thumb of one hand while the angular needle is inserted vertically in the center, until it meets resistance from the steel wall at the bottom of the port (Fig. 8.4; Pakumed medical products, gmbh, Germany). It is worth to notice that the needle only penetrates the soft silicone at the top of the subcutaneous port. The "gripper needle" has a built-in short plastic tube, on which the syringe is fitted, as mentioned above. After use, the needle is removed and an antiseptic is applied at the point of entry. The skin remains uncovered until the next session.

8.2.2 Advantages of the Port System After the Implemented Catheterization of the Hepatic Artery

The port is an invisible device that does not restrict the day-to-day activities and does not require frequent special care (for instance the patient can even fearlessly swim). The risks of catheter contamination, infection, or thrombosis are very low, and its effective life can last as up to

years. Its use is indicated on MRI as up to 1.5 T for most devices, and as up to 3 T for specific devices. The patient avoids the inconvenience of the repeated catheterizations and the 12-h immobilization of the catheterized limb, obligatory to circumvent a hematoma.

Purpose of this Chapter is to evaluate the feasibility and benefits to the patients of this temporary port system implementation to perform Peptide Receptor Radionuclide Therapies (PRRT). Furthermore, it is attempted to appraise the effects of the ^{111}In-DTPA^0-Octreotide energy absorption by this port system in order to maximize the tumor radioactivity uptake and absorbed dose compared to the internationally applied intravenous injection, minimizing the dose to other tissues and especially to the critical organs, such as the kidneys and bone marrow.

Temporary installation of the port system outweighs the technique of hepatic artery catheterization as it avoids the use of contrast agents and the patient's fatigue due to the 24 h leg immobilization after the catheterization of the femoral artery to evade a possible hematoma, having an optimal quality of life.

8.3 Material and Methods

8.3.1 Selection of Patients

The feasibility study cohort included a total of nine patients [five males and four females] with an age range of 51–78 years (Table 8.2), with unresectable liver metastases, confirmed by biopsy, originated from lung (one case), pancreas (three cases), small intestine (three cases), liver (one HCC-case with multiple bilobar lesions, of neuroendocrine character), and one case of unknown origin. A total of 108 infusions were performed (Fig. 8.5) via the subcutaneously installed port system, using ^{111}In-DTPA^0-Octreotide ranging from 24 GBq (648.6 mCi) to 77 GBq (2849.0 mCi). A 6–8 weeks time interval between the sessions, according to the protocol, was followed to avoid any possible stunning

Table 8.2 Patient characteristics and therapeutic response according to the RECIST criteria

a/a	Patient/sex	Age	Primary origin	Cumulative dose (GBq)	RECIST criteria	PFS (months)	OS (months)
1	K.A./f	65	Unknown origin	65	PR	122	>142
2	K.F./m	73	Small intestine	74	PR	49	79
3	G.G./m	75	HCC	77	PR	34	55
4	S.S./f	78	Small intestine	58	SD	27	32
5	B.S./m	59	Lung	48	SD	58	105
6	M.V./f	51	Pancreas	67	PR	61	86
7	K.A./f	61	Pancreas	65	PR	60	60
8	G.I./m	69	Small intestine	63	PR	22	46
9	F.G./m	59	Pancreas	24	PR	20	34

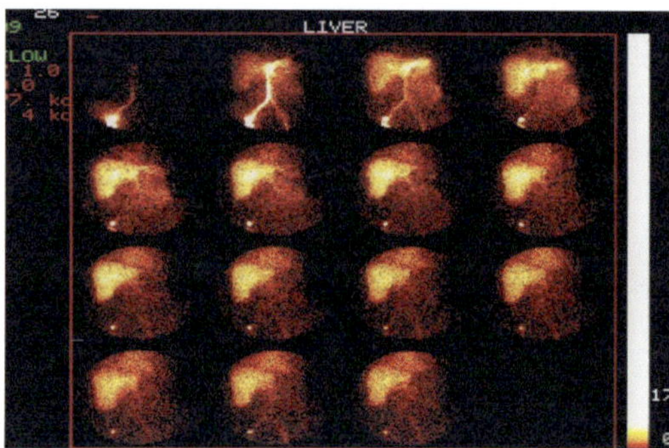

Fig. 8.5 Dynamic scintimages (anterior view) of intra-arterial infusion via an implanted port system

effect; the median cumulative activity for this nine-patient cohort was 65.0 GBq, based on the following eligibility criteria: (1) liver lesions of neuroendocrine character, confirmed by biopsy (irrespective of number), (2) failure of an earlier therapeutic modality or discontinuation due to unacceptable toxicity, (3) hemoglobin level >10 g•dL^{-1}, white blood cell count >3•10^3 cells•dL^{-1} and platelet count >75•10^9 cells•L^{-1}, (4) serum creatinine ≤1.2 mg•dL^{-1} or creatinine clearance >60 mL•min^{-1}, (5) presence of high density of somatostatin receptors in metastatic liver foci, as presumed by an initial diagnostic scintigraphy, with simultaneous uptake of >130% of the metastatic foci relative to normal liver parenchyma corresponding to visual score 4 [10], (6) a Karnofsky index [11] greater than 40 (Table 8.3), and (7) a progressive disease status, according to the RECIST 1.1 criteria [12, 13].

Patient's written consent prior to any diagnostic or therapeutic practice was obtained. The study protocol was approved by the Research and

Table 8.3 Karnofsky performance status scale definitions rating (%) criteria

100	Normal no complaints; no evidence of disease
90	Able to carry on normal activity; minor signs or symptoms of disease. Able to carry on normal activity and to work; no special care needed
80	Normal activity with effort; some signs or symptoms of disease
70	Cares for self; unable to carry on normal activity or to do active work
60	Requires occasional assistance, but is able to care for most of his personal needs. Unable to work; able to live at home and care for most personal needs; varying amount of assistance needed
50	Requires considerable assistance and frequent medical care
40	Disabled; requires special care and assistance. 30 severely disabled; hospital admission is indicated although death not imminent. 20 very sick; hospital admission necessary; active supportive treatment necessary
30	Severely disabled; hospital admission is indicated although death not imminent
20	Very sick; hospital admission necessary; active supportive treatment necessary
10	Moribund; fatal processes progressing rapidly. Unable to care for self; requires equivalent of institutional or hospital care; disease may be progressing rapidly
0	Dead

Ethics Committee of the "Aretaieion" University Hospital. Patients, being under repeated Sandostatin—LAR treatment (30 mg per 20 days), did not discontinue the dosage but they were intramuscularly injected 15–20 days prior to the radioactive session.

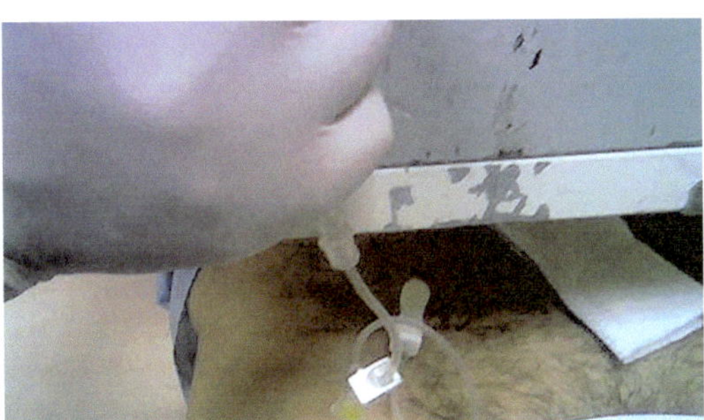

Fig. 8.6 Intra-arterial Radiopeptide Injection transdermally at the point where the drum is subcutaneously installed

8.3.2 Methodology

Prior to the initiation of the treatment and the installation of the catheter port system, patients were subjected to an OctreoScan diagnostic scintigraphy that allowed the radiopeptide treatment to be initiated ("theragnostic principle")[1]. Of the aforementioned eligibility criteria, the following three predetermined the infusion: (a) the intensity of the radioactive tumor uptake (had to have a visual score 4) according to a predetermined optical scale, where the radioactive tumor concentration had to be equal or higher of the half of the patient's spleen and kidney sum, (b) Karnofsky index to be above 40 [patients with Karnofsky index less than 40 were excluded due to poor life expectancy], and (c) hematological, hormonal and biochemical tests had to be within normal ranges.

Size and location of neuroendocrine tumors were determined using the Couinaud [14] classification, according to which the liver is subdivided into eight independent sections, each with its own vascular irrigation (inflow/outflow) and cholangiogenic outflow. Radiopeptide Injection of ^{111}In-DTPA^0-Octreotide was injected with a 20 mL syringe (Fig. 8.6) of a custom-made infusion needle transdermally, at the location where

---

[1]Linguistically the optimal approach is a synergy of the two words diagnosis and therapy, where "diagnosis" should precede "therapy" according to GS Limouris ("Gnosti-Thera" principle, Chap. 7).

the port was subcutaneously located, by the nuclear physician over a period of 20–30 min. The procedure finishes/ends with 10 mL saline rinsing to remove any radioactive residues on the drum walls and catheter.

At the end of treatment, patients stayed for 24 h mandatorily in a specially designed and appropriately shielded single-room radiotherapy unit of the hospital for follow-up and also for dosimetric calculations [blood-sample collection 30 min 2 h, 4 h, 8 h, and 24 h post-infusion and 24-h urine collection, as well] and radiobiological reasons, according to the international radiation protection regulations. The discharge provided oral and written instructions on the precautions that patients had to follow, in order to reduce the radiological burden on adjacent members and the environment, based on the radiation rate ($\leq$20µSv/h), at a distance of 1 m from patients' body.

8.3.3 Evaluation/Dosage Protocol

The feasibility study involved nine patients with confirmed hepatic neuroendocrine metastases. Each of them received 4.070 GBq (110 mCi) to 5.920 GBq (160 mCi) of ^{111}In-DTPA^0-Octreotide through a special catheter port-system, directly into the common hepatic artery and consequently to the feeding tumor artery. This method compared to the repeated infusions after catheterization of the femoral artery is incomparably convenient and well tolerated by the patients because the port is used for all subsequent sessions. Whole body acquisitions were performed for each patient 30 min, 24 h, 48 h, 72 h, and 94 h post-infusion, using an Elscint, APEX SPX4 γ-camera, equipped with a medium-energy, parallel-hole collimator. Both ^{111}In photoelectric peaks (172 and 247 keV) were used in this protocol. Anterior and posterior views of the whole body and regions of interest (ROIs) are obtained. (Fig. 8.7). The areas of organs that were superimposed were excluded from the delineation and evaluation. The accumulated dose in normal and neoplastic tissues are converted into time–activity curves to calculate the absorbed dose. The bone marrow residence time was calculated from the blood samples, assuming that the radioactive distribution in marrow and blood is homogeneous (MIRD, leaflet No. 11); furthermore, due to the small size of the radiopeptide, the specific radioactivity for bone marrow was considered to be equal to the specific radioactivity for blood [15, 16]. Additionally, for the dosimetry, the 24 h urine collection was taken into account [15, 16]. To assess the therapeutic response, the tumor size and number were compared before and after the sessions, according to the RECIST 1.1 criteria as previously described [12, 13].

8.3.4 Results

Side effects during the infusions [e.g. slight discomfort in the abdomen, in almost all patients, nausea, and fever] were transient and treated with simple symptomatic intervention. In 7 patients a partial response (PR) was achieved with a significant decrease of tumor diameter, while disease stabilization in 2 was noticed. None of the nine treated patients showed complete response (CR). Late side effects (WHO II to III hematological toxicity) erythropoietin (40,000 units subcutaneously) was given in weekly baseline, while two patients had blood transfusions. WHO I hematological toxicity observed in two women (Table 8.2, patient no 6 and 7), which was however reversible. None of the patients showed hepatotoxicity during the overall survival period. GFR and creatinine levels were within normal contexts. A clear decrease in serum Cr-A in all patients was observed. The absorbed dose in liver, kidneys, and tumor intravenously, intra-arterially, and with the intraarterial port system is tabulated in Fig. 8.4. The mean PFS in months was 49.0 and for OS 60.0 (Table 8.4, Fig. 8.8).

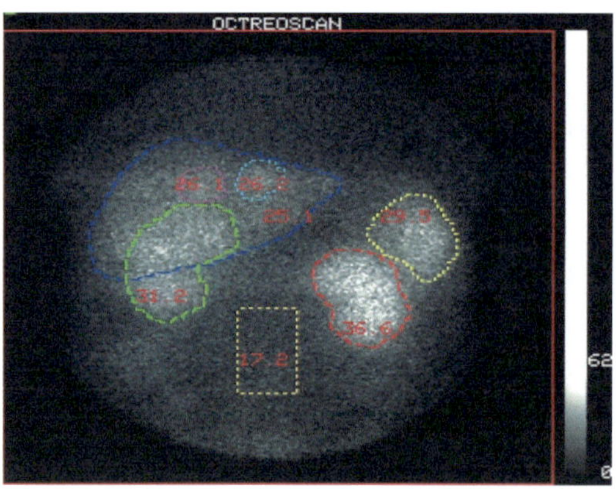

Fig. 8.7 ROIs created for dosimetry from a planar ^{111}In-DTPA^0-Octreotide scan

Table 8.4 Comparison of absorbed dose (a) after simple i.v. administration, (b) after simple intra-arterial administration, and (c) after intra-arterial administration through the mounted catheter port-system

Organ	Intravenous implementation mGy/MBq	Intra-arterial implementation mGy/MBq	i.a. port-system implementation[a] mGy/MBq
Liver	0.399	0.14	0.090–0.240
Kidneys	0.45–0.52	0.41	0.28–0.961
Liver tumor	11.20	15.2	2.2–19.6

[a]Liver, liver tumor or kidney dose fluctuations depend of the activity amount aroused from the port-tip, fixed before or after the outgrowth of the common or proper hepatic artery. I is intended to be set after the outgrowth of the splenic artery of the celiac trunk, otherwise the dose in the liver-kidney-spleen will be increased. Thus, the closer to the tumor the port-tip the higher the tumor dose

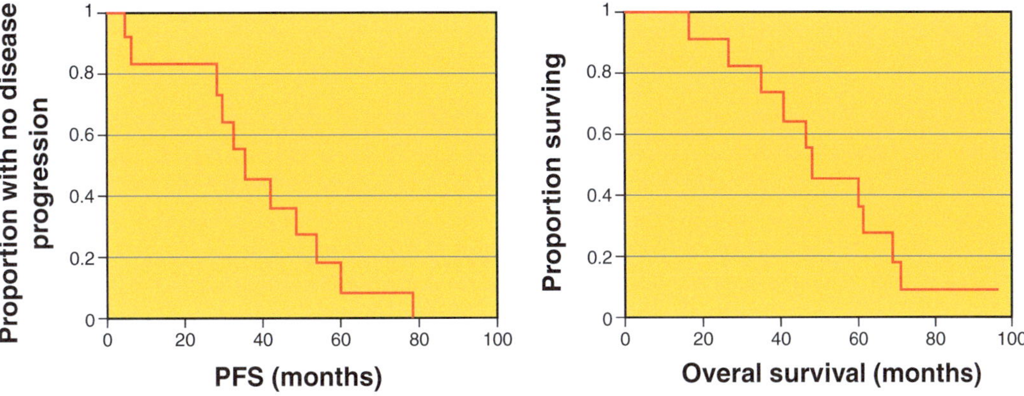

Fig. 8.8 Kaplan-Meier curves for progression-free (left) and overall survival (OS) (right) of the nine NETs, intra-arterially treated with ^{111}In-DTPA^0-Octreotide through the temporally implemented "drum"-port system

8.4 The Personalized Treatment Concept in the Peptide Receptor Radionuclide Therapeutic Schemes

It is certain that personalized dosimetry on the course of the therapeutic applications of radiopharmaceuticals significantly improves its quality, provides maximum safety in clinical radioisotope application, and maximizes the chances of a positive therapeutic effect. The necessity of personalized dosimetry is demonstrated by the present study as well from patient to patient; large differences were observed in the absorbed dose to tumors and healthy organs. The personalized dosimetry is a demanding process and requires the presence of specialized scientific potential, specialized equipment and availability time on the γ-camera. In clinical practice every nuclear medicine department when is involved in therapeutic applications, develops its own protocol of internal dosimetry based on its needs, available equipment, the crowd of specialized staff, and its inherent peculiarities. Pan-European efforts try to homogenize dosimetric methods aiming to reduce the uncertainty of the results. The basis for personalized dosimetry in therapeutic applications with radiopharmaceuticals is the calculation of cumulative radioactivity. The only one method which is suitable for the personalized calculation of the cumulative radioactivity is the acquisition of scintigraphic images at various times after the administration of the radiopharmaceutical. The simplest case of imaging is taking anterior and posterior scintigraphic images. It takes the least time possible on the γ-camera, it gives reliable results but limits the detail illustration of the distribution of the cumulative radioactivity. When there are overlaps between organs with significant radiopharmaceutical uptake, a precise determination of the quantity corresponding to each instrument is impossible. This phenomenon usually leads to an underestimation of the dose to the cancer tumor and overestimation in healthy tissues. The topographic scintigraphic images give a more detailed illustration of the cumulative activity. Although tomography imaging requires more time for the acquisition, this should be preferred whenever possible since significantly increases the accuracy of the calculations. After the cumulative radioactivity has been determined, the calculation of the absorbed dose in cancerous and healthy organs follows. Usually, a program in computer is mandatory since the number of computations is huge. The MIRDOSE and OLINDA are suitable for these calculations. They give reliable results and are often used in many studies. They have the disadvantage to perform calculations on specific anthropomorphic models and not on the real patient's anatomy and they give the choice of a suitable model that fits the anatomy of most patients; however, in cases of patients with anatomical features, the calculations can have significant uncertainties. Another disadvantage of such software is that they consider the distribution of cumulative activity as homogeneous in organs and cancers that often is not the case. This consideration greatly facilitates the calculations but is far from the reality. The distribution of radioactivity in sensitive organs and tumors are heterogeneous, partly because of differences on the receptor density. Particularly in solid tumors there are areas with significantly lower radiopharmaceutical uptake which receive a lower absorbed dose and have increased chances of future relapse. Also a disadvantage of the software MIRDOSE and OLINDA is that they cannot calculate sizes smaller than those provided by the software. For example, these software calculate the median dose in the pancreas; however, they cannot calculate the dose in any part of it such as in its head or tail.

8.5   Therapeutic Evaluation/ Discussion

Until recently, the treatment of multiple, unresectable, non-functional, small or medium-sized metastasized liver tumors, of neuroendocrine character and positive for somatostatin receptors was based on various loco-regional therapeutic modalities like radiofrequency ablation and selective trans-arterial (chemo- or radio-) embolization [17]. These methods are still the classic way of NET management, preferred globally, though no without negligible side effects, i.e. myelotoxicity, peri-tumoral damage of healthy tissue and often severe pain and fever. About 30 years ago, Krenning and Kwekkeboom (in Amsterdam/Rotterdam) as well as Reubi and Maecke (in Basel) succeeded to compose, and further to systematically produce, both for diagnostic and therapeutic purposes, somatostatin analogues that they could be labeled with ^{111}In, ^{90}Y and ^{177}Lu. In addition, they modified the labeled peptide complex by replacing the chelator DTPA with DOTA molecule, in order to enhance the destructive action of radiopharmaceuticals, to increase carrier-receptor affinity and

to improve its stability molecule. Today, 30 years after the discovery, the synthetic construction and tactics use of the aforementioned radiopeptides, embolization and chemo-embolization are still the classic treatment of choice. For the management of unresectable, non-functional neuroendocrine tumors, Peptide-Receptor Radionuclide Therapy (PRRT) tends to be often a one-way street to tackle this tumor histotype. The results of the NETTER-1 study [18] (the first randomized multicenter study of phase III), where the included patients received four carrier added (c.a) ^{177}Lu-DOTATATE intravenous injections plus standard doses of Sandostatin-LAR (vs. continuous high doses of Sandostatin-LAR), demonstrate a median progression free survival that exceeded 40 months in patients treated with PRRT (vs. 8.4 months in patients receiving only Sandostatin-LAR). Thus, NETTER-1 consists of a landmark study in Nuclear Medicine, highly forwarding—PRRT in the first lines of the therapeutic pharetra, probably as a second treatment line in cases where somatostatin analogs fail.

The "Aretaieion Protocol" [1, 19] consists of intra-arterial administration of high doses of ^{111}In-DTPA^0-Octreotide plus the intravenous DTPA co-infusion. Its use not only intra-arterially but also after a temporal implementation of a catheter port-system was evaluated in this chapter and we consider it to be a promising therapeutic development. The objective relationship disease-response after PRRT and progressive deterioration is straightforward analogous; the best response is more likely to occur in patients with progressive disease rather than being in a stagnant disease state (Table 8.4).

The side effects of ^{111}In-DTPA^0-Octreotide therapy are few and far transient, with mild bone marrow suppression as the most common finding. In none of the patients any impairment in the kidney or pituitary gland function was observed. The side effects are based on the experience we have obtained from over than 40 months follow-up period; in this small series of nine patients, except a WHO I to II grade transient myelotoxicity, as the common side effect, no other adverse reaction could be observed. We faced early and acute side effects during the process of radiopeptide infusion, such as blood pressure drop, nausea, abdominal discomfort, which occurred after the end of the administration; furthermore, immediately after the radiopeptide treatment, vomiting and fever could happen, where symptomatic treatment was sufficient. As late side effect in 2/9 patients we account a WHO III myelotoxicity, successfully managed by blood transfusions. It is worth noting that these two patients have had chemotherapy in their medical history, a fact that advocates that bone marrow become vulnerable to the effect of the previous chemotherapy schemes. From the deduced therapeutic effects of intra-arterial use of ^{111}In-DTPA^0-Octreotide through a temporary, intravascularly mounted port, a 70% (7/9) of the study patients had partial response (PR) and only in a 30% (2/9) a stabilization disease (SD) was observed. Consequently, all nine patients as a whole had an objective benefit from the effect of the radiopeptide. Analogous radiopeptide treatment with port is not available internationally, so our results were compared with intravenous n.c.a. ^{111}In-DTPA^0-Octreotide administration by Valkema et al. [20], where 8% (2/26) showed PR, by Buscombe et al. [21] with a 17% (2/17) PR, by Tiensuu Janson et al. [22] with a 40% (2/5) PR, by Anthony et al. [23] with an 8% (2/26) PR and by Delpassand et al. [24] with a 7% (2/29) PR. On the contrast to our low, 30% stabilization rate, the corresponding rate of SD of worldwide authors was 60% (3/5) for Tiensuu Janson [22], 87% (13/15) and 87.5% (7/8) for Nguyen [25] and Caplin [26] respectively [who had zero partial response (PR)], 58% (15/26) for Valkema et al., also 58% (7/12) for Buscombe et al. [21], 81% (21/26) for Anthony et al. [23] and 55% (16/29) for Delpassand et al. [24]. This could be explained due to two reasons: (a) because of the different method of administration [intra-arterial vs. intravenous] treatment, where the mean absorbed dose per session by volume is higher compared with those intravenously administered [1, 27] and those referred by Krenning et al. [28], Kwekkeboom et al. [29] and Stabin et al. [30] as "first passage effect" and (b) because the total

dose administered at our study was on average 67GBq per patient, while internationally is lower and only in excellent rare cases, it exceeded 27GBq [29, 30] a dose that is totally inadequate for an effective DNA damage. As far as a possible nephrotoxicity, recent studies by de Jong et al. [31] have shown that the concentration of the radiopharmaceutical is distributed in the inner zone of the kidney cortex, while the radiation-sensitive glomeruli are in the outer zone of the cortex and therefore the ^{111}In electron range cannot reach to offend them. So far, no patient has developed any degree of renal toxicity to date, according to the latter monitoring data.

8.6 Conclusion

In unresectable neuroendocrine metastatic liver lesions, intra-hepatic, high-dose administration of ^{111}In-DTPA^0-Octreotide results in promising therapeutic effects ("Aretaieion Protocol"—intra-arterial administration plus co-administration of DTPA). Given the loco-regional nature of the technique as well as the extremely short transmission range of ^{111}In Auger and Internal Conversion electrons, after the temporary implementation of a catheter (port) system up to the proper hepatic artery, no renal, hepatic, or bone marrow toxicity were observed. The subcutaneous implant port-system provides stable drum–catheter coupling mechanism, high flow rate in a thin lumen, secure placement of the puncture needle in the chamber diaphragm, easy puncture site, and excellent quality of life. This implantation system did not cause any problems to the patients after an average of 16 months.

References

1. Limouris GS, Chatziioannou A, Kontogeorgakos D, et al. Selective hepatic arterial infusion of In-111-DTPA-Phe1-octreotide in neuro-endocrine liver metastases. Eur J Nucl Med Mol Imaging. 2008;35:1827–37.
2. Lorenz M, Müller HH. Randomized, multicenter trial of fluorouracil plus leucovorin administered

either via hepatic arterial or intravenous infusion versus fluorodeoxyuridine administered via hepatic arterial infusion in patients with nonresectable liver metastases from colorectal carcinoma. J Clin Oncol. 2000;18:243–54.

3. Allen-Mersh TG, Earlam S, Fordy C, et al. Quality of life and survival with continuous hepatic artery floxuridine infusion for colorectal liver metastases. Lancet. 1994;344:1255–60.

4. Yamagami T, Nakamura T, Yamazaki T, et al. Catheter tip f4xation of a percutaneously implanted port-catheter system to prevent dislocation. Eur Radiol. 2002;12:443–9.

5. Wacker FK, Boese-Landgraf J, Wagner A, et al. Minimally invasive catheter implantation for regional chemotherapy of the liver: a new percutaneous trans-subclavian approach. Cardiovasc Intervent Radiol. 1997;20:128–32.

6. Clouse ME, Ahmed R, Ryan RB, et al. Complications of long term transbrachial hepatic arterial infusion chemotherapy. AJR Am J Roentgenol. 1977;129:799–803.

7. Oberfield RA, McCaffrey JA, Polio J, et al. Prolonged and continuous percutaneous intra-arterial hepatic infusion chemotherapy in advanced metastatic liver adenocarcinoma from colorectal primary. Cancer. 1979;44:414–23.

8. Herrmann KA, Waggershauser T, Sittek H, et al. Liver intraarterial chemotherapy: use of the femoral artery for percutaneous implantation of catheter-port systems. Radiology. 2000;215:294–9.

9. Strecker EP, Boos IB, Ostheim-Dzerowycz W. Percutaneously implantable catheter-port system: preliminary technical results. Radiology. 1997;202:574–7.

10. Zaknun JJ, Bodei LJ, Mueller-Brand J, et al. The joint IAEA, EANM, and SNMMI practical guidance on peptide receptor radionuclide therapy (PRRNT) in neuroendocrine tumors. Eur J Nucl Med Mol Imaging. 2013;40(5):800–16.

11. O'Toole DM, Golden AM. Evaluating cancer patients for rehabilitation potential. West J Med. 1991;155:384–7.

12. Therasse P, Arbuck SG, Eisenhauer EA, et al. New guidelines to evaluate the response to treatment in solid tumors. European Organization for Research and Treatment of Cancer, National Cancer Institute of the United States, National Cancer Institute of Canada. J Natl Cancer Inst. 2000;92:205–16.

13. Eisenhauer EA, Therasse P, Bogaerts J, et al. New response evaluation criteria in solid tumours: revised RECIST guideline (version 1.1). Eur J Cancer. 2009;45:228–47.

14. Couinaud C. Le foie: Etudes anatomiques et chirurgicales. Paris: Masson et Cie; 1957.

15. Sgouros G. Dosimetry of internal emitters. J Nucl Med. 2005;46(S1):18S–27S.

16. Forrer F, Krenning EP, Kooij PP, et al. Bone marrow dosimetry in peptide receptor radionuclide therapy with [177Lu-DOTA(0),Tyr(3)]octreotate. Eur J Nucl Med Mol Imaging. 2009;36:1138–46.

17. Kress O, Wagner HJ, Wied M, et al. Transarterial chemoembolization of advanced liver-metastases of neuroendocrine tumours; a retrospective single center analysis. Digestion. 2003;68:94–101.

18. Strosberg J, Wolin E, Chasen B, et al. 177-Lu-Dotatate significantly improves progression-free survival in patients with midgut neuroendocrine tumors: results of the phase III NETTER-1 trial. Pancreas. 2016;45:483.

19. Limouris GS, Karfis I, Chatziioannou A, et al. Super-selective hepatic arterial infusions as established technique ('Aretaieion' protocol) of 177 Lu DOTA-TATE inoperable neuroendocrine liver metastases of gastro-entero-pancreatic tumors. Q J Nucl Med Mol Imaging. 2012;56:551–8.

20. Valkema R, De Jong M, Bakker WH, et al. Phase I study of peptide receptor radionuclide therapy with [111In-DTPA°]-octreotide: the Rotterdam experience. Semin Nucl Med. 2002;32:110–22.

21. Buscombe JR, Caplin ME, Hilson JW. Long term efficacy of high activity 111In-pentetreotide therapy in patients with disseminated neuroendocrine tumors. J Nucl Med. 2003;44:1–6.

22. Tiensuu Janson E, Eriksson B, Oberg K, et al. Treatment with high dose [(111)In-DTPA-D-PHE1]-octreotide in patients with neuroendocrine tumors evaluation of therapeutic and toxic effects. Acta Oncol. 1999;38:373–7.

23. Anthony LB, Woltering EA, Espanan GD, et al. Indium-111-pentetreotide prolongs survival in gastroenteropancreatic malignancies. Semin Nucl Med. 2002;32:123–32.

24. Delpassand ES, Samarghandi A, Zamanian S, et al. Peptide receptor radionuclide therapy with 177Lu-DOTATATE for patients with somatostatin receptor–expressing neuroendocrine tumors: the first US phase 2 experience. Pancreas. 2014;43:518–25.

25. Nguyen C, Faraggi M, Giraudet A-L, et al. Long-term efficacy of radionuclide therapy in patients with disseminated neuroendocrine tumors uncontrolled by conventional therapy. J Nucl Med. 2004;45:1660–8.

26. Caplin ME, Mielcarek W, Buscombe JR, et al. Toxicity of high activity In-111 octreotide therapy in patients with disseminated neuroendocrine tumours. Nucl Med Commun. 2000;21:97–102.

27. Kontogeorgakos DK, Dimitriou PA, Limouris GS, et al. Patient specific dosimetry calculations using mathematic models of different anatomic sizes during therapy with 111In-DTPA-D-Phe1-octreotide infu-

sions after catheterization of the hepatic artery. J Nucl Med. 2006;47:1476–82.

28. Krenning EP, Bakker WH, Kooij PPM, et al. Somatostatin receptor scintigraphy with indium-111-DTPA-D-Phe-1-octreotide in man: metabolism, dosimetry and com-parison with iodine-123-tyr-3-octreotide. J Nucl Med. 1992;33:652–8.

29. Kwekkeboom DJ, Bakker WH, Kooij PP, et al. [177Lu-DOTA0,Tyr3]octreotate: comparison with [111In-DTPA0]octreotide in patients. Eur J Nucl Med. 2001;28:1319–25.

30. Stabin M, Kooij PP, Bakker WH. Radiation dosimetry for indium-111-pentetreotide. J Nucl Med. 1997;38:1919–22.

31. De Jong M, Valkema R, Van Gameren A, et al. Inhomogeneous localization of radioactivity in the human kidney after injection of [111In-DTPA]octreotide. J Nucl Med. 2004;45(7):1168–71.

Non-invasive Radiological Modalities for the Evaluation of Neuroendocrine Liver Tumors

Athanasios G. Zafeirakis and Georgios S. Limouris

9.1 Introduction

The comparison and response assessment of U/S, CT, or MRI in patients with hepatic neuroendocrine secondaries after a therapy is an important and highly relevant area of diagnostic imaging due to the large number of patients presented with liver disease. The purpose of imaging must be accurate regarding the number, size, and location of these lesions. The therapeutic planning is usually highly dependent on the degree of liver parenchyma involvement, because only a limited number of the patients can be subject to surgical resection or often tandem managed with local ablative therapies. Multifocal metastases require a different approach, not only as monotherapy with Peptide Receptor Radionuclide Therapeutic approach (PRRT) but also often combined with systemic chemotherapy or mTOR agents.

9.2 The Radiological Evaluation of Patients with Hepatic Tumors of Neuroendocrine Character

9.2.1 Computed Tomography

Computed Tomography (CT) is widely used for the localization of pancreatic neuroendocrine tumor primaries as well as for their metastases. On noncontrast CT, most neuroendocrine tumors appear isodense. As most of them are hypervascular, they are presented as a hyper-attenuating, enhancing mass after the i.v. contrast implementation. Delayed imaging of very small tumors proves to be helpful, since it is unclear which from the arterial or portal venous phase imaging is the best for their identification. Thus, the multiphase imaging technique is suggested in order to increase sensitivity and to use the narrow window-level settings in order to increase the contrast between the tumor and healthy pancreas.

CT has markedly evolved with the advent of multidetector technology (MDCT), particularly at the abdominal area, where movement artifacts are disturbing due to respiratory movement and intestinal peristalsis. While scanners with 64 or more detector lines are still the most common ones, scanners with 2–16 layers are still widely used. With the advent of multidetector CT (MDCT), bi- or even tri-

A. G. Zafeirakis (✉)
Nuclear Medicine Department, Army Share Fund Hospital of Athens, Athens, Greece
e-mail: a.g.zafeirakis@army.gr

G. S. Limouris
Nuclear Medicine, Medical School, National and Kapodistrian University of Athens, Athens, Greece

© Springer Nature Switzerland AG 2021
G. S. Limouris (ed.), *Liver Intra-arterial PRRT with ^{111}In-Octreotide*,
https://doi.org/10.1007/978-3-030-70773-6_9

phase liver examinations can be combined into a thoraco-abdominal CT scan without conciliation in spatial or temporal resolution. It takes only a few seconds to record. It can be noticed that even in monolayer spiral CT scanners, adequate image quality of the liver can be obtained (Fig. 9.1).

The recently developed Positron Emission Tomography/Computed Tomography (PET/CT) scans combine the advantages of positron emission tomography (high-sensitivity functional imaging) and the benefits of computed tomography (high-spatial resolution morphological imaging) into a single real-world imaging in oncology patients.

An optimal examination technique is essential for a sensitive detection and specific characterization of focal liver lesions. A bi-phase liver examination with a late phase and a venous-venous phase can be considered standard imaging practice today, particularly as is in the case of the follow-up of liver neuroendocrine metastases after trans-arterial radionuclide infusion. The value of delayed protocols (e.g., 5 min after contrast agent injection) is reported to be controversial, in which the other authors do not see any added value [2, 3]. Contrast agent timing is regarded crucial due to the short acquisition time of MDCT since the optimal enhancement phase has to be included within a very short acquisition window. Therefore, according to Schima et al. [4]

the use of modern contrast agent power injectors and bolus timing are mandatory.

In focal liver lesions due to neuroendocrine tumors, biphasic spiral CT detection rates range from 60 to 75% and for benign and malignant lesions are about 70% [5–9] CT imaging, even with the latest MDCT technology, has been shown to be inferior in lesion detection compared to gadolinium-enhanced MRI [10] or liver-specific MRI [7] and also regarding their characterization [8, 9] mainly observed in lesions less than 1 cm in diameter.

According to the literature, liver metastases can be detected by spiral CT, with a sensitivity of 58–85% [11–13]. Data from single-breasted spiral CT and MDCT indicate that the optimal reconstructed slice thickness for reading CT liver examinations on transverse sections should be in the range of 2.5–5 mm [14, 15]. Depending on the primary tumor, liver metastases may have different morphological and enhanced characteristics, which are mainly consistent in histological characteristics, e.g. cystic, mucinous, and solid, and vascularity (hypovascular or hypervascular). Some primary tumors such as thyroid carcinomas, carcinoids, neuroendocrine tumors, and renal cell carcinomas usually present hypervascular liver metastases [16]. Metastases of pancreatic carcinoma, breast carcinoma, and colon carcinoma can sometimes also be hypervascular [16] (Fig. 9.2). In liver metastases from an unknown primary (UP), occasionally hypervas-

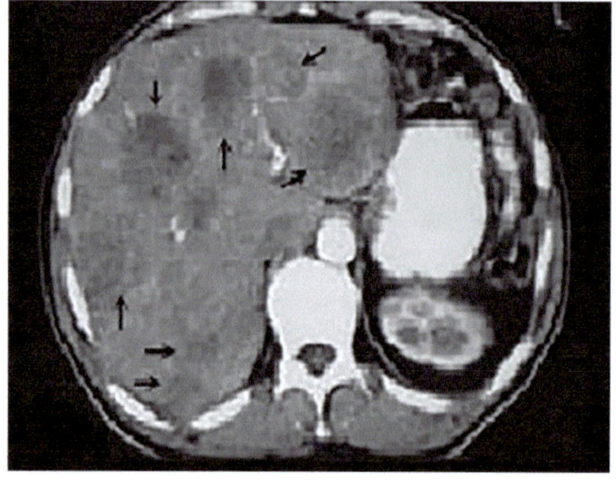

Fig. 9.1 Multiple liver metastases from a small intestine carcinoid in a 55-year-old woman. Trans-axial contrast-enhanced CT [1]

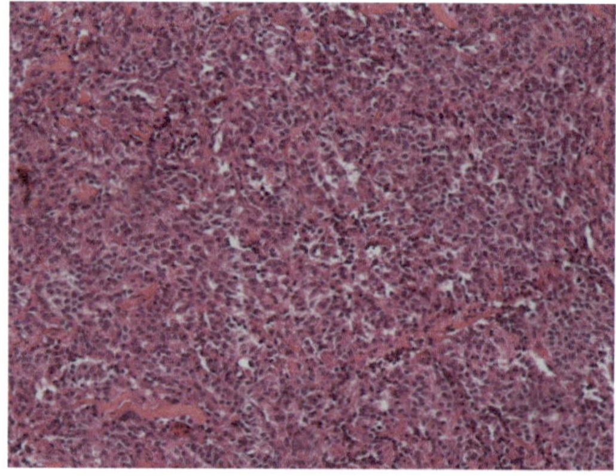

Fig. 9.2 Histological section of a well-differentiated pancreatic NET (Hematoxylin Eosin ×10)

cular lesions can be seen. The hypervascularity of these lesions is best recognized in the late arterial phase of the liver. The pronounced vascularity results in rapid wash-out of the contrast agent in later phases [8].

CT is also widely used in identifying primary carcinoid tumors According to Jeung et al. [17] carcinoid tumors are also hypervascular and therefore avidly enhance following the administration of intravenous contrast. Central bronchial carcinoid typically appears as a smooth, enhancing mass within the bronchial lumen (often with an extra-luminal component) with associated airway obstruction, collapse, or recurrent infection. On the other hand, peripheral bronchial carcinoid presents as a solitary pulmonary nodule. In contrast to bronchial carcinoids, the primary carcinoid tumor within the GI tract may not be identified on imaging, usually due to its small size and inability to differentiate from the adjacent bowel wall. Yet, according to Mehta et al. [18] they may present as a hypervascular mass or as bowel wall thickening with avid enhancement. The standard morphologic modality for NET imaging is MDCT due to its high spatial resolution, generally <1 mm with recent MDCT scanners [19]. MDCT can localize the primary tumor, assess the extent of disease, characterize the architectural relationships with the surrounding structures and be used to reassess the disease following treatments [20–23].

The multiplanarity of this technique (transaxial, coronal, sagittal, and curved planes can be reconstructed) and the three-dimensional maximum intensity projection and volume rendering techniques, which delineate the organ and vascular anatomy in 3D, improve accuracy and image interpretation [24–26]. MDCT is reproducible and allows for comparison between baseline and follow-up images. CT is the method of choice to guide the biopsy of thoracic lesions.

9.2.2 Magnetic Resonance Imaging

Since the early 1990s, Magnetic Resonance Imaging (MRI) has been used as the classical procedure of choice for abdominal and liver imaging. Since then the three technical evolu-

tions which increased its diagnostic value and improved the image quality mainly in the abdominal presentation were the achievement of (α) the gradient-echo (GRE) sequence, (β) the single shot techniques, and (γ) the phased-array coils. However, besides the aforementioned technical evolutions, MRI has only recently reached its popularity, where respiratory or motion artifacts can be considered as negligible and the spatial resolution sufficient. Furthermore, the development of 3D sequences, the respiratory triggering, and the parallel imaging strategies were strong evolutions towards a robust, high-quality liver imaging module as is MRI [27]. The development of 3D sequences is of particular value for applications requiring high spatial resolution and dedicated postprocessing as is the case of MRI angiography. Furthermore, for viewing in multiple anatomical planes, enabling accurate image interpretation the three-dimensional acquisition is recommended [26]. According to Lee et al. [28] dynamic studies following bolus injection of contrast agents with T1-weighted (w) 3D gradient echo sequences are necessary in liver imaging. In this sequence type, the entire liver can be scanned within an acceptable breath holding time of 15–20 s with a layer thickness of up to 2 mm [29]. As aforementioned, MRI has the advantage of a high spatial resolution ranging from 2 to 4 mm, amplified at higher field strength in a 3-Tesla scanner [30], in parallel shortening the acquisition time. Additionally, the absence of radiation exposure renders MRI the technique of choice especially in the young or those with long-standing disease who require repeated assessments [23, 25, 31].

The better soft tissue contrast of MRI, as compared to CT, is particularly useful to detect liver metastases for which MRI represents the most sensitive technique [32, 33]. MRI has similar indications as CT and is generally used as a problem-solving technique [32, 34].

Furthermore, due to its high soft tissue contrast, it has the ability to discriminate different tissue compounds (e.g., fat from mucin or blood, water and also hepatocytes, bile ducts) based on different signal behaviors in T1- and T2-weighted (w) sequences as well as on the tissue-specific

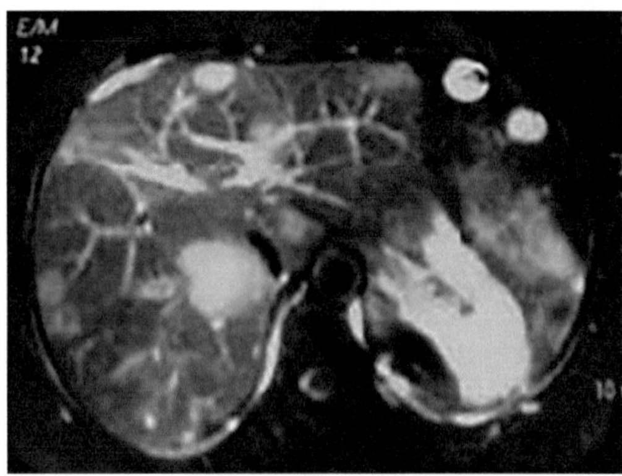

Fig. 9.3 MRI images of the liver. High-signal intensity foci of the in MRI T2 sequence image [1]

MR contrast agents (Fig. 9.3). MRI is considered superior to CT for lesion assessment in the solid visceral organs [35]. As with CT, multiphase CE MRI is recommended, with fat-suppressed CE T1-weighted (T1W) imaging providing the best accuracy, with an area under the receiver-operating curve (AUROC) of 0.98 [36, 37].

Liver-specific contrast agents can basically be categorized into two groups (a) the iron oxide particles (Super-paramagnetic Particles of Iron Oxides = SPIO), targeting the Reticulo-Endothelial-System (RES) aligned to the so-called Kupffer cells, causing a signal decrease in T2/T2*-weighted sequences by inducing local in-homogeneities of the magnetic field, and (b) the hepatobiliary contrast agents, directed to the hepatocytes and excreted via the bile, causing a signal increase in T1-weighted sequences by shortening the T1 relaxation time.

In malignant liver tumors there are usually no Kupffer cells, in contrast to normal hepatic parenchyma and solid benign liver lesions which contain variable amounts of them [38]. Accordingly, a high contrast is achieved between malignant liver lesions and normal liver parenchyma, where, due to signal loss in normal liver tissue, the malignant lesions in T2*w and T2w sequences are highlighted as "hyper-intense" lesions vs. the "dark" normal liver tissue.

In hepatobiliary contrast agents a specific uptake directly from the hepatocytes takes place. Since these agents shorten the T1-relaxation times cause a signal increase in normal liver parenchyma and in solid benign lesions. In malignant lesions, primaries and secondaries lack specific uptake of hepato-biliary contrast agents and appear as hypo-intense lesions against the bright liver parenchyma.

According to Del Frate et al. [39] and Matsuo et al. [40] the sensitivity of liver metastases detection with MRI ranges from 54 to 81%. Semelka et al. [41] reported that in a direct comparative trial, gadolinium-enhanced MRI was superior to biphasic spiral CT in lesion detection and lesion characterization, thus this superior diagnostic value of MRI adds a significant impact on patient treatment. Liver-specific contrast agents lead to a significant increase in the detection rate of true positive lesions in patients with suspected metastases. An established part of a sophisticated liver MRI protocol is the diffusion-weighted MRI. Its superiority regarding the detection of lesions over other simple sequences has been emphasized by Zech et al. [42]. Bartolozzi et al., Lowenthal et al., Huppertz et al., and Bluemke et al., by using hepatobiliary contrast agents achieved detection rates ranging from 70 and 90% [8, 43–45].

Hepatobiliary phase images are crucial for lesion detection, particularly in hypervascular metastases, despite the value of the early arterial phase for lesion characterization in identifying signs of hypervascularity. Hypervascular lesions can sometimes be poorly detected in the arterial phase of dynamic gadolinium standard chelates, whereas hepatobiliary phase images, after administration of liver-specific contrast agents, allow reliable detection irrespective of the contrast agent time [12, 46, 47]. The latter authors suggest that combined reading of early dynamic phase images (obtained with standard gadolinium chelates) and delayed phase images of liver-specific agents give the highest detection rate. Using liver-specific and super-paramagnetic contrast media, the soft-tissue contrast can be further increased [48]. Within a single-dose injection of liver-specific contrast medium, Primovist® or MultiHance® both an early dynamic phase and a liver-specific phase can be achieved. Nowadays, the above contrast agents are considered to be the best noninvasive choice for the detection of liver metastases, especially if additional diffusion-weighted sequences are acquired [21].

The use of MRI in the detection of typical primary neuroendocrine tumors classically demonstrates low signal intensity on T1-weighted images and high signal intensity on T2-weighted images [49]. It also demonstrates avid enhancement after the administration of gadolinium, reflecting their hypervascular nature. Additionally, T1-weighted GRE (gradient recalled echo) sequences have shown to be of value in the identification of these tumors. Larger lesions tend to demonstrate necrosis. Gadolinium-based contrast may be especially useful in cases where noncontrast MRI techniques are negative or equivocal. Characteristics suggesting malignancy include large primary tumor, central necrosis, locally aggressive features such as vascular invasion, and calcification. According to Semelka et al. [50] MRI examinations of primary carcinoid tumors reveal two different morphologies: either a well-defined nodular mass or a regional, relatively uniform bowel wall thickening. Both patterns of tumors are difficult to be detected; however, in both cases the late gadolinium-enhanced T1-weighted fat-suppressed images reveal moderately hyper-intense masses, reflecting the tumoral larger interstitial space compared to the adjacent bowel. Furthermore, the same author [51] reports on a positive predictive value of 96% for MRI in pancreatic NETs. MRI is particularly advantageous in localizing primary pancreatic tumors and for staging and restaging liver lesions [10]. Moreover, cholangiopancreatic sequences (magnetic resonance cholangio-pancreato-graphy), specified at studying the involvement of the biliary and pancreatic ducts, are useful for surgical planning and should always precede resection of a pancreatic NET [52]. Gastrinomas morphologically tend to show ring or peripheral enhancement, while most other subtypes of NETs demonstrate a diffuse pattern of enhancement. Finally, for gastrointestinal NETs, MRI is able to detect around two-thirds of lesions [53] with fat-suppressed T1-weighted imaging yielding maximal results.

Metastatic lesions appear similarly to the primary neoplasm, therefore typically presenting as hypervascular lesions with or without central necrosis. In unenhanced MR images, the signal intensity of liver metastases is typically low in T1w-GRE images and moderately high in T2w sequences. Thus, due to the relatively high image contrast between metastases and unaffected liver parenchyma in unenhanced T1-w-GRE images, many metastases can be detected in this sequence. T2-w images contribute not only to lesion detection but also to lesion characterization. Burrel et al. [54] showed this finding in 75% of cases. Interestingly, 15% of cases showed increased enhancement only in the arterial phase. Nevertheless, T2-weighted imaging and hepatic arterial phase T1-weighted fat-suppressed imaging have been shown to be the most sensitive [32, 34]. Furthermore, some of the metastases may display T2-weighted hyper-intensity approaching that of hemangiomas [55]. Solid benign lesions are often nearly iso-intense to normal liver tissue on unenhanced T2-w images, while cysts and hemangiomas are markedly hyper-intense. With gadolinium-enhanced MRI, hypo- and hypervascular metastases can be differentiated. In contrast to hemangiomas with their "cotton-wool" enhancement and centripetal fill-in, hypervascular metastases tend to be more homogeneous and with "blurred" edges on imaging. According to Taouli et al. [56] diffusion-weighted MRI was found to be particularly useful for differentiating metastases from small hemangiomas or cysts.

Advances in diffusion weighted imaging (DWI) have led to its widespread clinical use in abdominal imaging. Vossen et al. [57] showed that there was a statistically significant difference in apparent diffusion coefficient (ADC) values between hemangiomas and NET metastases (as well as other hypervascular liver lesions), with an AUROC of 0.91.

An added advantage of using DWI is its ability to reflect lesion changes in treatment response [58–60].

9.2.3 Ultrasound

Ultrasound (U/S) is indisputably a first-line imaging procedure to detect known or suspected liver lesions so as further investigations to be planned. This modality is easy to perform with quick access; meanwhile, with limitations based in the fact that (a) the diagnostic accuracy of the examination strongly depends on the skills and experience of the examiner and (b) that an overlay of extensive intestinal gas, often reduces visualization of the liver. According to Harvey et al. [61] and Bartolozzi et al. [62] when the grayscale ultrasound β-mode is used, detection rates only of 58–70% for liver tumors can be achieved. However, using new techniques, such as tissue harmonic imaging recording double-frequency echoes, a better delineation and detection of focal liver lesions can be achieved compared to conventional β-mode ultrasound [63]. Furthermore, other new techniques include 3D scanning mode, speckle reduction imaging, and crossbeam mode.

Gray-scale ultrasound is very useful in the differential diagnosis of the most common benign lesions. Besides the β-mode sonography, flow-depended techniques like power-Doppler sonography or color-coded duplex sonography are used for liver imaging. Although these techniques are employed in most cases to obtain information about the hepatic vasculature, according to Reinhold et al. [64] they also provide information about the characterization of focal liver lesions based on their perfusion patterns. Furthermore, for the study of focal liver injury enhanced contrast ultrasound is considered as an established component; according to Albrecht et al. [65] an increase in the detection rate of focal liver lesions from 63 to 91% was observed, by β-mode ultrasound or combined β-mode and enhanced contrast ultrasound, respectively. As far the characterization of the lesions, contrast-enhanced ultrasound allows a significant improvement in the diagnosis of the type of lesion.

Contrast products for ultrasound consist of micro-bubbles with a diameter of 2–6 μm [66]. They consist of an envelope of biocompatible materials, including proteins, lipids or biopolymers, and a filling gas. Zech et al. [67] reports that the first-generation contrast agents have almost completely disappeared from the market. Today, the approved means for second-generation ultrasound contrast agents are Optison® (GE Healthcare, Princeton, USA) or SonoVue® (Bracco Imaging, Milano, Italy). However, of these second-generation contrast agents, only SonoVue® is approved for liver imaging. Contrast ultrasound, in combination with CT and MRI scans allows a reliable evaluation of lesions and increases the detection rate of focal liver disease. Nowadays, this technology is widely available. According to our own experience [68] and being in concordance to international references [69–72] micro-bubbles sonoporation seems to be the appropriate method for enhancing the peptide internalization, for the benefit of the treated patient. On the course of tomosonography procedure, the dose received by the examiner—doctor from patient's body, previously treated with radiopeptides, is considerably high rate and should not be ignored.

9.2.3.1 Enhancement Results of ^{111}In-Octreotide Therapy After Sonoporation

In our institution, aimed to optimize the efficiency of Auger and Internal Conversion electron emission of ^{111}In-Octreotide by increasing its cell internalization, sonoporation in 29 NET cases was performed by administrating the contrast agent SonoVue®. It was attempted to estimate the uptake and distribution differentiation of ^{111}In-Octreotide in somatostatin receptor-positive tumors when contrast micro-bubbles and US are applied.

Thus, in patients with liver metastasized neuroendocrine tumors, treated with ^{111}In-Octreotide, after hepatic artery catheterization, a first whole body scintigraphy as well tomo-scintigraphy was performed, about 7 h post-infusion, focusing on the upper abdomen area, where liver, kidneys, and spleen are the dominant organs of interest. The same scintigraphic procedure was repeated at 24, 48, 72, and 96 h posttreatment, followed by tomo-U/S. Just after performing the second (24 h post-infusion) scintigraphy and tomo-U/S 2.4 mL of the contrast agent SonoVue® was i.v. administrated to each patient, in trip-trop, diluted in 100 mL normal saline. A second dosage of the contrast was administered 10 min later, followed by second tomo-U/S (sonoporation; U/S creates transient permeability of cell membranes in the presence of microbubbles allowing increased flow of foreign molecules to enter cell).

A second planar upper-abdomen scintigraphy (anterior/posterior view) was performed after sonoporation. Both scintiscans were qualitatively and semi-quantitatively compared.

SonoVue® is an aqueous suspension of stabilized microbubbles of 1 up to 10 μm diameter. One milliliter of the contrast agent contains 200–500 microbubbles. Liver ultrasonography usually lasts about 12–20 min. [111]In radiation burden of the examiner has to be pointed out and not to be ignored (Fig. 9.4).

Sonoporation procedure and evaluation Radionuclide uptake measurements are performed to the scinti-scans before and after the Ultrasound-microbubbles application and the differences of the relative activity (tissue/background) on the target area. Pre- and post-sonoporation gives an index called Treatment Enhancement Ratio (TER) in a range of 2.5–4.0 showing a statistically significant peptide internalization increase in the combined treatment of ^{111}In-Octreotide and Ultrasound-microbubble contrast application.

We approved that Ultrasound-microbubbles application increases and differentiates the uptake and distribution of ^{111}In-Octreotide in somatostatin receptor-positive tumors. After sonoporation, scintigraphic images analysis gives semi-quantitative data and a Treatment Enhancement Ratio (TER) specific for the tumor region. Radiopharmaceutical distribution before and after microbubbles application shows pattern differentiation of the mean counts on tumor selective regions. Furthermore, the internalization increment was observed to be directly analogue to the duration of the bubble treatment. Cell permeabilization enhancement by the ultrasound bubble contrast application leads to peptide internalization increase, in ^{111}In-Octreotide infusion, raising its tumoricidal effectiveness for the benefit of the treated patient.

9.2.4 Angiography

Today the role of diagnostic angiography is limited to specific indications, widely replaced by cross-sectional imaging modalities. The basic principle of angiography for the diagnostic

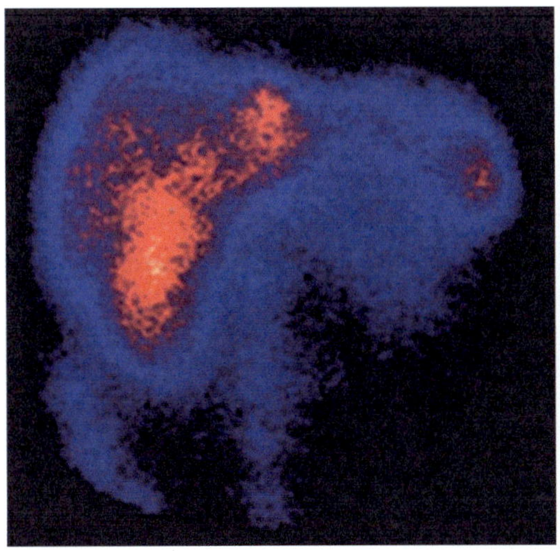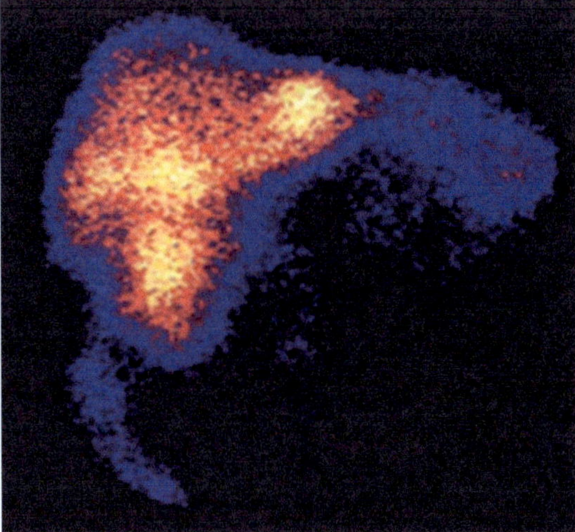

Fig. 9.4 Enhancement and pattern differentiation of the mean counts on tumor regions after sonoporation. Induced acceleration of intracellular motion of the receptors in the tumor after the microbubbles. Ultrasound application is estimated by the index T.E.R. (here = 3.75). Left scan, anterior view (before-) and right scan, anterior view (after sonoporation)

evaluation of liver tumors relies on the strong vascularity of some tumors as are neuroendocrine tumors, and, so that pathological tumor vessels and tumor regression on angiographic images to be visible [68]. Its sensitivity and specificity for the detection of lesions is limited to larger tumors, thus, it no longer plays a significant role in the diagnosis. However, angiography has recently redefined its value in radiology and has become a tool for the delivery of therapeutic agents to the liver. New technical developments allow the use of flat panel detectors in angiography systems with sufficient spatial resolution. Together with sophisticated C-arms of high mobility and fast rotation, transversal sections can be obtained during an angiographic examination, which contributes to a more precise assessment of the vascular supply of liver lesions and anatomical variants.

9.3 Summary and Conclusion

Liver-specific contrast MRI is definitively the modality of choice for dedicated liver examinations for the evaluation of NETs; however, the difference between diagnostic CT and MRI has been gradually diminished due to the ongoing evolution of the former. On the other hand, the superb contrast resolution of MRI permits highly sensitive detection of intrahepatic lesions. Assessment of vascularity and perfusion may well be efficiently performed by 3D dynamic gadolinium chelation scans. Hepatocyte-specific contrast agents and new techniques such as diffusion-weighted imaging further increase the sensitivity and specificity.

Furthermore, MDCT allows dedicated liver studies to be combined with whole-body staging (or thoracic and abdominal) to provide information about hepatic and extra-hepatic tumor burden within a single examination. For targeted examination of unclear, potentially benign liver lesions and for staging prior to liver surgery, MRI may be recommended as the method of choice. If a staging CT scan has already been performed, MRI should also not be omitted if intrahepatic findings have a direct impact on further treatment. MDCT is suitable for all emergency situations as it allows easy patient access and very short acquisition times so that noncooperative or clinically unstable patients can be easily examined. Ultrasonography will still be the first imaging modality in patients with liver tumors. Lesions appearing unclear in β-mode ultrasound can often be reliably characterized by using of contrast-enhanced ultrasound. However, U/S cannot replace MDCT and MRI in the pre-interventional or preoperative examination of patients with liver NETs. Pure diagnostic angiography is nowadays used for specific reasons; however, angiographic delivery of drugs (e.g., radio-embolization or trans-arterial chemoembolization and PRRT) and targeted pre-interventional vascular assessment have revived the use of angiography. Furthermore, the advantages of MRI over CT are the lack of ionizing radiation and the use of gadolinium chelate contrast agents, which have a better safety profile in terms of allergic reactions and nephrotoxicity, although the latter point is slightly mitigated by the concerns of nephrogenic systemic fibrosis.

9.4 Perspectives

The diagnosis, treatment, and follow-up of neuroendocrine tumors necessitate a large number of different imaging modalities, such as U/S, CT, MRI, Negatron-, and Positron Scintigraphy. Though U/S offers the possibility to perform guided biopsies from different lesions, a quick total body examination and a better staging of the disease, nowadays, it has been largely replaced by hybrid imaging systems with superior spatial resolution, particularly for high-grade tumors. Furthermore, tracers with higher specificity as ^{18}F-L-DOPA, ^{11}C-L-DOPA, and ^{11}C-5-hydroxy-tryptophan demonstrate better imaging results, the two latter necessitating a standby cyclotron.

References

1. Limouris GS, Chatziioannou A, Kontogeorgakos D, et al. Selective hepatic arterial infusion of In-111-DTPA-Phe1-octreotide in neuro-endocrine

liver metastases. Eur J Nucl Med Mol Imaging. 2008;35:1827–37.

2. Hwang GJ, Kim M-J, Yoo HS, et al. Nodular hepatocellular carcinoma: detection with arterial-, portal- and delayed-phase images at spiral CT. Radiology. 1997;202:383–8.

3. Schima W, Hammerstingl R, Catalano C, et al. Quadruple-phase MDCT of the liver in patients with suspected hepatocellular carcinoma: effect of contrast material flow rate. AJR Am J Roentgenol. 2006;186:1571–9.

4. Schima W, Kulinna C, Ba-Ssalamah A, et al. Multidetector computed tomography of the liver. Radiologe. 2005;45:15–23.

5. Kondo H, Kanematsu M, Hashi H, et al. Preoperative detection of malignant hepatic tumors: comparison of combined methods of MR imaging with combined methods of CT. AJR Am J Roentgenol. 1999;174:947–54.

6. Semelka RC, Cance WG, Marcos HB, et al. Liver metastases: comparison of current MR techniques and spiral CT during arterial portography for detection in 20 surgically staged cases. Radiology. 1999;213:86–91.

7. Reimer P, Jahnke N, Fiebich M, et al. Hepatic lesion detection and characterization: value of non-enhanced MR imaging, super-paramagnetic iron oxide-enhanced MR imaging, and spiral CT—ROC analysis. Radiology. 2000;217:152–8.

8. Bartolozzi C, Donati F, Cioni D, et al. Detection of colorectal liver metastases: a prospective multicenter trial comparing unenhanced MRI, MnDPDP-enhanced MRI, and spiral CT. Eur Radiol. 2004;14:14–20.

9. Oudkerk M, Torres CG, Song B, et al. Characterization of liver lesions with mangafodipir trisodium-enhanced MR imaging: multicenter study comparing MR and dual-phase spiral CT. Radiology. 2002;223:517–24.

10. Semelka RC, Martin DR, Balci C, et al. Focal liver lesions: comparison of dual-phase CT and multi-sequence multiplanar MR imaging including dynamic gadolinium enhancement. J Magn Reson Imaging. 2001;13:397–401.

11. Lencioni R, Donati F, Cioni D, et al. Detection of colorectal liver metastases: prospective comparison of unenhanced and ferumoxides-enhanced magnetic resonance imaging at 1.5 T, dual-phase spiral CT, and spiral CT during arterial portography. MAGMA. 1998;7:76–87.

12. Ward J, Guthrie JA, Scott DJ, et al. Hepatocellular carcinoma in the cirrhotic liver: double-contrast MR imaging for diagnosis. Radiology. 2000;216:154–62.

13. Vails C, Andia E, Sanchez A, et al. Hepatic metastases from colorectal cancer: preoperative detection and assessment of resectability with helical CT. Radiology. 2001;218:55–60.

14. Weg N, Scheer MR, Gabor MP. Liver lesions: improved detection with dual-detector-array CT and routine 2.5 mm thin collimation. Radiology. 1998;209:417–26.

15. Haider MA, Amitai MM, Rappaport DC, et al. Multidetector row helical CT in preoperative assessment of small (< or = 1.5 cm) liver metastases: is thinner collimation better? Radiology. 2002;225:137–42.

16. Danet IM, Semelka RC, Leonardou P, et al. Spectrum of MRI appearances of untreated metastases of the liver. AJR Am J Roentgenol. 2003;181:809–17.

17. Jeung MY, Gasser B, Gangi A, et al. Bronchial carcinoid tumors of the thorax: spectrum of radiologic findings. Radiographics. 2002;22(2):351–65.

18. Mehta P, Colletti PM. Neuroendocrine tumors: a review of CT and MRI findings. http://snmmi.files.cms-plus.com/ACNM/08_NeuroendocrineTumorsv5-version2.pdf.

19. Sundin A, Rockall A. Therapeutic monitoring of gastroenteropancreatic neuro-endocrine tumors: the challenges ahead. Neuroendocrinology. 2012;96:261–71.

20. Sundin A, Vullierme MP, Kaltsas G, et al. ENETS consensus guidelines for the standards of care in neuroendocrine tumors: radiological examinations. Neuroendocrinology. 2009;90:167–83.

21. Ganeshan D, Bhosale P, Yang T, et al. Imaging features of carcinoid tumors of the gastrointestinal tract. AJR Am J Roentgenol. 2013;201:773–86.

22. Arigoni S, Ignjatovic S, Sager P, et al. Diagnosis and prediction of neuro-endocrine liver metastases: a protocol of six systematic reviews. JMIR Res Protoc. 2013;2:e60.

23. de Mestier L, Dromain C, d'Assignies G, et al. Evaluating digestive neuro-endocrine tumor progression and therapeutic responses in the era of targeted therapies: state of the art. Endocr Relat Cancer. 2014;21:R105–20.

24. Sundin A. Radiological and nuclear medicine imaging of gastroentero-pancreatic neuroendocrine tumors. Best Pract Res Clin Gastroenterol. 2012;26:803–18.

25. Sahani DV, Bonaffini PA, Fernandez-Del Castillo C, et al. Gastroentero-pancreatic neuroendocrine tumors: role of imaging in diagnosis and management. Radiology. 2013;266:38–61.

26. Kim KW, Krajewski KM, Nishino M, et al. Update on the management of gastroenteropancreatic neuroendocrine tumors with emphasis on the role of imaging. AJR Am J Roentgenol. 2013;201:811–24.

27. Zech CJ, Schoenberg SO, Herrmann KA, et al. Modern visualization of the liver with MRT. Current trends and future perspectives. Radiologe. 2004;44:1160–9.

28. Lee VS, Lavelle MT, Rofsky NM, et al. Hepatic MR imaging with a dynamic contrast-enhanced isotropic volumetric interpolated breath-hold examination: feasibility, reproducibility, and technical quality. Radiology. 2000;215:365–72.

29. Rofsky NM, Lee VS, Laub G, et al. Abdominal MR imaging with a volumetric interpolated breath-hold examination. Radiology. 1999;212:876–84.

30. Hwang J, Kim YK, Park MJ, et al. Liver MRI at 3.0 tesla: comparison of image quality and lesion detectability between single-source conventional and dual-source parallel radiofrequency transmissions. J Comput Assist Tomogr. 2012;36:546–53.

31. Sundin A. Radiological and nuclear medicine imaging of gastroenteropancreatic neuroendocrine tumours. Best Pract Res Clin Gastroenterol. 2012;26:803–18.
32. Dromain C, de Baere T, Lombroso J, et al. Detection of liver metastases from endocrine tumors: a prospective comparison of somatostatin receptor scintigraphy, computed tomography, and magnetic resonance imaging. J Clin Oncol. 2005;23:70–8.
33. Schraml C, Schwenzer NF, Sperling O, et al. Staging of neuroendocrine tumours: comparison of [^{68}Ga] DOTATOC multiphase PET/CT and whole-body MRI. Cancer Imaging. 2013;13:63–72.
34. Dromain C, de Baere T, Baudin E, et al. MR imaging of hepatic metastases caused by neuroendocrine tumors: comparing four techniques. AJR. 2003;180:121–8.
35. Pisegna JR, Doppman JL, Norton JA, et al. Prospective comparative study of ability of MR imaging and other imaging modalities to localize tumors in patients with Zollinger-Ellison syndrome. Dig Dis Sci. 1993;38:1318–28.
36. Ichikawa T, Peterson MS, Federle MP, et al. Islet cell tumor of the pancreas: biphasic CT versus MR imaging in tumor detection. Radiology. 2000;216:163–71.
37. Herwick S, Miller FH, Keppke AL. MRI of islet cell tumors of the pancreas. AJR Am J Roentgenol. 2006;187:W472–80.
38. Namkung S, Zech CJ, Helmberger T, et al. Superparamagnetic iron oxide (SPIO)-enhanced liver MR imaging with ferucarbotran: efficacy for characterization of focal liver lesions. J Magn Reson Imaging. 2007;25:755–65.
39. Del Frate C, Bazzocchi M, Mortele KJ, et al. Detection of liver metastases: comparison of gadobenate dimeglumine-enhanced and ferumoxides-enhanced MR imaging examinations. Radiology. 2002;225:766–72.
40. Matsuo M, Kanematsu M, Itoh K, et al. Detection of malignant hepatic tumors: comparison of gadolinium- and ferumoxide-enhanced MR imaging. AJR Am J Roentgenol. 2001;177:637–43.
41. Semelka RC, Martin DR, Balci C, Lance T. Focal liver lesions: comparison of dual-phase CT and multi-sequence multiplanar MR imaging including dynamic gadolinium enhancement. J Magn Reson Imaging. 2001;13:397–401.
42. Zech CJ, Herrmann KA, Dietrich O, et al. Black-blood diffusion-weighted EPI acquisition of the liver with parallel imaging: comparison with a standard T2-weighted sequence for detection of focal liver lesions. Invest Radiol. 2008;43:261–6.
43. Lowenthal D, Zeile M, Lim WY, et al. Detection and characterization of focal liver lesions in colorectal carcinoma patients: comparison of diffusion-weighted and Gd-EOB-DTPA enhanced MR imaging. Eur Radiol. 2011;21:832–40.
44. Huppertz A, Balzer T, Blakeborough A, et al. Improved detection of focal liver lesions at MR imaging: multicenter comparison of gadoxetic acid-enhanced MR images with intraoperative findings. Radiology. 2004;230:266–75.
45. Bluemke DA, Sahani D, Amendola M, et al. Efficacy and safety of MR imaging with liver-specific contrast agent: US multicenter phase III study. Radiology. 2005;237:89–98.
46. Kettritz U, Schlund JF, Wilbur K, et al. Comparison of gadolinium chelates with manganese-DPDP for liver lesion detection and characterization: preliminary results. Magn Reson Imaging. 1996;14:1185–90.
47. Youk JH, Lee JM, Kim CS. MRI for detection of hepatocellular carcinoma: comparison of mangafodipir trisodium and gadopentetate dimeglumine contrast agents. AJR Am J Roentgenol. 2004;183:1049–54.
48. Morana G, Salviato E, Guarise A. Contrast agents for hepatic MRI. Cancer Imaging. 2007;7:S24–7.
49. Owen NJ, Sohaib SA, Peppercorn PD, et al. MRI of pancreatic neuroendocrine tumours. Br J Radiol. 2001;74:968–73.
50. Semelka RC, John G, Kelekis NL, et al. Small bowel neoplastic disease: demonstration by MRI. J Magn Reson Imaging. 1996;6:855–60.
51. Semelka RC, Custodio CM, Cem Balci N, et al. Neuroendocrine tumors of the pancreas: spectrum of appearances on MRI. J Magn Reson Imaging. 2000;11:141–8.
52. Schima W. MRI of the pancreas: tumours and tumor-simulating processes. Cancer Imaging. 2006;6:199–203.
53. Bader TR, Semelka RC, Chiu VC, et al. MRI of carcinoid tumors: spectrum of appearances in the gastrointestinal tract and liver. J Magn Reson Imaging. 2001;14:261–9.
54. Burrel M, Llovet JM, Ayuso C, et al. MRI angiography is superior to helical CT for detection of HCC prior to liver transplantation: an explant correlation. Hepatology. 2003;38:1034–42.
55. Debray MP, Geoffrey O, Laissy JP, et al. Imaging appearances of metastases from neuroendocrine tumours of the pancreas. Br J Radiol. 2001;74:1065–70.
56. Taouli B, Vilgrain V, Dumont E, et al. Evaluation of liver diffusion isotropy and characterization of focal hepatic lesions with two single-shot echo-planar MR imaging sequences: prospective study in 66 patients. Radiology. 2003;226:71–8.
57. Vossen JA, Buijs M, Liapi E, et al. Operating characteristic analysis of diffusion-weighted magnetic resonance imaging in differentiating hepatic hemangioma from other hypervascular liver lesions. J Comput Assist Tomogr. 2008;32:750–6.
58. Liapi E, Geschwind JF, Vossen JA, et al. Functional MRI evaluation of tumor response in patients with neuroendocrine hepatic metastasis treated with transcatheter arterial chemoembolization. AJR. 2008;190:67–73.
59. Lee SS, Byun JH, Park BJ, et al. Quantitative analysis of diffusion-weighted magnetic resonance imaging of the pancreas: usefulness in characterizing solid pancreatic masses. J Magn Reson Imaging. 2008;28:928–36.

60. Anaye A, Mathieu A, Closset J, et al. Successful preoperative localization of a small pancreatic insulinoma by diffusion-weighted MRI. JOP. 2009;10:528–31.
61. Harvey CJ, Albrecht T. Ultrasound of focal liver lesions. Eur Radiol. 2001;11:1578–93.
62. Bartolozzi C, Lencioni R, Caramella D, et al. Small hepatocellular carcinoma. Detection with US, CT, MR imaging, DSA, and Lipiodol-CT. Acta Radiol. 1996;37:69–74.
63. Tanaka S, Oshikawa O, Sasaki T, et al. Evaluation of tissue harmonic imaging for the diagnosis of focal liver lesions. Ultrasound Med Biol. 2000;26:183–7.
64. Reinhold C, Hammers L, Taylor CR, et al. Characterization of focal hepatic lesions with duplex sonography: findings in 198 patients. Am J Roentgenol. 1995;164:1131–5.
65. Albrecht T, Hoffmann CW, Schmitz SA, et al. Phase-inversion sonography during the liver-specific late phase of contrast enhancement: improved detection of liver metastases. AJR Am J Roentgenol. 2001;176:1191–8.
66. Quaia E. Microbubble ultrasound contrast agents: an update. Eur Radiol. 2007;17:1995–2008.
67. Zech CJ, Reiser MF. Radiological evaluation of patients with liver tumors. In: Bilbao JI, Reiser MF, editors. Liver radioembolization with ^{90}Y microspheres. Berlin Heidelberg: Springer; 2014. p. 15–26.
68. Limouris GS, Lyra M, Lamprakos L, et al. Pharmacokinetic differences before and after sonoporation during In – 111 – DTPA – Phe Octreotide therapy in man. J Nucl Med. 2006;47(Suppl 1):419. [abstr].
69. Moosavi-Nejad S, Hosseini H, Akiyama H, Tachibana K. Reparable cell sonoporation in suspension: theranostic potential of microbubble. Theranostics. 2016;6(4):446–55.
70. Wrenn SP, Dicker SM, Small EF, et al. Bursting bubbles and bilayers. Theranostics. 2012;2:1140–59.
71. Tachibana K, Uchida T, Ogawa K, et al. Induction of cell-membrane porosity by ultrasound. Lancet. 1999;353:1409.
72. Hwang JH, Brayman AA, Reidy MA, et al. Vascular effects induced by combined 1-MHz ultrasound and microbubble contrast agent treatments in vivo. Ultrasound Med Biol. 2005;31:553–64.

Angiographic Anatomy on the Course of Liver Intra-arterial Infusion

Athanasios G. Zafeirakis and Georgios S. Limouris

10.1 Introduction

Liver interventional radiologists and surgeons are acquainted with the plethora of variations of the mesenteric and the hepatic arterial bed to perform in an efficient manner any kind of therapeutic trans-arterial procedure; particularly, on the course of radiopeptides infusion after catheterization of the celiac trunk in unrecognized collateral vessels. The radiobiological burden from the intra-artrial radiopeptide infusions does not result in severe side effects (i.e., gastrointestinal ulceration, cholecystitis, pacreatitis, skin necrosis) as in the case of microspheres radioembolization [1]. On the contrary, it is medically unfair to infuse not targeted organs and tissues. Despite the advantages in vascular techniques i.e., Computed Tomography (CT)- or Magnetic Resonance Imaging (MRI)-angiography, at present, there is no substitute for conventional digital subtraction angiography (DSA) because many of the small vessels are beyond the resolution capabilities of CT or MR angiography. Furthermore, DSA provides not only anatomical but also flow characteristics.

10.2 Liver Arterial Anatomy

10.2.1 Classical Description and Anatomical Variations

The celiac trunk arising from the abdominal aorta trifurcates into the common hepatic, left gastric, and splenic artery, the former divided consequently into the gastro-duodenal and proper hepatic artery (Fig. 10.1). The latter bifurcates into the right (RHA) and left hepatic artery (LHA) to supply the corresponding hepatic lobes. The right hepatic artery further divides into the right anterior and right posterior hepatic artery, while the left hepatic artery divides into branches supplying segments II and III. The supply of segment IV originates from one or more branches arising from the proper, right or left hepatic artery. This classical description of the hepatic arterial bed refers to only 55–65% of the population. Any hepatic arterial anatomy that deviates from what has been so far described is considered to represent an anatomical variation. The data necessary for the study of such variations may be obtained from direct observation of large autopsies, surgical series, or from radiological studies, initially by conventional angiography including DSA or more recently CT or MR angiography.

A. G. Zafeirakis (✉)
Nuclear Medicine Department, Army Share Fund Hospital of Athens, Athens, Greece
e-mail: a.g.zafeirakis@army.gr

G. S. Limouris
Nuclear Medicine, Medical School, National and Kapodistrian University of Athens, Athens, Greece

© Springer Nature Switzerland AG 2021
G. S. Limouris (ed.), *Liver Intra-arterial PRRT with ^{111}In-Octreotide*,
https://doi.org/10.1007/978-3-030-70773-6_10

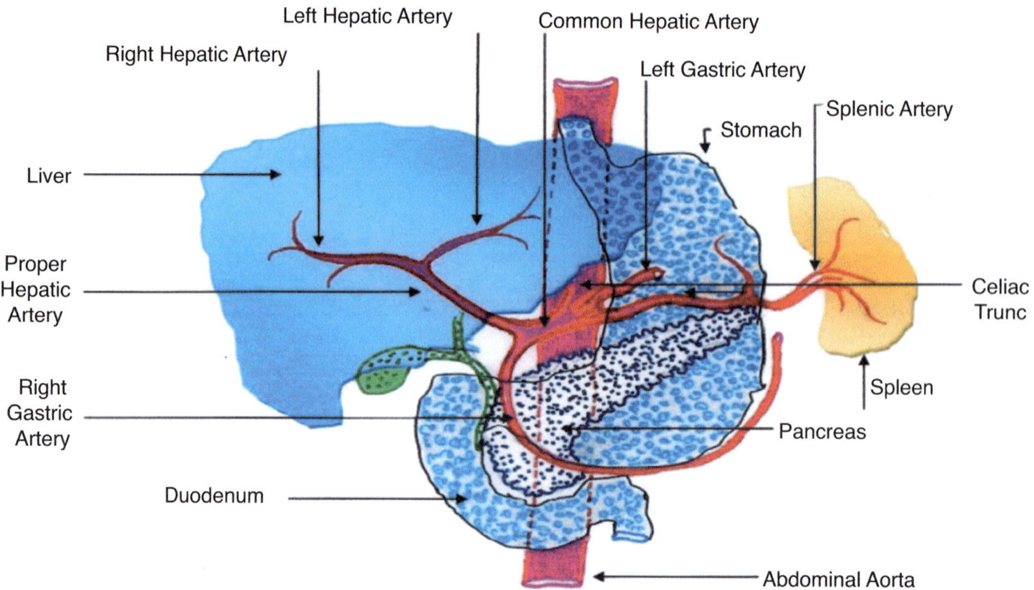

Fig. 10.1 Celiac trunk

10.2.2 Terminology

Often, either the left or the right branch of the hepatic artery arises from another origin than the proper hepatic artery of the celiac trunk. Such a vessel arise is called "aberrant" (an irregular variation). Two types of aberrant hepatic arteries can be observed, the replacing and the accessory. If a branch substitutes an absent hepatic artery, we refer to it as an aberrant "replaced" hepatic artery. In case when an additional artery to one normally present is observed, we refer to it as an aberrant "accessory" artery.

10.2.3 Michels' Classification of Anatomical Variants

Albrecht von Haller (Fig. 10.2) first de-scribed in 1756 aberrant hepatic arteries; it was not earlier than two centuries later, when Michels published his classical study of hepatic arterial anatomy, analyzing in detail the results following the dis-

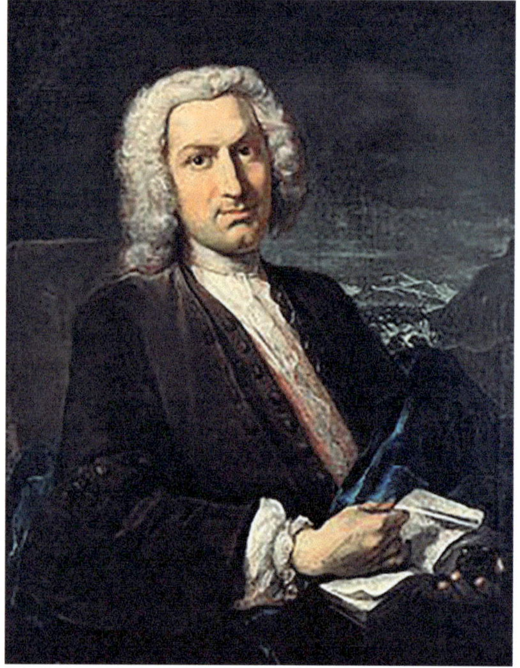

Fig. 10.2 Albert von Haller (1708–1777)

Table 10.1 Relevant anatomic variants according to Michaels' study of 200 cadavers

Type I	Standard (55%)
Type II	Replaced LHA (10%)
Type III	Replaced RHA (11%)
Type IV	Replaced RHA and LHA (1%)
Type V	Accessory LHA from LGA (8%)
Type VI	Accessory RHA from SMA (7%)
Type VII	Accessory RHA from LHA (1%)
Type VIII	Accessory RHA and LHA and replaced RHA or LHA (2%)
Type IX	CHA replacedfrom SMA (2.5%)
Type X	CHA replacedfrom LGA (<1%)

LHA left hepatic artery, *RHA* right hepatic artery, *LGA* left gastric artery, *SMA* superior mesenteric artery, *CHA* common hepatic artery [3]

Table 10.2 Anatomic variants not mentioned by Michels

CHA	From aorta
LHA	From LGA + RHA from CHA
CHA	From aorta + aberrant LHA from LGA + aberrant RHA from SMA
LHA	From CHA + RHA from GDA
CHA	From CT + aberrant LHA from LGA + aberrant RHA from aorta
CMT + LHA	From LGA
RHA	From GDA
LHA	From CHA + RHA from SMA
RHA	From CT

CHA common hepatic artery, *LHA* left hepatic artery, *LGA* left gastric artery, *RHA* right hepatic artery, *SMA* superior mesenteric artery, *GDA* gastroduodenal artery, *CT* celiac trunk [3]

section of 200 cadavers [2]. He defined ten anatomical variations (Table 10.1) of the hepatic artery [3]. Later on, in 1966, he proposed an internationally re-cognized classification of these hepatic abnormalities, which only very later, in 1994, was further modified by Hiatt et al. [4]. In the conventional anatomy, defined as type I according to Michels' classification, the main hepatic artery originates from the celiac trunk, gives off the gastro-duodenal artery and the proper hepatic artery that continues as the right hepatic artery. The right hepatic artery further splits into its anterior and posterior branch, and the left hepatic artery further splits into branches that feed segments II and III. Segment IV is fed by the branch or branches originating from the proper, the right or the left hepatic artery. The left hepatic artery arising from the left gastric artery is defined as type II variation, while the right hepatic artery originating from the superior mesenteric artery is defined as type III variation; the coexistence of both aberrants is defined as type IV variation. In type V variation the left lobe is supplied by the accessory left hepatic artery, originating from the left gastric artery. In type VI variation, the right lobe is supplied by the accessory right hepatic artery, originating from the superior mesenteric artery. In type VII variation, both the right and left accessory arteries exist. In type VIII variation, the aberrant right hepatic artery and the accessory left hepatic artery or the accessory right hepatic artery and the aberrant left hepatic artery coexist. The hepatic trunk originates from the superior mesenteric artery, and finally in type X variation, it originates from the left gastric artery.

10.2.4 Other Anatomical Variants

The frequency of anomalies not included in Michels' system is reported to be 1.8% [5] and 16.6% [6], respectively. The knowledge of these aberrant vessels is useful on the course of the catheterization in radiopeptide therapy. Further clinically relevant anatomical variants are summarized in Table 10.2.

10.3 Extrahepatic Vessels Originating from the Hepatic Vasculature

When performing radiopeptide therapy, it is of high importance to identify any vessel that supplies blood to liver tumors, as this may result in radiopeptide burden in healthy tissues. According to Carratero et al. [7] this is one of the most serious complications affecting the GI tract, which seldom might lead to gastritis, even rarely to ulceration in case that an unwished infusion occurs via the gastro-duodenal and right gastric artery.

10.3.1 Vessels Originating from the Common- (CHA) and Proper Hepatic Artery (PHA)

10.3.1.1 Gastro-Duodenal Artery (GDA) and Pancreato-Duodenal Arcade (PDA)

The importance of GDA and PDA lies in the fact that there are not only the largest extra-hepatic vessels but also two of the most constantly present, having many possible origins. They both supply blood to the duodenum, pancreas, and stomach and form the most important part of the anastomotic system between the celiac axis and the superior mesenteric artery. According to Liew et al. [1] and Song et al. [8] they also have the potential to become important collateral vessels in cases of celiac stenosis, thus providing alternative routes of flow. For optimizing the ^{111}In-Octreotide infusions, this is of highest importance to obtain the proper angiographic assessment.

10.3.1.2 Peribiliary Plexus Arteries (PPA)

According to Arias Fernandez et al. [9] there is a vascular network distributed around the intra- and extra-hepatic bile duct [10], also known as "communicating arcades"; based on studies of Uchikawa et al. [11] the peri-biliary plexus connects the hepatic arteries with the portal venous system through the bile duct walls. In cases of segmental arterial or portal occlusion, communicating arcades function as a col-lateral pathway allowing the revascularization of hepatic segmental territories [10, 11].

10.3.2 Vessels Originating from the LHA

10.3.2.1 Right Gastric Artery (RGA)

The RGA arises from any site of the hepatic artery, although most frequently from the left hepatic artery, often anatomizing with LGA via an arterial arcade [12]. Yamagami et al. [13] and Cosin et al. [14] report that this anatomical disposition may be useful in those cases where anterograde catheterization and occlusion of the GRA cannot be performed, thus allowing access to it from the left gastric artery. Although there is a minor contribution of the blood supply to the stomach, the right gastric artery plays an important role in radiopeptide infusions since passage of the radio-pharmaceutical through it may result in an increased gastric radiobiological burden.

10.3.2.2 Falciform Artery (FA)

More than two and a half centuries ago, in 1753, Albrecht von Haller (Fig. 10.2) was the first who described the falciform artery (FA). According to Williams et al. [15] and Baba et al. [16] it arises as a terminal branch of the middle or left hepatic artery and runs within the falciform ligament together with the umbilical vein. It follows a characteristic course by running in an oblique plane, from the left intersegmental fissure to the anterior abdominal wall. In selective catheterization of the hepatic artery, failure to identify the FA may result in the delivery of ^{111}In-Octreotide radiopharmaceutical to the anterior abdominal wall, which may further result in unwished increased radiobiological burden.

10.3.2.3 Accessory Left Gastric Artery (aLGA)

According to Song et al. [17] the accessory left hepatic artery is present in up to 21% of the population. It originates from the arteries of the hepatic segments II or III or the proper hepatic artery and connects with the esophagus and gastric fundus [18]. Arias Fernandez et al. reported recently [9] that it is best visualized during the venous phase of the left hepatic angiogram. If present, on the course of ^{111}In-Octreotide infusion, an increased radiobiological burden has to be taken into account.

10.3.2.4 Accessory Left Phrenic Artery (aLPA)

It rarely arises from the left hepatic artery, with negligible incidence according to Piao et al. [19] and Song et al. [17] of 0% and 2%, respectively, usually originating from the celiac trunk.

10.3.3 Vessels Originating from the Right Hepatic Artery (RHA)

10.3.3.1 Cystic Artery (CA)

According to Ottery et al. [20], the cystic artery at a 95% typically arises from the right hepatic artery; however, in an about 18% it may originate from the replaced or accessory right hepatic artery, from the left hepatic artery (7%), the double cystic artery (2–15%) [21, 22], the common hepatic artery (3%), the gastro-duodenal artery (1%) or the superior mesenteric artery [21, 23–25].

Perforating arteries arising from the GDA, hepatic parenchyma arteries, and cystic artery consist of the gallbladder blood supply; the latter acting as the origin of parasitic supply to tumors located in the gallbladder fossa, in the right lobe or the medial segment of the liver [26].

10.4 Hepatic Vessels Originating from the Extrahepatic Vasculature

Since there are many hepatic vessels originating from non-hepatic sources, it is important for both the interventional radiologist and the nuclear physician to be acquainted with the hepatic arterial net as well as the degree of the extra-hepatic collaterals for an optimum vessel hyper-selective catheterization. Based on our experience we have to emphasize that collaterals should be adequately recognized for an effective catheter management since they often are the main feeding tumor vessels, where without them a proper and accurate treatment would not be successfully achieved. In Table 10.3 are tabulated the most often intra-hepatic tumor locations and the likely origin of the parasitic arteries.

Table 10.3 Intra-hepatic tumor location and the likely origin of the parasitic arteries

Tumor location	Likely origin
• Liver right lobe (posterior surface) near the diaphragm	• Right inferior phrenic artery • Right intercostal arteries • Lumbar arteries
• Liver right lobe (anterior surface) • Liver lower edge of the medial segment	• Omental artery • Colic artery
• Liver left lobe	• Right gastric artery • Left gastric artery • Left inferior phrenic artery
• Liver caudate lobe	• Right inferior phrenic artery • Right renal capsular artery • Gastric artery

References

1. Liu DM, Salem R, Bui JT, et al. Angiographic considerations in patients undergoing liver directed therapy. J Vasc Interv Radiol. 2005;16:911–35.
2. Michels NA. Collateral arterial pathways to the liver after ligation of the hepatic artery and removal of the celiac axis. Cancer. 1953;6:708–24.
3. Saiz-Mendiguren AJ, Vivas I, Bilbao JI. Vascular anatomy and its implication in radioembolization. In: Bilbao JI, Reiser MF, editors. Liver radioembolization with ^{90}Y micro-spheres. Berlin Heidelberg: Springer; 2014. p. 27–40.
4. Hiatt JR, Gabbay J, Busuttil RW. Surgical anatomy of the hepatic arteries in 1000 cases. Ann Surg. 1994;220:50–2.
5. Koops A, Wojciechowski B, Broering DC, et al. Anatomic variations of the hepatic arteries in 604 selective celiac and superior mesenteric angiographies. Surg Radiol Anat. 2004;26:239–44.
6. Coskun M, Kayahan EM, Uzbek O, et al. Imaging of hepatic arterial anatomy for depicting vascular variations in living related liver transplant donor candidates with multidetector computed tomography: comparison with conventional angiography. Transplant Proc. 2005;37:1070–3.
7. Carretero C, Munoz-Navas M, Betes M, et al. Gastroduodenal injury after radioembolization of hepatic tumors. Am J Gastroenterol. 2007;102:1216–20.
8. Song SY, Chung JW, Kwon JW, et al. Collateral pathways in patients with celiac axis stenosis: angiographic-spiral CT correlation. Radiographics. 2002;22:881–93.

9. Arias Fernandez J, Martin Martin B, Pinheiro da Silva N, et al. Extrahepatic vessels depending on the hepatic artery. Identification and management. Radiologia. 2011;53(1):18–26.
10. Kan Z, Madoff DC. Liver anatomy: microcirculation of the liver. Semin Intervent Radiol. 2008;25(2):77–85.
11. Uchikawa Y, Kitamura H, Miyagawa S. Portal blood flow via the peribiliary vascular plexus demonstrated by contrast enhanced ultrasonography with Sonazoid. J Hepatobiliary Pancreat Sci. 2011;18(4):615–20.
12. Van Damme JP, Bonte J. Vascular anatomy in abdominal surgery. New York: Thieme; 1990.
13. Yamagami T, Nakamura T, Iida S, et al. Embolization of the right gastric artery before hepatic arterial infusion chemotherapy to prevent gastric mucosal lesions: approach through the hepatic artery versus the left gastric artery. AJR Am J Roentgenol. 2002;179:1605–10.
14. Cosin O, Bilbao JI, Alvarez S, et al. Right gastric artery embolization prior to treatment with yttrium-90 microspheres. Cardiovasc Intervent Radiol. 2007;30:98–103.
15. Williams DM, Cho KJ, Ensminger WD, et al. Hepatic falciform artery: anatomy, angiographic appearance, and clinical significance. Radiology. 1985;156:339–40.
16. Baba Y, Miyazono N, Ueno K, et al. Hepatic falciform artery. Angiographic findings in 25 patients. Acta Radiol. 2000;41:329–33.
17. Song SY, Chung JW, Lim HG, et al. Non-hepatic arteries originating from the hepatic arteries: angiographic analysis in 250 patients. J Vasc Interv Radiol. 2006;17:461–9.
18. Song SY, Chung JW, Yin YH, et al. Celiac axis and common hepatic artery variations in 5002 patients: systematic analysis with spiral CT and DSA. Radiology. 2010;255(1):278–88.
19. Piao DX, Ohtsuka A, Murakami T. Typology of abdominal arteries, with special reference to inferior phrenic arteries and their esophageal branches. Acta Med Okayama. 1998;52:189–96.
20. Ottery FD, Scupham RK, Weese JL. Chemical cholecystitis after intra-hepatic chemotherapy. The case for prophylactic cholecystectomy during pump placement. Dis Colon Rectum. 1986;29:187–90.
21. Daseler EH, Anson BJ, Hambley WC, et al. The cystic artery and constituents of the hepatic pedicle: a study of 500 specimens. Surg Gynecol Obstet. 1947;85:47–63.
22. Loukas M, Fergurson A, Louis RG Jr, et al. Multiple variations of the hepatobiliary vasculature including double cystic arteries, accessory left hepatic artery and hepatosplenic trunk: a case report. Surg Radiol Anat. 2006;28:525–8.
23. Mlakar B, Gadzijev EM, Ravnik D, et al. Anatomical variations of the cystic artery. Eur J Morphol. 2003;41:31–4.
24. Molmenti EP, Pinto PA, Klein J, Klein AS. Normal and variant arterial supply of the liver and gallbladder. Pediatr Transplant. 2003;7:80–2.
25. Sarkar AK, Roy TS. Anatomy of the cystic artery arising from the gastroduodenal artery and its choledochal branch—a case report. J Anat. 2000;197(Pt 3):503–6.
26. Wagnetz U, Jaskolka J, Yang P, et al. Acute ischemic cholecystitis after trans-arterial chemoembolization of hepatocellular carcinoma: incidence and clinical outcome. J Comput Assist Tomogr. 2010;34(3):348–53.

Intra-arterial Radiopeptide Infusions: Identifying Anatomic Variants

Georgios S. Limouris and Athanasios G. Zafeirakis

11.1 Normal, Variant, and Parasitized Extrahepatic Arterial Supply to the Liver

Standard hepatic arterial anatomy and its variants were first described by Michels as mentioned in Chaps. 9 and 10, based on his study of 200 cadavers [1], where he defined ten configurations of hepatic arterial variants. Of these, the most common one is the trifurcation of the celiac artery into the splenic (SA), the left gastric (LGA), and the common hepatic artery (CHA). Then, the CHA bifurcates into the proper hepatic (PHA) and gastro-duodenal artery (GDA). The PHA in turn bifurcates into the right hepatic (RHA) and the left hepatic artery (LHA). The segment IV artery that arises from the RHA is termed middle hepatic artery (MHA). The segment IV can also originate from the LHA.

Although the abovementioned configuration is called "standard" or "normal", this is the case in only 55% of subjects. Other common variants include a replaced left hepatic artery (rLHA) arising from the left gastric artery found in 11% of patients, a replaced right hepatic artery (rLHA)

arising from the superior mesenteric artery (SMA) found in 10% of patients, and an accessory left hepatic artery (aLHA) arising from the LGA, observed in another 8% of patients. Table 11.1 shows a complete list of anatomic variants according to Michel's classification.

Special attention should be paid to several suspected vessels consisting the most common parasitized arterial source of tumor supply, observed in about 18% of patients. According to Chung et al. [2] the most common one used to be the

Table 11.1 Relevant anatomic variants of the hepatic artery according to Michels's classification [1]

Type I	Standard anatomy with right, middle, and left HA arising from the CA (55%)
Type II	Replaced LHA from the LGA (10%)
Type III	Replaced RHA from SMA (11%)
Type IV	Replaced RHA from SMA, LHA from LGA and MHA from CA (1%)
Type V	Accessory LHA from LGA (8%)
Type VI	Accessory RHA from SMA (7%)
Type VII	Accessory RHA from SMA (1%)
Type VIII	Accessory RHA and LHA and replaced RHA or LHA (2%)
Type IX	CHA replaced from SMA (2.5%)
Type X	CHA replaced from LGA (<1%)

HA hepatic artery, *CA* celiac axis, *LHA* left hepatic artery, *RHA* right hepatic artery, *LGA* left gastric artery, *SMA* superior mesenteric artery, *CHA* common hepatic artery

G. S. Limouris (✉)
Nuclear Medicine, Medical School, National and Kapodistrian University of Athens, Athens, Greece
e-mail: glimouris@med.uoa.gr

A. G. Zafeirakis
Nuclear Medicine Department, Army Share Fund Hospital of Athens, Athens, Greece

© Springer Nature Switzerland AG 2021
G. S. Limouris (ed.), *Liver Intra-arterial PRRT with* ^{111}*In-Octreotide*,
https://doi.org/10.1007/978-3-030-70773-6_11

right inferior phrenic artery, which was found in almost 50% of patients. The same study found that the left and right gastric artery, the superior mesenteric, and pancreatic-duodenal arteries were much less frequent.

The importance of extrahepatic blood supply of the liver was noticed by Michels who categorized 16 different routes, apart from the hepatic arterial variants, from which blood could supply parts of the liver [1], including the inferior phrenic, internal mammary, and intra-costal arteries. Furthermore, according to Seki et al. [3] tumors near the surface of the liver are more likely to recruit extrahepatic blood supply. Also, parasitized extrahepatic arteries frequently supply tumors at the bare area of the liver, (Fig. 11.1) and according to Miyayama et al. [4] they consist a main cause of recurrence after treatment. Therefore, these potential routes require close attention and appropriate recognition in the evaluation of radio-infusion patients, since they can lead to incomplete treatment and recurrence after treatment.

Similar findings were reported by Covey et al. in 2002 in a study evaluating 600 patients that had undergone angiography, where the "standard" anatomy was observed in only 61.3% of cases [5]. He further found that the most common variant was a LHA arising from LGA in 10.7%, a rRHA originated from the SMA in 8.7% of patients and several other variants not mentioned in Michals's study as a CHA directly arose from the aorta, and a "double hepatic" artery, where one or both of the left and the right hepatic arteries originated directly from the aorta or from the celiac artery. Michals's and Covey's studies reflect the wide variability of the hepatic arterial anatomy.

According to Tohma et al. [6], the liver perihilar plexus includes arteries providing a communicating arcade between the right and left hepatic artery, connecting the segment IV branch or the main LHA with the main or anterior trunk of the RHA. Consequently, in cases where branch hepatic arteries are occluded, intrahepatic communications between segments are in existance, providing collateral flow. In studies of Mays and Wheeler in 1974 and Charnsangavej et al. in 1982 interruptions of any major hepatic artery, such as is the RHA or LHA, results in immediate filing via cross collaterals of the occluded branch [7, 8]. To be familiar and to appropriately evaluate these arcades, it is very important to expand options concerning catheter placement for radionuclide infusions [9].

11.2 Extrahepatic Arterial Anatomy: Identification and Treatment

Apart from the intrahepatic collateral vessels that supply arterial flow to tumors across segments or lobes, extrahepatic arteries, termed "parasitized", are found in about 17% of patients, either in cases undergoing chemo-embolization [2] or individuals undergoing radio-embo-lization [10]. Thus, they should be carefully screened in all diagnostic cross-sectional CT or MRI imaging required before treatment. Again, thin-section arterial phase breath-held images yield the useful information. All these variants of the hepatic arterial vasculature have to be identified during hepatic angiography before the PRRT treatment for two main reasons: (a) in case of vascular abnormalities, to prevent inappro-priate placement of the catheter into the hepatic artery, and (b) because if not identified properly may lead to radiopeptide temporary housing in excess amounts and burden the hepatic parenchyma or other neighboring to

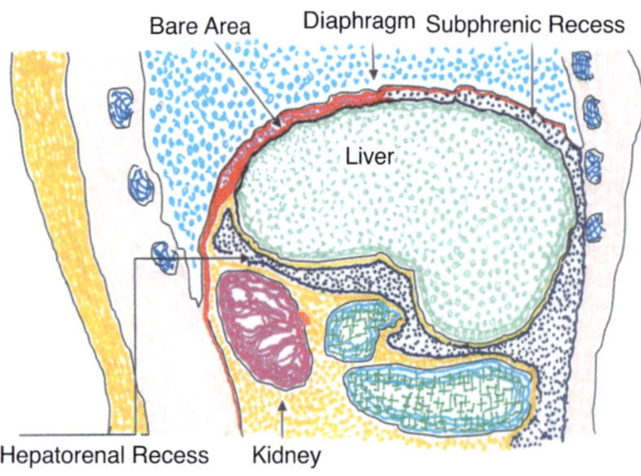

Fig. 11.1 Schematic sagittal section of the abdomen. Bare area in tight proximity to the diaphragm

the liver organs. Superficial [3] or larger than 5 cm size tumors [2] or in contact with the bare area [4] (Fig. 11.1), the right or inferior border of the liver are prone to the aforementioned variants. Angiography is initiated with abdominal aortography with flush-injection of the mid- to lower-thoracic aorta (T8 to T11) to identify any extrahepatic vessel that could supply the liver tumor.

11.3 Conclusion

Variant hepatic arterial anatomy and parasitized extrahepatic arteries can guarantee for an intended sufficient degree of destruction of intrahepatic tumors. The carefully consecutive screening of the arterial extrahepatic anatomy on the course of the initial angiography, performed before each radiopeptide infusion, assesses the therapeutic efficacy of the radiopeptide treatment.

References

1. Michels NA. Newer anatomy of liver and its variant blood supply and collateral circulation. Am J Surg. 1966;112(3):337–47.
2. Chung JW, Kim HC, Yoon JH, et al. Transcatheter arterial chemoembolization of hepatocellular carcinoma: prevalence and causative factors of extrahepatic collateral arteries in 479 patients. Korean J Radiol. 2006;7(4):257–66.
3. Seki H, Kimura M, Yoshimura N, et al. Development of extrahepatic arterial blood supply to the liver during hepatic arterial infusion chemotherapy. Eur Radiol. 1998;8(9):1613–8.
4. Miyayama S, Yamashiro M, Okuda M, et al. The march of extra-hepatic collaterals: analysis of blood supply to hepatocellular imaging and implication for therapy. J Vasc Interv Radiol. 2010;19(10):1490–149.
5. Covey AM, Brody LA, Maluccio MA, et al. Variant hepatic arterial anatomy revisited: digital subtraction angiography performed in 600 patients. Radiology. 2002;224(2):542–7.
6. Tohma T, Cho A, Okazumi S, et al. Communicating arcade between the right and left hepatic arteries: evaluation with CT and angiography during temporary balloon occlusion of the right or left hepatic artery. Radiology. 2005;237(1):361–5.
7. Mays ET, Wheeler CS. Demonstration of collateral arterial flow after interruption of hepatic arteries in man. N Engl J Med. 1974;290(18):993–6.
8. Charnsangavej C, Chuang VP, Wallace S, Soo CS, Bowers T. Angiographic classification of hepatic arterial collaterals. Radiology. 1982;144(3):485–94.
9. Chuang VP, Wallace S. Hepatic arterial redistribution for intraarterial infusion of hepatic neoplasms. Radiology. 1980;135(2):295–9.
10. Abdelmaksoud MHK, Louie JD, Kothary N, et al. Consolidation of hepatic arterial inflow by embolization of variant hepatic arteries in preparation tumors before yttrium-90 radioembolization. J Vasc Interv Radiol. 2011;22(10):1355–62.

Dosimetry and Dose Calculation: Its Necessity in Radiopeptide Therapy

Maria I. Paphiti

Abbreviations

CSDA	Continuous Slowing Down Approximation
CT	Computed Tomography
D	Dimensional
DPK	Dose Point Kernels
DVH	Dose Volume Histograms
EBRT	External Beam Radiation Therapy
EGS	Electron Gamma Shower
i.a	Intra-arterial
i.v.	Intravenous
IC	Internal Conversion
ICRP	International Commission on Radiological Protection
ICRU	International Commission on Radiation Units
LET	Linear Energy Transfer
MC	Monte Carlo
MCNP	Monte Carlo N-Particle Transport code
MIRD	Medical Internal Radiation Dose
MRI	Magnetic Resonance Imaging
OAR	Organs at Risk
p.i.	Post injection
PD	Progression Death
PET	Positron Emission Tomography
PR	Partial Response
PRRT	Peptide Receptor Radionuclide Therapy
R	Range
RBE	Relative Biological Effect
RECIST	Response Evaluation Criteria in Solid Tumors
RILD	Radiation-Induced Liver Disease
ROI	Region of Interest
SD	Stable Disease
SPECT	Single Photon Emission Tomography
$t1/2$	Half-Life
TAC	Time-Activity Curves
TD	Tolerance Doses
US	Ultrasound
VOI	Volume of Interest

12.1 Introduction

Two components relate to the topic of *dosimetry* in radiopeptide therapy (PPRT). *Dose* (Gy) is specifically defined as that energy absorbed in tissue; and *activity* (GBq) is the amount of the isotope delivered to the target organ. Radiopeptide *infusion*, as a radio-molecular therapy, can be considered as low-dose rate brachytherapy and at the present time is best described by the Committee on Medical Internal Radiation Dose (MIRD) which is a committee within the Society of Nuclear Medicine. The infusion of high activities of $[^{111}In]$ In$^+$ octreotide

M. I. Paphiti (✉)
National Health System, Athens, Greece

© Springer Nature Switzerland AG 2021
G. S. Limouris (ed.), *Liver Intra-arterial PRRT with ^{111}In-Octreotide*,
https://doi.org/10.1007/978-3-030-70773-6_12

to the liver neuroendocrine lesions after catheterization of the hepatic artery requires experience and knowledge of many factors. More important is to find a way of achieving an adequate long normal liver function, optimizing kidney protection, and avoiding the development of any myelodysplastic or myelo-hyperplastic syndromes. This is difficult with any treatment involving radiation, and strict clinical protocols should be followed, with careful control of the maximum tolerance dose at each organ. Chemotherapy, as a long-term alternative therapy, has demonstrated mediocre results to the lesions with severe side effects. Unfortunately, no single laboratory test is considered as a sensitive valid index of liver function. Surrogates include nonspecific liver enzymes, transaminases, and bilirubin levels. The liver's complex and varied functions are a challenge for the clinician as they strive to assess the risk of a liver burden and determine the suitability of each patient separately for this type of therapy. Clinical experience with nonradioactive arterial-based therapy has established patient selection criteria attempting to minimize side effects that might be likely to result. Although these guidelines might be a helpful point for these intra-arterial radiopeptide infusion schemes, they represent in some way stringent standards based on the injected activity per session, the pharmacokinetics related to the intrahepatic arterial net pattern, and the neo-angiogenesis extension.

12.2 Liver Tolerance to Ionizing Radiation

Nearly all experimental and clinical data up to date have been based on external beam radiation. Even animal models are not optimal surrogates for human hepatic radiation response. Whole liver radiation by external beam causes radiation-induced liver disease (RILD) in 5–10% of patients [1–3]. RILD is a clinical syndrome of anicteric hepatomegaly, ascites, and elevated liver enzymes (especially alkaline phosphatase) which occurs usually from 2 weeks up to 90 days post radiotherapy.

Preexisting liver disease may render patients more susceptible to RILD, and for those patients the mean liver dose should be ≤ 28 Gy, a figure quite similar to the published tolerance doses (TD) by Emami et al. in 1991 [4], suggesting a 5% probability in 5 years [$TD_{5/5}$ (Gy)] of liver failure at 30 Gy, whereas at 40 Gys the probability is 50% in 5 years' time [$TD_{5/5}$ (Gy)].

Observations for liver tolerance in nuclear medicine have been noted in preclinical studies employing animal models, by various infusion methods (vein, heart aorta, hepatic artery and portal vein) with and without liver tumors in order to study radiopeptide infusion to normal and tumor tissue. Common observation point, in animal and humans, confirmed that arterial infusion of radiopeptide is distributed according to the somatostatin tissue density in rather uniform homogeneity.

12.2.1 Neuroendocrine Tumor Imaging

Hepatocellular carcinoma is a major cause of death. Gastro-hepatic neuroendocrine tumors (NETs) are a heterogeneous group of neoplasms with different degrees of malignancy. Reubi et al. [5] demonstrated in 1985 the presence of receptors for the somatostatin on the surface of intestinal NET cells. This finding was initiated for the identification of the mechanism of action of octreotide. Reubi's team coupled this analog to the iodine isotope [^{125}I] I, but, later, in 1990 Krenning's team in cooperation with colleagues at Sandoz Research Institute developed [^{111}In]In-pentetreotide (OctreoScan, Mallinckrodt). In 1993 Krenning et al. [6] published the data "… The Rotterdam experience with more than 1000 patients…" and in 1994 FDA approved [^{111}In] In-pentetreotide as an imaging radiopharmaceutical.

12.2.2 Hepatic Cancer, "Aretaieion" Protocol

In recent years, the introduction of [^{111}In] In-pentetreotide, peptide-based radiopharmaceutical, started a new era "from bench to bedside" to treat NETs with radiolabeled peptides. A variety of radionuclides ($[^{111}In]In$, $[^{137}Lu]Lu$, $[^{90}Y]Y$, $[^{166}Ho]Ho$, $[^{188}Re]Re$) have been explored by binding them with peptides such as DOTA-TATE, DOTA-TOC, DOTA-NOC, DOTA-LAN, etc. by employing different administration routes (i.v., i.a.) or even more, intra-arterially by radioembolization with $[^{90}Y]Y$-, $[^{166}Ho]Ho$-, or $[^{188}Re]$ Re-labeled microspheres [7]. According to Limouris et al. ("Aretaieion" protocol) [8, 9], $[^{111}In]In$-DTPA-Phe1-octreotide has been administered intra-arterially based on the fact that since the liver has double blood supply (portal vein and hepatic artery), tumors receive blood supply primarily from the arterial hepatic than the portal circulation. Injection via the hepatic artery allows preferential delivery of therapeutic radionuclides, but, such a procedure requires interventional radiology, as this activity must be administered directly into the common, left, or right hepatic artery with the help of an angiographic catheter under radiological control. Sufficient delivery of high activities straight to the tumor may be achieved by that way, offering a great advantage of high tumor uptake with less perfusion in healthy tissues.

12.3 Peptide Receptor Radionuclide Therapy (PRRT)

Peptide receptor radionuclide therapy (PRRT) is a site-directed target therapeutic strategy that specifically employs radiolabeled peptides as biological targeting vectors designed to deliver radiation doses to cancer cells, which overexpress specific receptors. Peptides are characterized by their small size and low molecular weight (compared to proteins or antibodies) achieving rapid penetration into target tissues, and by their low molecular weight they accomplish consequently, rapid diffusion into target tissue. Upon binding with the radioligand, they internalized, resulting in long retention in tumor cells, permitting thereafter the emission of ionizing radiation, from the attached radionuclide, destroying thus

selectively and simultaneously all the whole-body metastases.

Criteria for successful use of radiolabeled peptides are:

- High target specificity
- High binding affinity
- Long metabolic stability
- High target to background ratio

12.3.1 Radionuclide Selection

The success of PRRT relies on the selection of the appropriate radionuclide, which is based on several considerations as the following:

1. Particle-emitting radionuclides, such as α-particles, radionuclides that emit Auger, conversion electrons, or β's, are suitable for radionuclide therapy due to their high energy transfer (LET) within a small volume.
2. The choice of emission type depends on the size of the tumor to be treated and the degree of heterogeneity in order to figure out the intra-tumoral distribution of radionuclide.
3. The physical half-life of the radionuclide should be matched with peptides' pharmacokinetics in order to be long enough for tumor irradiation during the time of peptides' bio-localization within tumor.
4. Energy of emission: The LET of α-particles is $\approx 80\ keV/\mu m$, whereas for β^- particle emitters, it is $0.2\ keV/\mu m$ and consequently alphas may produce lethal damage to cancer cells. The clinical application of β^- particles is dependent on their energy; low-energy β's are suitable for medium to large homogeneous tumors, whereas the high energy ones are preferred for large heterogeneous tumors.
5. Specific activity is another important parameter to consider for radionuclide selection. For effective and efficient radiolabeling, high specific activity is needed for the radionuclide.
6. The radionuclide should be available with high purity, non-carrier added, i.e., free from any contaminants.

Table 12.1 Therapeutic radionuclide characteristics according to emission type, energy, range, etc.

Characteristics	Alpha decay	Beta decay	Low-energy electron decay
Emission	α-particles	β-particles	Auger, Coster-Kronig electrons
Energy	2–10 MeV	0.05–2.5 MeV	10 eV–10 keV
Range	50–100 μm	0.2–15 mm	2 nm–0.5 μm
Path track	Straight	Tortuous	Contorted
Ionizations	Dense	Less dense	Relatively dense in vicinity area
LET	80–300 keV/μm	0.2 keV/μm	4–26 keV/μm
Mechanism	In the cell nuclei, oxygen independent	Cross-fire effect, many cells, oxygen dependent	Breaks in DNA strands, bystander effect
RBE	High	Low	Low
Necessity	Binding to cancer cell	Close to target/cell surface	Incorporation into nucleus
Cross-fire effect	No	Yes	No

7. In order to proceed for dosimetry applications, the radionuclide should have a γ-emission in order to acquire scintigraphic images. High-energy β's may produce a bremsstrahlung image, but for low-energy β's, that is not possible.
8. Low cost of the radionuclide is always desirable.

Table 12.1 summarizes radionuclide characteristics promoting for therapy applications. (Data from Dash A et al. 2015 [10].)

Some up-to-date suitable radionuclides for PRRT are [^{111}In]In, [^{90}Y]Y, [^{177}Lu]Lu, and [$^{186/188}$Re]Re. Obviously, the list of therapeutic radionuclides is longer considering those β emitters for bone pain palliation, such as [^{32}P]P, [^{89}Sr]Sr, [$^{186/188}$Re]Re, [^{153}Sm]Sm, [^{223}Ra]Ra, etc.

12.4 Indium-111 as a Therapeutic Isotope

12.4.1 Indium-111 Properties

[^{111}In]In$^+$ is an electron capture nuclide, i.e., it does not emit a beta particle but instead captures one of the orbital electrons (usually the K electron, the Kronig-Auger) in the indium atom. Following the capture of this electron, the resulting cadmium nucleus is left in an excited state and immediately rids itself of this excess energy by emitting gamma ray photons with energies of 173 and 245 keV, and x-ray photons of energy approximately 23 keV, as a result from the de-excitation of the daughter cadmium atom. In a small percentage of disintegrations, the cadmium-111 nucleus uses its excess energy to eject an orbital electron from the atom; this is called an internal conversion (IC) electron, and, it emerges from the atom with kinetic energy equal to the original energy of the photon minus the binding energy of the electron in the atom.

The transformation process may be written as

$$^{111}_{49}\text{In} + e \rightarrow {}^{111}_{48}\text{Cd} + \gamma$$

(see Table 12.2, data from http://www.nucleide.org/DDEP_WG/DDEPdata.htm) [11].

The range for electrons with $E = (0.25–100)$ KeV has been calculated using Cole's equation [12] R (μm) $= 0.043 (E + 0.367)^{1.77}–0.007$

For electrons with $E = (0.5–2.5)$ MeV calculations based on [13] to equation

R (mm) $= 2.4E + 2.86 E^2 - 0.14$

12.4.2 Production of Carrier-Free [^{111}In] In$^+$

[^{111}In]In$^+$ is a cyclotron-produced radionuclide and it can be produced via nuclear reactions such as

Table 12.2 The properties of emitted radiation during the decay of indium-111

$T1/2$ phys	Type of decay	Emissions	Energy (KeV)	Range in tissue
2.83 days	Electron capture (100%)	γ	$E\gamma$: 173 (87%), 247 (94%)	
		e - Auger	E_{Auger}: 0.5–25 (95%)	R_{max}: 0.02–13 µm
		e - IC	E_{ic}: 144 (10%) 245 (6%)	R_{max}: 200–620 µm

$$Cd\left(p,n\right)^{111} In, Cd\left(d,2n\right)^{111} In, and\, ^{109}Ag\left(\alpha,2n\right)^{111} In$$

The production yield of ^{111}In from the nuclear reaction on silver is much lower than that from the irradiation of cadmium targets with protons, and both cadmium reactions remain the most widely used for ^{111}In production methods.

However, activity at the end of bombardment contains undesirable radionuclide contaminants such as ^{109}In ($t1/2 = 4.3$ h), ^{110m}In ($t1/2 = 4.9$ h), and ^{114m}In ($t1/2 = 49$ days) that are not possible to spare from ^{111}In due to their similar chemical characteristics. The first two radionuclides of indium have a relatively short half-life, and hence cooling for 24 h after the end of bombardment will reduce their contaminants.

Alternative, ^{111}In obtained from irradiation of a natural silver target with an energetic α-beam is free from the long lived ^{114m}In ($T1/2 = 49.5$ days), which emits high energy gamma radiation. Radiochemical separation of ^{111}In from the irradiated target can be performed by various techniques such as coprecipitation with Fe (OH)$_3$ or La (OH)$_3$, ion exchange, and extraction chromatography. Each of these techniques has its own advantages and disadvantages. Liquid extraction and ion exchange chromatography are widely used for radiochemical separation of ^{111}In on the commercial scale. However, despite the development of robust separation and purification technology, low production yields are major impediment concerning large-scale production of ^{111}In [14].

12.4.3 ^{111}In-DTPA-Phe-Octreotide

^{111}In-DTPA-Phe1-octreotide was the first approved radiopharmaceutical (introduced by Mallinckrodt Pharmaceuticals, plc) for diagnostic imaging of somatostatin receptor (sstr)-positive tumors. In 1994, Eric Krenning and Dik Kwekkeboom [15] first implemented ^{111}In-DTPA-Phe1-octreotide in peptide receptor radionuclide therapies (PRRT) taking advantage of the specific characteristics of the Auger and conversion electron emission of ^{111}In. Three years later Limouris et al. [8] first introduced the use of ^{111}In-DTPA-Phe-octreotide after permission of the Scientific and Ethical Committee of the "Aretaieion" University Hospital of the National and Kapodistrian University Medical School in Athens, routinely as first-line therapy (a treatment scheme that only lately in 2017, by Strosberg et al. and for Netter-1 project with ^{177}Lu-Dotatate [16], was officially established) in high doses for the treatment of patients with liver metastasized neuroendocrine tumors. This scientific procedure was encouraging regarding symptom relief but, for tumor size shrinkage, was mainly successful for small-diameter liver lesions. The recommended administered activity ranged from 110 mCi (4.07 GBq) to 160 mCi (5.920 GBq), and the whole scheme of therapy was given up to 12 cycles. Major drawback of ^{111}In-coupled peptides is the limited range of Auger electrons and consequently their short tissue penetration (~10 µm). By replacing Phe3 with Tyr^3 in the octapeptide sequence, its receptor affinity was improved, and by replacing in turn DTPA with DOTA, the radionuclide chelator stability strengthened.

12.5 Internal Dosimetry

12.5.1 The Basics of Internal Dosimetry

The basic physical quantity to study ionization radiation effects to biological tissues is the *absorbed dose*, D, which is defined as the mean energy imparted $d\varepsilon$ into a volume of tissue with mass dm, that is,

$$D = \frac{d\varepsilon}{dm}$$

The unit of measure for absorbed dose is JKg^{-1} in base units and in International System of Units, it is known as Gray (Gy) ($1\ JKg^{-1} = 1$ Gy).

The mean absorbed dose to an organ from an internally administered radiopharmaceutical is dependent on the characteristics of both the radionuclide and the pharmaceutical itself in terms of the type of radiation emitted as well as the spatial and temporal distribution of the radionuclide within the body.

In other words, the absorbed dose rate can be described by

$$\dot{D} = \frac{kA \sum_i n_i E_i \Phi_i}{m}$$

where $\dot{D}$ is the absorbed dose rate (Gy/s), A is the activity (MBq), n is the number of radiations with energy E emitted per nuclear transition, E is the energy per radiation (MeV), Φ is the fraction of energy emitted from the source that is absorbed in the target and equals from zero up to one (0–1), m is the mass of the target (g or Kg), and k is a kind of proportionality constant (Gy-Kg/MBq-s-MeV).

Hint 1. Absorbed dose rate is more familiar to radiotherapy applications than to internal dosimetry. In radiomolecular radiotherapy the dose rate is not constant during the session but rises from zero up to a maximum point and drops slowly back to an almost zero level. Radiation distributions irradiate simultaneously all the tumor sites from hours up to several days.

Hint 2. Both of them, either internal or external radiation therapy, are interested to find out the relationship between the absorbed dose and the biological effect.

Hint 3. In internal dosimetry, cumulated dose and cumulated activity over a time period are more appropriate as terms for calculating the absorbed dose in a source target.

$$D = \frac{k\tilde{A} \sum_i n_i E_i \Phi_i}{m}$$

D is the absorbed dose and $\tilde{A}$ is the cumulated activity.

In order to measure the distribution of the radiopharmaceutical in vivo and derive the absorbed dose to different organs and tumors, the following methodologies have been developed, each of them having its own assumptions, advantages, and drawbacks.

12.5.2 Method 1: The MIRD Formalism and *S* Values

The Medical Internal Radiation Dose Committee (MIRD) of the Society of Nuclear Medicine has tried to establish a common nomenclature in the calculus process of absorbed dose estimation from internal emitters. From 1968, following the MIRD PRIMER [17], where the MIRD schema was published in a didactic form, and up-to-date, MIRD formalism is the most widely accepted one for internal dose calculations, with several revisions published in a series of pamphlets numbered from MIRD No.1 [18] up to MIRD No.26. According to MIRD the mean absorbed dose $\bar{D}$ (Gy) can be calculated from the equation

$$\bar{D} = \tilde{A} \cdot S$$

where $\tilde{A}$ is the cumulated activity (MBq s), expressing the total number of decays during a specific time interval taken place within the organ,

$$\tilde{A} = \int_0^t A(t)\,dt$$

and *or S − value* is the other important parameter of the MIRD scheme: it carries information about the way energy is transferred to an organ, and it is related to the nuclei as well as to the geometry of the system (i.e., source-target organ). The equation for *S − factor* becomes

$$S = \frac{k\tilde{A}\sum_i n_i E_i \Phi_t}{m}$$

12.5.2.1 The Cumulated Activity $\tilde{A}$ and Effective Half Time t_e

The meaning of cumulated activity in a source is in fact the number of decays in the source over a certain time and thus activity A is expressed by

$$A(t) = A_0\, e^{-\lambda t}$$

Here, A_0 is the initial activity, A is the activity over a period (t), and λ is the decay constant.

In the case of administration of radiopharmaceutical in the body, a certain amount of radioactivity could be removed by a first-order exponential decay, and two parameters should be considered in mind: the radioactive decay constant λ and the biological disappearance of activity λ_b

The radioactive decay constant λ is in other words the physical decay constant λ_p, and for the complete activity disappearance both the two components are added to give the effective disappearance constant, λ_e

$$\lambda_e = \lambda_p + \lambda_b$$

And the effective half time could be estimated by

$$t_e = \frac{t_p \times t_b}{t_p + t_b}$$

In conclusion cumulated activity could be evaluated form the time-activity curves (TAC)

$$\tilde{A} = \int_0^\infty A(t)\, dt = \int_0^\infty (f\, A_0)\, e^{\lambda_e}\, dt = \frac{(fA_0)}{\lambda_e} = 1.443\, fA_0$$

t_e where f is the absorbed fraction in a source region or in other words it is the uptake fraction.

S Value

The absorbed dose rate per unit activity, the S value, could be defined by summing all the energy emissions **i** of the relevant isotope's nuclear decay chart

$$S(r_k \leftarrow r_h) = \frac{k\sum_i n_i E_i \Phi_t (r_k \leftarrow h)}{m_h}$$

where $\Phi = 1$ for non-penetrating emissions such as electrons and alphas and for penetrating, i.e., photons $\Phi = 0$, $k = 2.13$ the proportionality constant, and m_h the source mass.

The dose to target organ r_k from a source organ r_h can be written in the form of $\overline{D}(r_k \leftarrow r_h) = \tilde{A} \bullet S(r_k \leftarrow r_h)$ and for multiple sources the dose to the same target may be calculated by summing the dose from each separate source organ and thus,

$$\overline{D}(r_i) = \sum_h \tilde{A}_h\, S(r_k \leftarrow r_h)$$

In consequence, S value (or S factor) is simply the absorbed dose conversion factor (Gy MBq^{-1} s^{-1}), and generally such factors have been calculated, by many scientists, from geometrical models using Monte Carlo simulations for a variety of nuclei and source-target organs [19–24]. Specifically, MIRD Pamphlets 5 and 11, respectively [25, 26], published S values for a model of reference man for 117 radionuclides including combinations of 25 source and target regions, whereas each organ is considered as both "a target" and "a source." Additionally S value tables could be found in the OLINDA/EXM software [27] and on the RADAR web site (www.doseinfo-radar.com) [28]. Bolch W E et al., in 1999, presented in MIRD Pamphlet 17 "the dosimetry of nonuniform activity distributions—radionuclide S values at the voxel level." [29]

Later, it became a necessity for a common nomenclature, so the MIRD committee published in 2009 the MIRD Pamphlet No. 21: "A generalized schema for radiopharmaceutical dosimetry-standardization of nomenclature" by Bolch WE et al. [30]

OLINDA/EXM: Organ Level Internal Dose Assessment/exponential modelling. It is a software for the calculation of absorbed dose to different organs in the body, being MIRDOSE [31] its predecessor.

Hint 1. The principle of reciprocity law holds in S value tables, and it is approximately the same for a given combination of source and target regions.

$$S\left(r_k \leftarrow r_h\right) \approx S\left(r_h \leftarrow r_k\right)$$

Although this is valid only under ideal conditions for regions with a uniform distribution of radionuclide, within a material that is infinite and homogeneous or absorbs the radiation without scatter, the reciprocity principle holds in S value tables for human phantoms.

Hint 2. It is to notice that the tabulations of S factors are in relation to the reference man. In order to adjust these values to the true specific data of any patient, measurements by the help of

CT, MRI, or US could be proceeded and S factors could be scaled by mass according to

$$S_{\text{patient}} \approx S_{\text{reference}} \frac{m_{\text{reference target organ}}}{m_{\text{patients target organ}}}$$

This linear scaling holds for α- and β–particles since the absorbed fraction for such emissions and self-irradiation equals to 1.0.

Hint 3. The validity of the previous assumptions is dependent on the energy of the radiation in relation to the source size and mass. According to Siegel JA and Stabin MG (1994) [32] in beta-particle emitters with average energy greater than 0.5 MeV, in spheres having masses less than 10 g, the absorbed fraction drops below 0.9, indicating that the error will be no greater than 10% without the correction for larger spheres or lower energies. For average electron energies the absorbed fraction for spheres with intermediate size, more than 10gr, the approximation is also valid and linear interpolation could be applied in the tables of absorbed fraction over the matrix of energies and sphere sizes, with reasonable values.

Hint 4. For photons, the absorbed fraction is less than 0.1 for sphere masses less than 100 g and energy more than 50 keV; as the mass increases this approximation is no more valid [33]. Linear interpolations of S factor tables could not be applied for photons. In MIRD Pamphlet No.11 [26], Snyder showed that for the case of self-irradiation (i.e., source and target is the same organ), the absorbed dose for photons will vary according to $m^{2/3}$ where m is the mass for the target organ and the scaling is becoming,

$$S_{\text{patient}} \approx S_{\text{reference}} \left[\frac{m_{\text{reference target organ}}}{m_{\text{patients target organ}}}\right]^{2/3}$$

12.5.2.2 The Residence Time τ

Another quantity used in MIRD methodology is the residence time, τ, which could be defined from the quotient of cumulated activity over the initial activity,

$\tau = \dfrac{\tilde{A}}{A_0}$ and thus, the dose equation could be expressed as

$$D = \tilde{A}\,S = A_0\,\tau\,S$$

But cumulated activity is $\tilde{A} = 1.443\,fA_0\,t_e$ and therefore, the residence time is calculated from the equation,

$$\tau = 1.443\,f\,t_e$$

Both cumulated activity and residence time are calculated from time-activity curves.

12.5.3 Method 2: Dose Voxel Kernel Dosimetry

Although many studies have been developed to validate and improve quantification with planar imaging, it was a necessity for the MIRD schema to be extended in order to consider nonuniform source distributions. A new era of hybrid equipment such as SPECT/CT, PET/CT, and PET/MRI has been developed offering 3D visualization of the internal structures of the body. Medical images could be stored and digitized providing thus a direct realistic way of describing the human anatomy. Moreover, different approaches for data simulation and quantification have been developed, and medical image data could be converted to voxel, and MIRD Pamphlet No. 17 [29] became thereafter a continuity to introduce voxel dosimetry allowing dosimetry calculations at the voxel level. The cumulative activity could be defined at the voxel level and derived from patient-specific SPECT or PET image data. In the same pamphlet, Bolch describes the MIRD schema in a 3D mode by introducing three principal methods for handling nonuniform dosimetry at the voxel level:

- Dose point kernels
- Application of direct Monte Carlo radiation transport
- Voxel S value approach

12.5.3.1 Dose Point Kernels

A dose point kernel (DPK) is defined as the radial distribution of absorbed dose around an isotropic point source in an infinite homogeneous propagation medium. DPKs for monoenergetic electrons have been calculated analytically in the Continuous Slowing Down Approximation (CSDA) by Berger MJ 1971 MIRD Pamphlet No. 7 [34] and later by Monte Carlo technique (Berger 1973) [35].

DPKs for electrons and photons can be used to produce 3D-absorbed dose distributions from cumulated activity maps. This requires the integration of kernels over the voxel geometry defined by the cumulated activity map available.

12.5.3.2 The Voxel S Value Approach

This approach allows the application of the MRD formalism in order to quantify nonuniform distributions of activity within target and source organs. The absorbed dose to a target voxel vox_k due to the cumulated activities in source voxels vox_h can be expressed as:

$$\bar{D}_{vox} = \sum_{h=0}^{N} \tilde{A}_{vox}\, S\left(vox_k \leftarrow vox_h\right) \text{ where } \quad \text{the}$$

sum is extended to all source voxels. The voxel S value is defined as the absorbed dose to the target voxel per unit decay in the source voxel, whence both are contained in an infinite homogeneous medium.

In analogy to S *value* in the MIRD scheme, voxel S *values* can be calculated using direct Monte Carlo radiation transport simulations, and such tabulations are available only for a limited number of radionuclides and voxel dimensions.

Even more, 3D dose distributions of mean absorbed dose per voxel allow the creation of iso-dose lines and dose volume histograms (DVHs) in the region of the organ of interest (something similar and familiar in external beam radiotherapy) which is very important for radiobiological assessment of the therapy treatment. At the time, several scientists (Bolch et al. 1999 in MIRD 17 [29], Lanconelli et al. 2012 [36], Amato et al. 2013 [37]) have published tabulations of voxel *S values* for most radionuclides commonly used in radiomolecular therapy and few voxel sizes.

> - There are two types of DVHs, the differential DVH and the cumulative DVH. Both are basic concepts from external beam radiotherapy.
> - Differential DVH: shows the %volume that has received a certain absorbed dose as a function of the fractionated absorbed dose.
> - Cumulative DVH: shows the %volume that has received an absorbed dose less than the figure given on the horizontal *x*-axis.
> - DVHs clinically usually include all structures and targets of interest in the radiotherapy plan and might be assist a correlation between absorbed dose and biological effect.

12.5.4 Method 3: Monte Carlo

In principle, the most accurate dosimetry can be obtained by performing a full MC (Monte Carlo) radiation transport program in voxel geometries considering patient-specific anatomy and radiopharmaceutical distribution in 3D images. This kind of calculations is based in fact on the acquisition of 3D voxel images from SPECT/CT or PET/CT systems describing both tissue density and radioactivity heterogeneity. Typically, the radioactivity distribution is assessed at different times in order to obtain time-activity curves (either at the voxel or at the organ level) that are employed to build a cumulated activity voxel image. This image acts as an emission probability chart for the definition of virtual voxel sources in the Monte Carlo simulation: homogeneously distributed, isotropic radioactive sources in each voxel. For each radionuclide decay chart, a transport code is created taking into account all possible interactions of the emitted radiation (electrons, photons, bremsstrahlung, and α-particles) within the transmitted medium such as scattering, absorption, and cross fire effect; the interactions between the various tissues are simulated as well as their path lengths through the different materials. In overall the main strength of MC simulations, the accuracy, is becoming through all these estimations of interactions between all various tissue types on the specific patient data. May be it's difficult and labyrinthine, may be it's not yet applicable for routine work, but it's the actual absorbed dose and codes such as EGSnrc (Kawrakow and Rogers 2003 [38]), MCNPX (Briesmeister 2000 [39]), Geant4 from CERN (European Organization for Nuclear Research) (Agostinelli et al. 2003 [40]), and GATE that are being increasingly used and trusted more and more by medical physicists.

12.5.5 Strengths and Limitations of the Dosimetry Methods

The MIRD formalism is based on the use of radionuclide-specific S values defined as the mean absorbed dose to a target organ per radioactive decay in a source organ. The use of standard anatomic models and S values at the organ level is the major limitation of this approach. Analytical models for adult man, nonpregnant female, pregnant woman for each trimester of pregnancy, and children (from the newborn and up to 15 years) as well as models of the brain and kidneys and unit density spheres exist, but tumor dosimetry is not included in all these models. However these drawbacks, the main advantage of this methodology relies on the simplicity and acceptance for most clinical applications.

The voxel S value approach provides a tool for fast calculation of the absorbed dose on a voxel level. Drawback of this method is that a DPK is only valid in a homogeneous medium, where it is commonly assumed that the body consists of uniform soft tissue density.

The Monte Carlo method offers accuracy of measurements with too many simulations but its good from time to time to run such code in order to validate the dosimetry work (Table 12.3).

12.5.6 Problems and Uncertainties

Absorbed dose calculations according to MIRD are depending on quantification of activity A and the S value. Activity measurements rely upon measurements from scintigraphic, planar, and/or tomographic data on a certain area, regions of interest (ROIs), or volumes of interest (VOIs), respectively. On the other hand, S value comes from simulating data, such as from models that approximately estimate any region of interest or organ.

Human models, however, are based on standardized phantoms according to ICRP 89 reference man adult/female at different ages (see appendix ICRP models), but in fact, there is a discrepancy between the actual body geometry of the patient and that of the model, resulting in inaccuracies of the absorbed dose calculation; what about the overweight or slim patient? How realistic are these models? So, in order to have greater accuracy in dosimetry calculations and not an overall estimation, the model should be more detailed and realistic.

Hint: Nowadays, by the help of hybrid imaging, voxel-based phantoms have been developed, offering the opportunity for more detailed models of patient anatomy (Fig. 12.1).

As might be expected, practical applications introduce several uncertainties [41] and errors that need to be accounted in order to extract accurate quantitative information, and these are related with:

1. *The physical principles associated with the detection (attenuation, scatter):* One of the major quantification problems with planar scintillation cameras relies between the detected count rate and activity measurements. The absorption of photons in the patient (atten-

Table 12.3 Lists the assumptions, strengths, and limitations that identify the three dosimetry methods

Dosimetry methods	Assumptions	Strengths	Limitations
MIRD formalism	Uniform activity distributions in the source region	Simple and easy to use for organ and lesion dosimetry without superposition	Absorbed dose may vary throughout the region
	Homogeneity of densities in source and target regions	Commonly accepted in most clinical and therapy applications	Does not consider patient-specific data
	Calculation of the mean absorbed dose to the target region		
Voxel S value	Uniform activity distributions within the voxel	3D distributions no superposition problem	Calculations of S value for each radionuclide and voxel dimensions
	Homogeneous medium of soft tissue	Isodose lines, DVHs	
Monte Carlo	TACs from SPECT/PET	Accuracy	Many simulations
	Density heterogeneity from CT	Measurements include heterogeneity and cross fire effect	Time-consuming

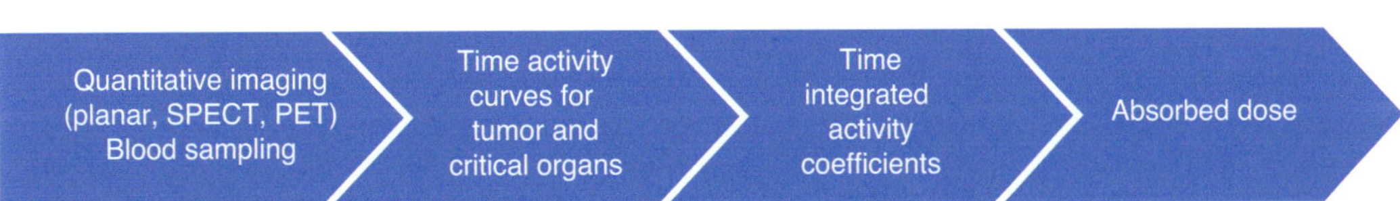

Fig. 12.1 Flow chart indicating the stages up to calculate absorbed dose

uation) reduces the expected number of detected events whereas there's always a part of scattered photons from the patient, with enough energy accepted by the energy window, resulting to an image with poor spatial resolution. Additionally, detection problems are associated with photons coming from overlapping tissues and from septal penetration by high-energy radionuclides such as in the case of ^{90}Y (due to bremsstrahlung radiation). All these difficulties are valid for both planar and SPECT imaging, except the problem of overlapping tissues which is greatly reduced in SPECT, and the organ activity that could be more accurately determined.

2. *The performance of the imaging systems (resolution, dead time)*: With PRRT the acquired imaging during the ongoing therapy is related with patients receiving high administered activities. The performance of the camera regarding the count rate and resolution is important. If large count losses occur due to dead time, etc., the scaling from counts to activity by the calibration factor will underestimate the activity and thereby the absorbed dose calculation.

3. *The acquisition protocols (patient's respiratory and movement problems)*: For both planar and SPECT cameras, the setup of the acquisition protocol is important because all images for dosimetry rely on the good quality of acquired data. However, the total acquisition time is quite limited by the time that a patient may stay comfortably immobilized, introducing thus movement and respiratory artifacts. Particularly for SPECT, the acquisition setup requires a sufficient number of projections so as to avoid reconstruction artifacts due to non-circular angular sampling.

4. *Post-processing errors (registration, segmentation, ROIs, TAC fitting)*: Multiple image acquisitions of the patient are needed for quantification, but patient position may differ at each time of measurement. The purpose of image registration is to transform the sequence of these images geometrically so that in the end, the pixel values in each of the images are associated with the same position in the patient. Although this is difficult, sometimes it might be helpful to remember the external beam radiation therapy techniques (EBRT) such as lasers, etc. Background-corrected ROIs should be drawn and copied for all images. The amount and rates of radiopharmaceutical uptake and excretion for an individualized treatment need to be determined for each patient by the help of TACs for different organs and tissues at several time points post administration. The number of measurements for the TACs is of importance to catch up the peak (max value of activity accumulation) as well as the excretion rate. Data points should be followed for at least three effective half-lives.

5. *Absorbed dose calculations (human dosimetric models are of average size, although there are age- and sex-specific models available)*: The general way of calculating the absorbed dose from planar images is to use organ-based S values multiplied by the time-integrated activity obtained from the TAC. The most used S values are those derived from the Cristy-Eckerman phantom [42], also included in the OLINDA software and online from the Radar web site. For patient-specific dosimetry, these phantoms should be used with caution since they represent a reference of an "average" male, female, or young person. Nevertheless, for individual patient, scaling of these S values can be obtained knowing the individual organ masses (Fig. 12.2).

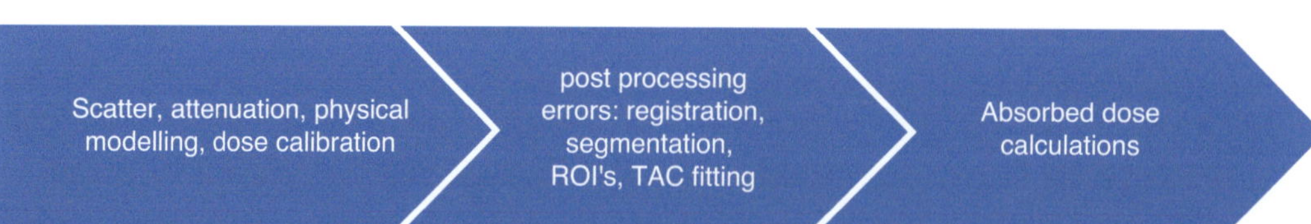

Fig. 12.2 Flow diagram including difficulties during dosimetry procedures

12.5.7 Internal Dosimetry in Clinical Practice

12.5.7.1 Dosimetry on an Organ Level

Dosimetry on an organ level is accessible by activity quantification of sequential 2D or 3D imaging.

Planar Scintigraphy: Conjugate View Method

Following the MIRD 16 scheme [43] the first step for an organ dosimetry is to estimate the cumulated activity by measuring the organ activity at different time points: by taking both anterior and posterior images and combining them with a geometrical mean, the so-called conjugate view images. Cumulated activity could be obtained by the following equation:

$$A = \frac{1}{K} \sqrt{\frac{C_A C_p}{e^{-\mu L}}} \frac{(\mu.l/2)}{\sinh(\mu.l/2)}$$

where:

$C_A C_p$ are the measured tumor counts over a period in a region of interest (ROI) in the anterior and posterior images respectively.

K is the calibration factor which converts counts to activity (cps MBq^{-1}).

T is the patient thickness over the ROI.

l is the source thickness.

μ is the effective attenuation coefficient for the employed radionuclide, camera, and collimator.

The expression $e^{-\mu L}$ is in fact the transmission factor across the patient thickness T through the ROI.

This method in theory is independent of the source depth and gives a reasonable dose estimate for those large organs without position overlapping and background activity. The main limitations of this method are the organ-organ or organ-background overlap in the projections which may lead to errors in the activity estimation for the OAR. In order for this method to be valid, additional corrections should be included such as correction for scatter, background, and overlapping organs.

Table 12.4 Examples of self S factors for In-111 vs tumor mass

Tumor ϕ (cm)	Tumor mass (g)	Self S factors (mGy/MBq-s)
1.23	1	6.31E − 3
1.54	2	3.25 E − 3
1.94	4	1.71 E − 3
2.22	6	1.17 E − 3
2.45	8	8.97 E − 3
2.64	10	7.23 E − 3
3.32	20	3.89 E − 3
4.18	40	2.10 E − 3

Tumor dosimetry is possible and S values for unit density spheres could be applied for the calculation of the self-absorbed dose to the tumor.

The drawback is that neither the contribution from the cross-absorbed dose from activity of nearby organs to the tumor nor the cross-absorbed dose from activity in the tumor to normal organs can be included in the calculations so we may consider them as "self S factors" and the absorbed dose as "self-absorbed dose."

Table 12.4 represents examples of "self S factors" for ^{111}In nuclide in relation to tumor mass (g) and diameter (cm). Tumors are simulated as spheres of various masses composed of homogeneous soft tissue with uniform distribution of radiopharmaceutical, and such self S factors are available from OLINDA/EXM software [27].

However, sometimes a tumor can be imaged only in one view anterior or posterior, such as a superficial tumor with poor uptake or high background activity. Automatically we cannot speak about a geometric mean of count rate. An approximate solution for these cases is given by the single effective point source method, and the activity is given by

$$A = C_x \, e^{\mu d} \, F / K$$

where C_x is the count rate from anterior or posterior view, K is the system calibration factor, and F is the background correction coefficient (Buijs WC et al. 1998) [44] which depends on organ and body thickness

$$F = 1 - (l/T)$$

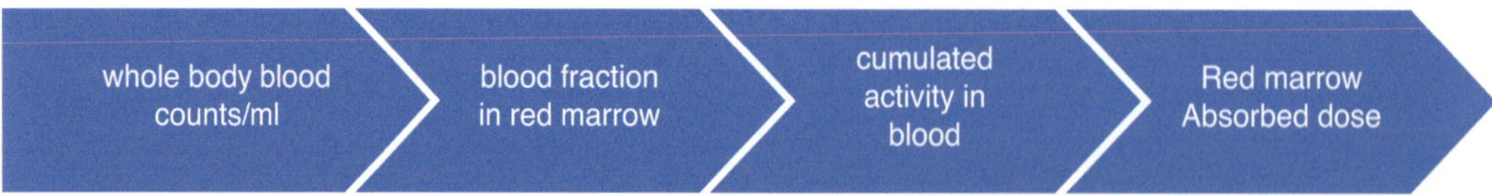

Fig. 12.3 Scheme of stages for red marrow absorbed dose calculation from blood sampling

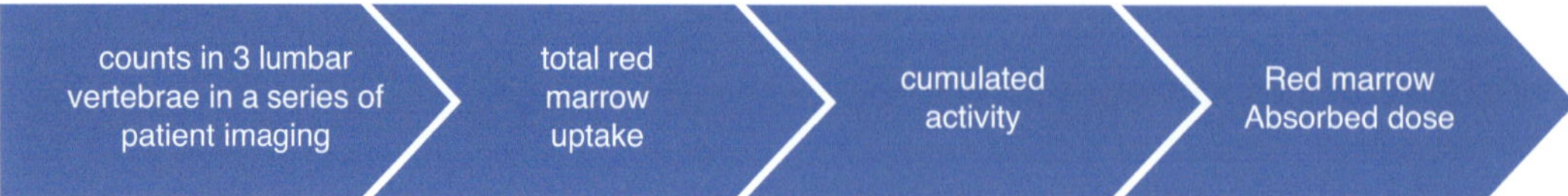

Fig. 12.4 Scheme of stages for red marrow dosimetry from imaging of three lumbar vertebrae

12.5.7.2 Red Marrow Dosimetry

Red marrow is the first organ at risk, and a safety threshold of 2Gy for absorbed dose is generally recommended to reduce the probability of severe marrow depression [4].

According to MIRD formalism three sources are assumed for red marrow dose calculation which is expressed as the activities of marrow, bone, and residual body.

$$D_{rm} = D_{rm \leftarrow rm} + D_{rm \leftarrow bone} + D_{rm \leftarrow RB}$$

Two main approaches are used for evaluation of red marrow dose: the imaging-based methods and the blood-based methods.

Blood method: This is the most familiar one, just blood sampling at various time points and using blood concentration (Siegel et al. 1990) [42]. According to Shen S et al. [45] if there is no specific radiopharmaceutical binding in blood or red marrow, the cumulated activity concentration in blood C_{blood} can be used to assess the activity concentration in red marrow using the red marrow-to-blood ratio (RMBLR)

$$\tilde{A}_{RM} = RMBLR \times C_{blood} \times m_{RM}$$

where m_{RM} = 1500 g. Sgouros et al. [46] introduce the quantity *RMBLR* which depends on RMECFF and the hematocrit (*HCT*) and thus $\tilde{A}_{RM}$ is equal to

$$\tilde{A}_{RM} = C_{blood} \frac{RMECFF}{(1 - HCT)} \times m_{RM}$$

where RMECFF is the vascular and extracellular fluid volume in the marrow and its working value was suggested to be 0.19.

HCT is the patient's hematocrit leading to RMBLR = 0.36 for a normal value of HCT.

(*RMBLR* ranges from 0.2 to 0.4 but a general value of 0.36 is the working one and is based on a hematocrit of 0.47 and red marrow extracellular fluid fraction of 0.19) (Fig. 12.3).

Imaging-based method: The imaging method is based on ROIs over some regions of marrow that can be clearly distinguished from other structures (as, e.g., L4 and L5 lumbar spine vertebra), and their measured counts should be normalized afterward to the gamma camera's imaging data. According to Christy et al. [19] the marrow in these vertebrae compromises 6.8% of the total body marrow skeleton, and hence by dividing their measured count rate with 0.068, the number of counts for the whole marrow could be estimated (Fig. 12.4).

In conclusion blood-based dosimetry approaches are obviously easier to perform in practice. They require only serial blood samples at various times after administration of the radiopharmaceutical and a patient-specific determination of the hematocrit.

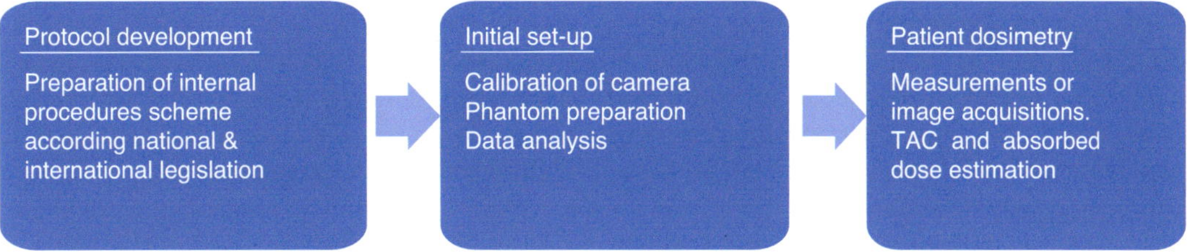

Fig. 12.5 Flow chart showing the main stages of absorbed dose estimation

12.6 Indium Dose Calculations

12.6.1 Treatment Protocol

When the therapy protocol is going to be organized, the following components should be considered regarding:

- Physics: decay data (values of n_i and E_i), LET of radiation, and deposition within the body
- Radiobiology such as biodistribution and retention of the radiopharmaceutical (Fig. 12.5)

12.6.1.1 Protocol Development

The first stage of patient dosimetry performance requires a protocol to set up all required procedures and clinical documentation needed to carry out the initial setup for the therapy scheme. These protocols must be harmonized on national and international guidelines and reference documents.

12.6.1.2 Gamma Camera Setup

The equipment used for dosimetry such as SPECT camera or SPECT/CT needs some initial setup measurements to be ready for collecting data. This is accomplished by a series of measurements and image acquisitions for which additional material such as phantoms and laboratory equipment will be needed. Images acquired must be processed using appropriate software in order to specify the calibration factor and the effective attenuation coefficient.

Phantom Preparation

A great variety of phantoms can be used. The simplest phantoms are a point source, a syringe, or a Petri dish. Additionally, acrylic phantoms of different shapes or even 3D-printed phantoms can be used. The better the patients' body simulating phantoms, the higher the absorbed dose accuracy.

Determination of Effective Attenuation Coefficient μ

The basic procedure involves the measurement of an ^{111}In source of activity approximately 230 µCi, for a fixed time (e.g., 5–6 min), at first in air without attenuating material and thereafter by adding sheets of tissue equivalent material (e.g., polymethyl methacrylate, PMMA) between the source and the gamma camera detector. Regions of interest must be drawn in order to obtain the source counts at all those various depths, and after subtraction of the background counts, the net transmission data should be statically analyzed by an exponential least-squares fitting regression method.

The effective attenuation coefficient found equal to 0.1185 (cm^{-1}) with Elscint SPECT camera and 0.14(cm^{-1}) has been established by Pereira et al. (2010) [47].

System Calibration Factor K

The final conversion of count rate to activity can be achieved using the calibration factor. The system sensitivity is determined by measuring the total count rate of a source of known activity which is called "standard" under the same acquisition and reconstruction parameters as the study data.

The activity of the standard dose is usually, but not restrictively, few tens of MBq if sufficient counts (e.g., 200.000 c/min) are obtained. The standard source should be counted in air at such a distance from the collimator that is approximately the midline used in the patient imaging study (e.g., 10 cm). In conclusion, the calibration factor K can be estimated, but ideally these measurements should be repeated to define mean value and standard deviation, SD.

System calibration factor was 84.067 (counts/s/MBq) compared to 80.0 ⟨MBq⟩, according to Pereira et al. 2010 [47].

12.7 Clinical Results from Patient Dosimetry

Once the initial gamma camera setup has been completed, the next step of acquiring and analyzing biokinetic data for patient dosimetry could proceed. The following dosimetry scheme is an example of dosimetry estimation in conventional planar or SPECT scintigraphy applications.

12.7.1 i.a and i.v. Administration

^{111}In-DTPA-Phe1-octreotide with i.a. administration has been performed in most of the patients using a catheter placed angiographically via the femoral artery. The average activity administered per session to patients was 5.4 ± 1.7 GBq, in slow i.a. infusion, lasting approximately 30 min. In parallel, dropwise i.v. infusion of 75 mg DTPA [TechneScan® DTPA (Mallinckrodt Medical catalogue number: DRN 4362)] in 200 mL normal saline solution was given, starting 30 min before the initialization of the catheterization procedure, lasting for about 4 h ("Aretaieion" Protocol) [8, 9]. Twelve sessions with treatment intervals of 7 up to 8 weeks were applied to the patients. Occasionally, for those patients wishing to avoid the catheterization procedure, a temporary port system (Pakumed, Germany) was installed (Chap. 7). Rarely, ^{111}In-DTPA-Phe^{1-} octreotide was infused intrave-

nously, mainly whence the catheter's endpoint could not reach in an acceptable proximity the tumor feeding artery due to catheterization reasons and in other cases where patients did not consent to the whole catheterization scheme.

12.7.2 Image Acquisition

For all patients scintigraphic images (anterior and posterior planar acquisitions) and SPECT of the abdomen have been acquired at 30 min, 24 h, 48 h, and 72 h after the transhepatic administration. A 20% energy window around the two dominant photopeak energies of ^{111}In (245 and 171 KeV) were centered. Parallel hole medium energy general purpose collimators were employed for imaging.

12.7.3 Blood and Urine Measurements

Blood samples (5 mL) were drawn at 30 min and 2 h, 6 h, 24 h, and 48 h after the completion of the radionuclide infusion. The blood activity concentration was measured using a dose calibrator. Assuming that the activity concentration in the bone marrow is the same as in blood, the time integrated activity concentrations obtained for blood (Forrer et al. 2009) [48] were also applied for calculation of the bone marrow self-dose. Urine samples were collected up to 24 h and were quantified using a dose calibrator.

A general scheme is to include at least three measurements so as TAC should reach the highest uptake until the retention becomes negligible (Siegel et al. 1999; Lassman et al. 2010) [43, 49]. To characterize the long-term retention of the radiopharmaceutical for each biological uptake, ICRU n0. 67 2002 [50] proposed data acquisition at times equal to multiples of the effective half-life (such as 0.5, 0.75, 1.5, 3, and 5). Table 12.5

Table 12.5 Dose estimation protocol and required data

Biokinetic data acquired	Day 0	Day 1	Day 2	Day 3	Day 4
5 mL blood sample	1 h, 2 h, 4 h, 8 h p.i.	24 h			
Cumulated urine	0–6 h, 0–24				
Tumor/organ imaging	1 h	24 h	48 h	72 h	96 h

illustrates a typical design of dose estimation protocol and the relevant required data.

Hint: Poorly chosen timing of measurements could result in the elimination of crucial time points of therapy which in consequence may cause for both cumulated activity and absorbed dose lack in accuracy.

12.7.4 Absorbed Dose Determination

For each of the images acquired, ROIs or VOIs of tumors and OARs should be delineated in order to determine their count rate. The background region was placed close to the ROIs for background correction. Those parts of organs showing tumor infiltration or superposition were excluded from the activity uptake evaluation study. The geometric mean value derived from the anterior and posterior images was taken, and by the help of calibration factor, attenuation coefficient, and the rest of the collected data from the setup measurements, their activity should be determined. Once the activity is known for all time points, the time-integrated activity can be calculated.

Then, the absorbed dose to tumor and OARs can be determined, as the product of the time-integrated activity and the S value, which is dependent on the mass or the volume. Tumors were modeled as spheres according to the OLINDA/EXM code and their actual diameter was measured by CT, MRI, or US. For the blood, the time-integrated activity concentration can be obtained; however, to calculate the blood absorbed dose, the whole-body absorbed dose needs to be also determined.

[111]In dosimetry calculations were performed considering the dose-limiting organs, the kidneys and the bone marrow. Tolerance doses accepted according to EMAMI were 23 Gy for the kidneys and 2 Gy for the bone marrow.

12.7.4.1 Example of Dose Calculations

After the i.a. infusion, ^{111}In-DTPA-Phe1-octreotide diffuses throughout the circulation to the major organs, tissues, and tumors. Table 12.6

Table 12.6 %uptake of OAR vs time for i.a. measurements

Time (h)	Tumor %	Kidney %	Liver %	Spleen %
0.52	15.2	8.3	6.8	7.3
21.90	10.0	4.6	3.9	5.0
46.90	8.0	2.5	2.4	3.7

shows an example of percentage activity uptake for the OAR, from the decay corrected measurement data.

Time-activity curves can be directly created and analyzed thereafter by nonlinear regression model to fit mono- or double exponential curves (Figs. 12.6 and 12.7). Direct assessment of the maximum uptake of the radiopharmaceutical for tumor and organs can be derived as well as their residence time which can be used as input into the OLINDA/EXM radiation dosimetry code. Additionally, the red marrow residence time and uptake can be calculated from the blood activity concentration curve (Fig. 12.7).

The mean absorbed dose for tumors and OAR is presented in Table 12.7. As it might be observed, the tumor dosimetry from i.a. formalities is higher approximately × 1.4-fold than the i.v. ones.

12.7.4.2 Tumor Regression

Figure 12.8 demonstrates the tumor response per therapy cycle. Tumor diameters are measured according to RECIST 1.1 criteria using contrast-enhanced CT images. For three sessions, after the initiation of therapy, no regression of tumor size has been observed except for discomfort relief. The reduction was started later at the fourth and at seventh was ranging around 20%; at eighth session it was raised up to 25% and at the ninth session around 30%. The general outcome regarding tumor reduction resulting from our studies was approximately 25% (range, 10–30%).

12.7.4.3 Biochemical Response

The serum tumor marker chromogranin A (CgA) was determined at the beginning of therapy and then routinely at the end of three consecutive sessions during the course of the therapeutic scheme and also as the main index in the follow-up period, in the long term. For patients with partial

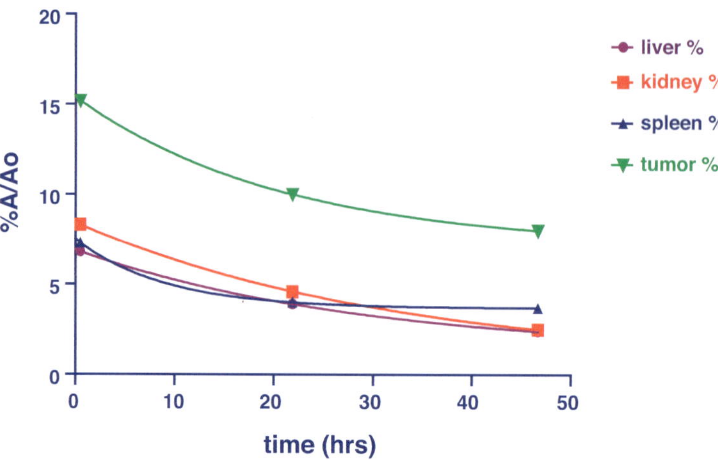

Fig. 12.6 Comparison of time-activity curves for tumor and OAR

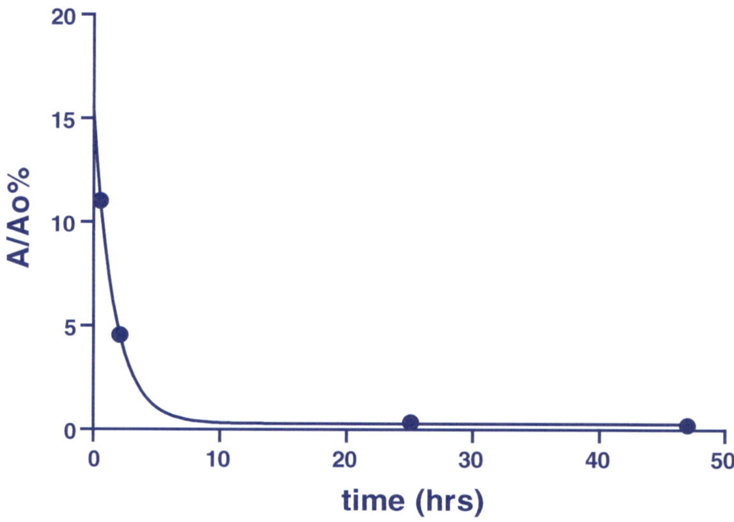

Fig. 12.7 Time-activity curve for blood after i.a. administration of ^{111}In-DTPA-Phe1-octreotide

response (PR), a marked decline was observed after the fifth session and at the end of eighth session a clear drop was seen; for those with stable disease (SD), a mediocre decline was shown after the sixth session, whereas in the group with progressive disease (PD), a continuous ascent of the serum Cr-A levels was noticed (Fig. 12.9).

12.7.4.4 Retreatment

Once the corresponding absorbed doses are determined, they should be embedded in an individualized therapeutic strategy. Often,

Table 12.7 Comparison of dosimetry between i.a. and i.v. applications

Organs	i.a. (mGy/MBq)	i.v. (mGy/MBq)
Liver	0.133 ± 0.04	0.399 ± 0.05
Spleen	1.77 ± 0.6	1.59 ± 0.6
Kidney	0.433 ± 0.08	0.499 ± 0.07
Tumor	15.2 ± 5.3	11.1 ± 4.3
Red marrow	0.0035 ± 0.0008	0.022 ± 0.002
	Tumor/organ ratio	
	i.a.	i.v.
Tumor/liver	114.3	27.8
Tumor/spleen	8.58	7.04
Tumor/kidney	35.1	22.2

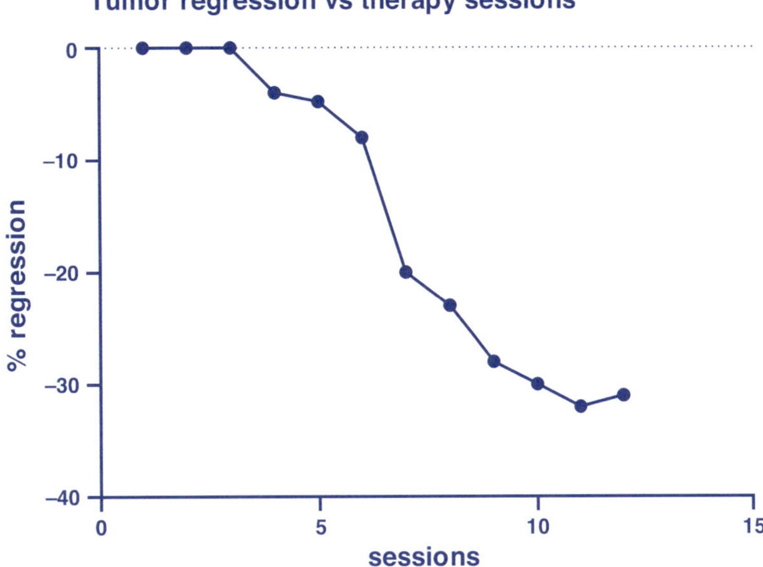

Fig. 12.8 Tumor reduction versus sessions: visible tumor consistency change start after the seventh session

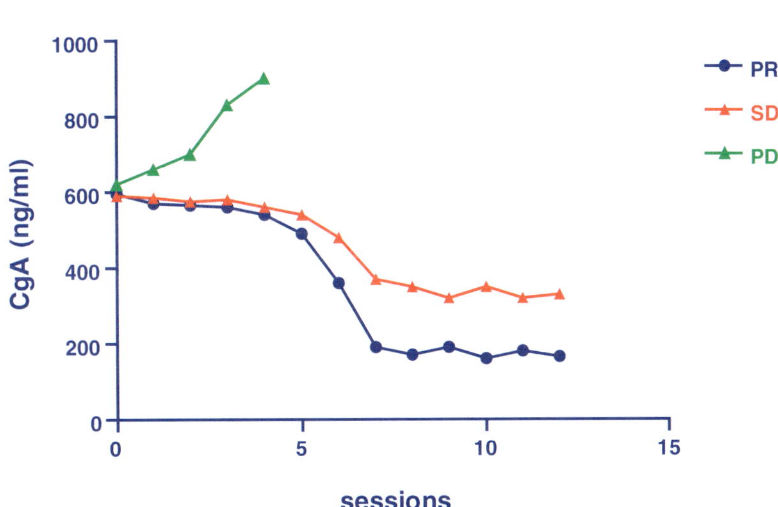

Fig. 12.9 Serum chromogranin A levels during ^{111}In-DTPA-Phe1-octreotide in patients with PR, SD, and PD response (*PR* partial response, *SD* stable disease, *PD* progression death)

tumors do not shrink immediately in response to therapy, so a delay in time should be allowed for therapy to be deemed efficient. Nonetheless, in some cases, despite the partial responses that have been already achieved, relapses of tumors could occur and thus retreatment becomes a necessity.

Extra sessions could well be tolerated and managed, by providing the preexisting personalized dosimetric data as well as all the relevant clinical data so as no severe cytotoxic reactions to OAR could be raised.

In overall excellent corporation of retreatment with radiation safety could be proceeded, and in some cases 14 cycles may apply in a mean time of 8 months after the end of 12th therapy session. Forrer et al. (2005) [51] established retreatments for those patients with disease relapsed after ^{90}Y-DOTATOC therapy, with ^{177}Lu-DOTATOC, and it was feasible, safe, and efficacious.

Table 12.8 Decay data of $[^{111}In]$ In$^+$ (from Fisher et al.) [52]

Principal radiation	E_i (keV)	n_i	Equilibrium dose const Gy kg Bq^{-1} s^{-1}
Auger electron	2.7	0.98	4.27E − 16
	19.3	0.156	4.82E − 16
Conversion electron	144.6	0.078	1.80E − 15
	167.3	0.0106	2.84 E − 16
	170.5	0.00203	5.54 E − 17
	171.2	0.000424	1.16 E − 17
	218.7	0.0493	1.73 E − 15
	241.4	0.00785	3.03 E − 16
	244.6	0.00151	5.91 E − 17
	245.3	0.000301	1.18 E − 17
x-ray	3.1	0.069	3.46 E − 17
	23.0	0.235	8.64 E − 16
	23.2	0.443	1.64 E − 15
	26.1	0.145	6.06 E − 16
γ-ray	171.3	0.902	2.47 E − 14
	245.4	0.904	3.69 E − 14

12.8 Conclusion

In this chapter, the main necessary steps to perform dosimetry with ^{111}In-DTPA-Phe1-octreotide were discussed and the most basic aspects of dosimetry by planar imaging have been dealt. Dosimetry is a sine qua non procedure for the optimal personalized radionuclide therapeutic strategy, aiming at the benefit of the oncologic patient.

Appendix

ICRP 89	
ICRP 89 Adult Male	**ICRP 89 15-year-old Male**
ICRP 89 Adult Female	**ICRP 89 15-year-old Female**
RPI ICRP 89 9 month Pregnant Woman	
RPI ICRP 89 6 month Pregnant Woman	
RPI ICRP 89 3 month Pregnant Woman	
	ICRP 89 10-year-old Male
	ICRP 89 10-year-old Female
	ICRP 89 5-year-old Male
	ICRP 89 5-year-old Female
ICRP 89 Newborn Male	
ICRP 89 Newborn Female	

References

1. Bolliger A, Inglis K. Experimental liver disease produced by X-ray irradiation of the exposed organ. J Pathol. 1933;36:19–30.
2. Dawson LA, Lawrence TS. The role of radiotherapy in the treatment of liver metastases. Cancer J. 2004;10:139–44.
3. Dawson LA, Ten Haken RK. Partial volume tolerance of the liver to radiation. Semin Radiat Oncol. 2005;15:279–83.
4. Emami B, Lyman J, Brown A, et al. Tolerance of normal tissue to therapeutic irradiation. Int J Radiat Oncol Biol Phys. 1991;21(1):109–22.
5. Reubi JC, Maurer R. Autoradiographic mapping of somatostatin receptors in the rat central nervous system and pituitary. Neuroscience. 1985;15(4):1183–93.
6. Krenning EP, Kwekkeboom DJ, Bakker WH, et al. Somatostatin receptor scintigraphy with [111In-DTPA-D-Phe1]- and [123I-Tyr3]-octreotide: the Rotterdam experience with more than 1000 patients. J Nucl Med. 1993;20:716–31.
7. IAEA Radioisotopes and radiopharmaceutical series No.5. Yttrium-90 and Rhenium-188 radiopharmaceuticals for radionuclide therapy.
8. Limouris GS, Chatziioannou A, Kontogeorgakos D, et al. Selective hepatic arterial infusion of In-111-DTPA-Phe1-octreotide in neuroendocrine liver metastases. Eur J Nucl Med Mol Imaging. 2008;35:1827–37.
9. Limouris GS, Karfis I, Chatziioannou A, et al. Superselective hepatic arterial infusions as established technique ('Aretaieion' protocol) of 177 Lu DOTA-TATE inoperable neuroendocrine liver metastases of gastro-entero-pancreatic tumors. Q J Nucl Med Mol Imaging. 2012;56:551–8.
10. Dash A, Chakraborty S, Pillai MRA, et al. Peptide receptor radionuclide therapy: an overview. Cancer Biother Radiopharm. 2015;30(2):47–71.

11. Laboratoire National Henri Becquerel. http://www.nucleide.org/DDEP_WG/DDEPdata.htm.

12. Cole A. Absorption of 20-eV to 50,000-eV electron beams in air and plastic. Radiat Res. 1969;38:7–33.

13. International Commission on Radiation Units and Measurements. Stopping powers for electrons and positrons, Report 37. Bethesda: International Commission on Radiation Units and Measurements; 1984. p. 1–271.

14. IAEA: "Technical Report Series no 468" Cyclotron produced radionuclides: physical characteristics and production methods.

15. Krenning EP, Kooij PP, Bakker WH, et al. Radiotherapy with a radiolabeled somatostatin analogue [111In-DTPA-D-Phe1] octreotide. A case history. Ann N Y Acad Sci. 1994;733:490–506.

16. Strosberg J, El-Haddad G, Wolin E, et al. Phase 3 trial of 177Lu-Dotatate for midgut neuroendocrine tumors. N Engl J Med. 2016;376:125–35.

17. Loevinger R, Berman M. A "Schema for absorbed-dose calculations for bio-logically-distributed radio-nuclides" MIRD Pamphlet No. 1. New York: Society of Nuclear Medicine; 1968.

18. Loevinger R, Berman M. A revised schema for calculating the absorbed dose from biologically distributed radionuclides. MIRD Pamphlet No. 1. Revised. New York: Society of Nuclear Medicine; 1976.

19. Cristy M, Eckerman K. Specific absorbed fractions of energy at various ages from internal photon sources. ORNL/TM-8381 V1-V7. Oak Ridge: Oak Ridge National Laboratory; 1987.

20. Stabin MG, Watson EE, Cristy M, et al. Mathematical models and specific absorbed fractions of photon energy in the nonpregnant adult female and at the end of each trimester of pregnancy. ORNL/T-12907. Oak Ridge: Oak Ridge National Laboratory; 1995.

21. Coffey JL, Cristy M, Warner GG. Specific absorbed fractions for photon sources uniformly distributed in the heart chambers and heart wall of a heterogeneous phantom. J Nucl Med. 1981;22(1):65–71.

22. Thomas SR, Stabin MG, Chen CT, et al. MIRD pamphlet No.14 revised: "a dynamic urinary bladder model for radiation dose calculations" Task Group of the MIRD Committee, Society of Nuclear Medicine. J Nucl Med. 1999;40(4):102S–23S.

23. Bouchet LG, Bolch WE, Weber DA, et al. MIRD pamphlet No.15 "Radionuclide S values in a revised dosimetric model of the adult head and brain". J Nucl Med. 1999;40(3):62S–101S.

24. Bouchet LG, Bolch WE, Blanco HP, et al. MIRD pamphlet No.19 "Absorbed fractions and radionuclide S values for six age-dependent multiregional models of the kidney". J Nucl Med. 2003;44(7):1113–47.

25. Snyder W, Ford M, Warner G. "Estimates of specific absorbed fractions for photon sources uniformly distributed in various organ of heterogeneous phantom" MIRD pamphlet No.5 revised. New York: Society of Nuclear Medicine; 1978.

26. Snyder WS, Ford MR, Warner GG, et al. "S", absorbed dose per unit cumulated activity for selected radionuclides and organs. MIRD pamphlet No.11. New York: The Society of Nuclear Medicine; 1975.

27. Stabin MG, Sparks RB, Crove E. OLINDA/EXM: the second-generation computer software for internal dose assessment in nuclear medicine. J Nucl Med. 2005;46(6):1023–7.

28. www.doseinfo-radar.com.

29. Bolch WE, Bouchet LG, Robertson JS, et al. MIRD pamphlet No.17 "the dosimetry of nonuniform activity distributions—radionuclide S values at the voxel level". J Nucl Med. 1999;40(1):11S–36S.

30. Bolch WE, Eckerman KF, Sgouros G, et al. MIRD Pamphlet No.21: a generalized schema for radiopharmaceutical dosimetry-standardization of nomenclature. J Nucl Med. 2009;50:477–84.

31. Stabin MG. MIRDOSE: personal computer software for internal dose assessment in nuclear medicine. J Nucl Med. 1996;37(3):538–46.

32. Siegel J, Stabin MG. Absorbed fractions for electrons and beta particles in spheres of various sizes. J Nucl Med. 1994;35:152–6.

33. Stabin MG, Konijnenberg MW. Re-evaluation of absorbed fractions for photons and electrons in spheres of various sizes. J Nucl Med. 2000;41(1):149–60.

34. Berger MJ. MIRD Pamphlet no 7—Distribution of absorbed dose around point sources of electrons and beta particles in water and other media. J Nucl Med. 1971;(Suppl 5):5–23.

35. Berger MJ. Improved point kernel for electrons and beta-ray dosimetry. Washington, DC: Atomic Energy Commission; 1973.

36. Lanconelli N, Pacilio M, Lo Meo S, et al. A free database of radionuclide voxel S values for the dosimetry of nonuniform activity distributions. Phys Med Biol. 2012;57:517–33.

37. Amato E, Minutoli F, Pacilio M, et al. An analytical method for computing voxel S values for electrons and photons. Med Phys. 2012;39:6808–17.

38. Kawrakow I, Rogers DWO. "The EGSnrc code system: Monte Carlo simulation of electron and photon transport" Report PIRS-701. National Research Council of Canada; 2003.

39. Briesmeister JF. "MCNPTM—a general Monte Carlo N-particle transport code", version 4C Report LA–13709–M. Los Alamos: Los Alamos National Laboratory; 2000.

40. Agostinelli S, Allison J, Amako K, et al. G4–a simulation toolkit. Nucl Instr Meth Phys Res Sect A. 2003;506:250–303.

41. Gear JI, Cox MG, Gustafsson J, et al. EANM practical guidance on uncertainty analysis for molecular radiotherapy absorbed dose calculations. EJNMMI. 2018;45:2456–74.

42. Siegel JA, Wessels BW, Watson EE, et al. Bone marrow dosimetry and toxicity for radioimmunotherapy. Antibody Immunoconjugate Radiopharm. 1990;3:213–33.

43. Siegel J, Thomas S, Stubbs J, et al. MIRD pamphlet No.16: techniques for Quantitative biodistribution Data Acquisition and Analysis for use in Human Radiation Dose Estimates. J Nucl Med. 1999;4:37S–61S.

44. Buijs WCAM, Siegel JA, Boerman OC, et al. Absolute organ activity estimated by five different methods of background correction. J Nucl Med. 1998;39:2167–72.

45. Shen S, DeNardo GL, Sgouros G, et al. Practical determination of patient specific marrow dose using radioactivity concentration in blood and body. J Nucl Med. 1999;4:2102–6.

46. Sgouros G. Bone marrow dosimetry for radioimmunotherapy: theoretical considerations. J Nucl Med. 1993;34:689–94.

47. Pereira JM, Stabin MG, Lima FRA, et al. Image quantification for radiation dose calculations-limitations and uncertainties. Health Phys. 2010;99(5):688–701.

48. Forrer F, Krenning EP, Kooij PP, et al. Bone marrow dosimetry in peptide receptor radionuclide therapy with 177 Lu-DOTA 0. Tyr3 octreotate. Eur J Nucl Med Mol Imaging. 2009;36:1138–46.

49. Lassman M, Chiesa C, Flux G, et al. EANM Dosimetry Committee guidance document good practice of clinical dosimetry. Eur J Nucl Med Mol Imaging. 2011;38(1):192–200.

50. ICRU Report 67, 2002, Absorbed dose specification in nuclear medicine.

51. Forrer F, Uusijarvi H, Storch D, et al. Treatment with 177Lu-DOTA-TOC of patients with relapse of neuroendocrine tumors after treatment with 90Y-DOTATOC. J Nucl Med. 2005;46:1310–6.

52. Fischer DR, Shen S, Meredith RF. MIRD Dose Estimate Report No. 20: radiation absorbed—dose estimates for [111]In- and ^{90}Y-ibritumomab tiuxetan. J Nucl Med. 2009;50:644–52.

Evaluation and Assessment of the Radio-Peptide Treatment Efficacy

Georgios S. Limouris and Athanasios G. Zafeirakis

13.1 Introduction/Historical Corner

An early attempt to define the objective response of a tumor was made in the 1960s [1]. However, more systematically defined response assessment criteria were made by WHO in 1979, which resulted in the WHO handbook for reporting results of cancer treatments [2, 3]. Though the distinction of solid tumor was apparent, the response pattern within solid tumors was not obvious. In 1994, several organizations involved in clinical research proposed guidelines with the term RECIST 1.0 [4]; however, their applicability in different neoplasms was less than optimal [5]. With the development of newer imaging modalities (PET scan, MRI, nuclear imaging, etc.), it became clear that response assessment estimation does not fit for all solid tumors since RECIST criteria, apart from size, do not take into account changes in various tumor characteristics like tumor viability, metabolic activity, and tumor density characteristics directly associated with tumor response.

This resulted in various specialized groups to define more suitable and specific tumor response criteria (Table 13.1) according to corresponding necessities.

Table 13.1 Main response assessment criteria

a/a	Criteria	References
1	WHO [World Health Organization]	[2, 3]
2	RECIST 1.0 [Response Evaluation Criteria In Solid Tumors]	[4]
3	RECIST 1.1 [Response Evaluation Criteria In Solid Tumors]	[6]
4	mRECIST [modified Response Evaluation Criteria In Solid Tumors]	[7]
5	PERCIST [PET Response Criteria in Solid Tumors]	[8]
6	irRC [immune-related Response Criteria]	[9]
7	Choi [Choi Criteria]	[10]
8	EASL [European Association for the Study of the Liver]	[11]
9	MDA [MD Anderson Criteria]	[12]
10	SWOG [Southwestern Oncology Group]	[13]
11	MacDonald [MacDonald Criteria]	[14]
12	RANO [Response Assessment in Neuro-Oncology]	[15]
13	EORTC [European Organization for Research and Treatment of Cancer]	[16]
14	RECICL [Response Evaluation Criteria in Cancer of the Liver]	[17]

G. S. Limouris (✉)
Nuclear Medicine, Medical School, National and Kapodistrian University of Athens, Athens, Greece
e-mail: glimouris@med.uoa.gr

A. G. Zafeirakis
Nuclear Medicine Department, Army Share Fund Hospital of Athens, Athens, Greece

© Springer Nature Switzerland AG 2021
G. S. Limouris (ed.), *Liver Intra-arterial PRRT with ^{111}In-Octreotide*,
https://doi.org/10.1007/978-3-030-70773-6_13

13.2 Response Assessment

13.2.1 WHO Criteria

The WHO criteria aim to standardize the response assessment mainly in prospective randomized cancer clinical trials [2, 3]. According to them, the lesions are classified into two groups as *measurable* and *non-measurable*. The size of the lesion derives as a two-dimensional measure by multiplying the longest diameter by its perpendicular (vertical one) one. Complete response (CR), partial response (PR), no change (NC), and progressive disease (PD) are defined separately for measurable and non-measurable disease and bone metastases. The rules for determining overall response (OR) and the concept of duration of response (RD) and disease-free interval (DFI) are described.

However, the inadequate description of details of measurement rules and handling of exceptions lead to development of many modifications to WHO criteria in various trials and often to loss of comparability. As a sequence, WHO criteria are widely replaced by RECIST one (Table 13.2).

13.2.2 RECIST Criteria

In late 1994, a new concept was presented as RECIST 1.0 guidelines [4] which subsequently after revision was released in 2009 as version 1.1 [6]. Table 13.3 provides at a glance the important features and major changes of RECIST 1.0 to RECIST 1.1. They later gained popularity and nowadays are accepted by the majority of investigation authorities in the assessment of treatment outcomes in solid tumor.

Table 13.2 Major differences between WHO and RECIST or RECIST 1.0 criteria

Parameter	WHO	RECIST or RECIST 1.0
CR (complete response)	Complete disappearance of all targeted lesions	Disappearance of all target lesions (up to 5 measurable liver lesions)
PR (partial response)	At least 50% decrease in tumor size	30% decrease of the sum of the greatest diameter of target lesions
SD (stable disease)	Meets neither PR nor PD criteria	Meets neither PR nor PD criteria
PD (progressive disease)	>25% increase of at least one lesion or a new lesion	20% increase of the sum of the greatest diameter of target lesions

Table 13.3 Major differences between RECIST 1.0 and RECIST 1.1 criteria

Parameter	RECIST or RECIST 1.0	RECIST 1.1
Minimum size of the measurable lesion	CT: 10 mm spiral, 20 mm non-spiral; clinical, 20 mm; lymph nodes, not mentioned	CT: 10 mm spiral; clinical, 10 mm; lymph nodes, ≥15 mm
Overall tumor burden	Up to 10 target lesions, maximum 5 per organ	Up to 5 target lesions, maximum 2 per organ
Complete response (CR)	Disappearance of all target lesions (up to 5 measurable liver lesions)	Disappearance of all target lesions (up to 2 measurable liver lesions); CR lymph nodes must be <10 mm short axis
Partial response (PR)	30% decrease of the sum of the greatest diameter of target lesions	At least 30% decrease of the sum of the greatest unidimensional diameters of target lesions, compared to baseline
Stable disease (SD)	Meets neither PR nor PD criteria	Meets neither PR nor PD criteria
Progressive disease (PD)	20% increase of the sum of the greatest diameter of target lesions	At least 20% increase of the sum of the diameters of target lesions, compared to baseline

13.2.3 MD Anderson Cancer Center Criteria for Bone Metastases

According to WHO and RECIST criteria, bone metastases were initially considered non-measurable lesions, because metastases located in irregularly shaped bones are difficult to be measured. Since NETs do not or rarely metastasize in bone, it is clinically important to appropriately manage the osseous spread of the neuroendocrine disease. Thus, in 2004 Hamaoka et al. [12] proposed new response assessment criteria for response assessment of bone metastasis, known as the MD Anderson (MDA) criteria. These allow the use of various radiologic techniques with baseline images obtained by x-ray (XR), CT, MRI, or by some other modalities. The recommended duration for follow-up imaging is 2–6 months (Table 13.4).

Vassiliou and Andreopoulos suggested MDA criteria may be improved by becoming more objective and accurate [18]. The implementation of CT to assess bone metastases would be very useful if the bone density in metastatic regions is measured in Hounsfield units (HU) after delineation of affected bone areas [18, 19].

13.2.4 Choi Criteria for Gastrointestinal Stromal Tumors (GISTs)

Choi et al. [10] in 2007 indicated that the RECIST 1.0 criteria underestimated the tumor response to imatinib in patients with metastatic GISTs; he aimed to develop criteria using CT scan as imaging modality as well as various tumor characteristics for the quantitative response evaluation in GISTs, beyond size measurement. In the meantime, EORTC criteria were available for response assessment using PET scan, but often the glucose uptake before treatment did not sufficiently detect them by FDG-PET (Table 13.5).

Choi criteria have been validated using time to progression endpoint. They are also used in assessing response in metastatic renal cell carcinoma [20], high-grade soft tissue sarcoma, solitary fibrous tumor [21], and hepatocellular carcinoma [22].

Table 13.4 MD Anderson Cancer Center criteria

Parameter	MD Anderson Cancer Center criteria
Complete response (CR)	Complete fill-in or sclerosis of a lytic lesion on x-ray and CT; disappearance of hot spots or tumor signal on SPECT/CT, CT, or MRI; normalization of osteoblastic lesion on x-ray and CT
Partial response (PR)	Sclerotic rim about initially lytic lesion or sclerosis of previously undetected lesion on x-ray or CT; partial fill-in or sclerosis of lytic lesion on x-ray or CT; regression of measurable lesion on x-ray, CT, or MRI; regression of lesion on SPECT/CT; decrease of blastic lesion on x-ray or CT
Stable disease (SD)	No change in measurable lesion on x-ray, CT, or MRI; no change in blastic/lytic lesion on x-ray, CT, or MRI; no new lesion on x-ray, SPECT/CT, CT, or MRI
Progressive disease (PD)	Increase in size of any existing measurable lesions on x-ray, CT, or MRI; new lesion on x-ray, SPECT/CT (excluding flares), CT, or MRI; increase in activity on SPECT/CT (excluding flares) or blastic/lytic lesion on x-ray or CT

Table 13.5 Choi criteria for the evaluation of treatment response in GISTs

Parameter	Choi criteria
Complete response (CR)	Disappearance of all lesions; no new lesions
Partial response (PR)	Decrease in size (sum of longest diameter as defined by RECIST criteria) of $\geq 10\%$ or a decrease in tumor density $\geq 15\%$ on CT; no new lesions, no obvious progression of non-measurable disease
Stable disease (SD)	No symptomatic deterioration attributes to tumor progression
Progressive disease (PD)	Increase in tumor size of $\geq 10\%$; on CT, new lesions, new intra-tumoral nodules or increase in the size of the existing intra-tumoral nodules

13.2.5 MacDonald and RANO Criteria for High-Grade Gliomas

In 1990, MacDonald et al. [14] published criteria for response assessment in high-grade gliomas, based primarily on contrast-enhanced computed tomography (CT) and the two-dimensional WHO oncology response criteria using enhancing tumor area including the use of corticosteroids and changes in the neurologic status of the patient.

However, it is obvious that there are significant limitations using only contrast-enhancing component of the tumor. Therefore, Wen et al. proposed new response criteria, commonly known as revised assessment in neuro-oncology (RANO) criteria [15].

RANO criteria provide (a) definitions and rules for standardization of imaging definitions, (b) number of lesions, and (c) definition of radiographic response. The sum of products of diameters (SPD) is calculated as products of maximal diameters, further adding them together. The responses are categorized as (a) contrast-enhancing lesions, (b) non-enhancing lesions, and (c) new lesions, based on thresholds defined in WHO criteria. The overall response (OR) is defined using response in enhancing lesions, non-enhancing lesions, new lesions, use of corticosteroids, and clinical status of the patient.

13.2.6 Response Assessment Criteria for Hepatocellular Carcinoma (HCC): EASL, mRECIST, and RECICL

The European Association for the Study of Liver (EASL) criteria is based on WHO criteria incorporating the concept of viable tumor tissue [11], quantifying the amount of enhancing (viable) tissue (Table 13.6).

Similarly, the American Association for the Study of Liver Disease (AASLD) developed a set of guidelines named as modifying RECIST criteria (mRECIST) [7] and aimed to accommodate the concept of viable tumor tissue, too (Table 13.6).

Table 13.6 Major differences between EASL and mRECIST criteria

Parameter	EASL	mRECIST
Complete response (CR)	Disappearance of any intra-tumoral enhancement in all lesions	Disappearance of any intra-tumoral enhancement in all target lesions (up to two measurable liver lesion)
Partial response (PR)	At least 50% decrease in the sum of the product of bidimensional diameters of viable (arterially enhancing) target lesions	At least a 30% decrease in the sum of unidimensional diameters of viable (arterially enhancing) target lesion, compared to baseline
Stable disease (SD)	Meets neither PR nor PD criteria	Meets neither PR nor PD criteria
Progressive disease (PD)	An increase of at least 25% in the sum of the diameters of viable (enhancing) target lesion	An increase of at least 20% in the sum of the diameters of viable (enhancing) target lesions compared to baseline

In 2009, the Liver Cancer Study Group of Japan proposed revisions to Response Evaluation Criteria in Cancer of the Liver (RECICL) [17]. The criteria consider the tumor necrosis as a direct effect of treatment, whereas the dense accumulation of lipiodol is regarded as necrosis, too. Tumors are measured in two dimensions.

Furthermore, in 2009 alpha-fetoprotein (AFP) and AFP-L3 and des-gamma-carboxyl protein (DCP) were added for the overall treatment response [17, 23].

13.2.7 PET Response Criteria in Solid Tumors (PERCIST)

In PERCIST criteria [8], response to therapy is expressed as percentage change in the sum of lesions (SULs) between the pre- and posttreatment positron emission tomography (PET) scans. A complete metabolic response (CmR) is considered as a visual disappearance of all metabolically active tumors (Table 13.7). A partial

Table 13.7 Major differences between RECIST 1.1 and PERCIST criteria

Parameter	RECIST 1.1	PERCIST
Complete response (CR)	Complete resolution of FDG uptake in all lesions	Complete resolution of FDG uptake in all lesions
Partial response (PR)	≥25% reduction in the sum of SUV max after more than one cycle of treatment	≥30% reduction of the UL peak of the FDG uptake and an absolute drop of 0.8 SUL peak units
Stable disease (SD)	Meets neither PR nor PD criteria	Meets neither PR nor PD criteria
Progressive disease (PD)	≥25% increase in the sum of SUV max or appearance of FDG-avid new lesions	≥30% increase in the SUL peak of the FDG uptake and an absolute increase of 0.8 SUL peak or appearance of FDG-avid new lesions

metabolic response (PmR) is defined as a visual disappearance of more than a 30% (and a 0.8-unit decline) in SULs between the most intense lesion before and after treatment, not necessarily of the same lesion. A stable metabolic disease (SmD) is characterized as no substantial visual metabolic change between the pre- and posttreatment scans. A progressive metabolic disease (PmD) is classified as more than a 30% (and 0.8-unit) visual increase in SULs or new lesions between the pre- and posttreatment scans. Wahl et al. proposed another metric of progression [8] in the case of a greater than 75% increase in total lesion glycolysis.

13.2.8 The European Organization for Research and Treatment of Cancer (EORTC) Criteria in Solid Tumors

Complete metabolic Response **(CmR)** would characterize a complete resolution of [18F]-FDG uptake within the tumor volume to be indistinguishable from surrounding normal tissue [16].

Partial metabolic response (PmR) would be defined as a reduction of a minimum of 15% ± 25% [18F]-FDG SUV in a tumor after one cycle of chemotherapy and greater than 25% after more than one treatment cycle.

Stable metabolic disease (SmD) is considered as an increase in tumor with [18F]-FDG SUV of less than 25% or a decrease of less than 15% and no visible increase in extent of [18F]-FDG tumor uptake (20% in the longest dimension).

Progressive metabolic disease **(PmD)** is classified as an increase in [18F]-FDG standardized uptake value (SUV) greater than 25% before and after treatment of the tumor defined on the baseline scan visible increase in the extent of [18F]-FDG tumor uptake (20% in the longest dimension) or the appearance of new [18F]-FDG uptake in metastatic lesions.

13.2.9 The Immune-Related Response Criteria (irRC) [9]

The immune-related response criteria arose out of observations that using the WHO or RECIST Criteria in immuno-oncology therapeutic schemes the delay (i.e., the time gap) between dosing (initial treatment) and the observed anti-tumor response failed to be taken into account. These observations first flagged in a key 2007 paper in the *Journal of Immunotherapy* [24], evolved into the immune-related response criteria (irRC), which was published in late 2009 in the journal *Clinical Cancer Research* [25]. The therapy results express four distinct response patterns: (a) immediate response (IR), durable stable disease (DSD), response after tumor burden increase, and response in the presence of new lesions. The first two patterns are conventional, whereas the latter two are novel and specifically recognized with immunotherapeutic agents [25].

Only measurable lesions are taken into consideration. Measures are taken bi-dimensionally for each lesion. To calculate total tumor burden, the sum of the perpendicular diameters of lesions at baseline is added to that of the new lesions.

Response categories under irRC are defined as immune-related complete response (irCR), immune-related partial response (irPR), immune-related stable disease (irSD), and immune-related progressive disease (irPD) using the same thresholds to distinguish between categories as defined in WHO criteria (Table 13.8).

According to irRC, the appearance of new lesions alone does not constitute irPD if they do not add to the tumor burden by at least 25%. Patients with new lesions but an overall tumor burden decrease qualifying for partial response ($\geq$50% decrease) or qualifying for stable disease (<50% decrease to >25% increase) are considered to have irPR or irSD, respectively [26].

13.3 The Southwest Oncology Group (SWOG) Criteria

In 1992, the Southwest Oncology Group (SWOG), in cooperation with the National Cancer Institute (NCI) in the USA and other major cooperative oncology groups, has participated in the development of new criteria for reporting the results of cancer clinical trial [13] (Table 13.9). Observing the three tabulated criteria and their differences, we can comprehend that a particular guideline may be useful in establishing uniformity of evaluation in a desired study population but may not be the best for that population during routine clinical practice. The comparison between them indicates that each of the guidelines has its own applicability and that no guideline can outweigh the other during routine clinical practice.

Table 13.8 Major differences between WHO and iRC criteria

Parameters	WHO	iRC
New measurable lesions (i.e., $\geq$5 × 5 mm)	Always represent PD	Incorporated into tumor burden
New non-measurable lesions (i.e., <5 × 5 mm)	Always represent PD	Do not define progression (but preclude irCR)
Non-index lesions	Changes contribute to defining BOR of CR, PR, SD, and PD	Contribute to defining irCR (complete disappearance required)
CR (complete response)	Disappearance of all lesions in two consecutive observations not less than 4 weeks apart	Disappearance of all lesions in two consecutive observations not less than 4 weeks apart
PR (partial response)	$\geq$50% decrease in SPD of all index lesions compared with baseline in two observations at least 4 weeks apart, in absence of new lesions or unequivocal progression of non-index lesions	$\geq$50% decrease in tumor burden com-pared with baseline in two observations at least 4 weeks apart
SD (stable disease)	50% decrease in SPD compared with baseline cannot be established nor 25% increase compared with nadir, in absence of new lesions or unequivocal progression of non-index lesions	50% decrease in tumor burden compared with baseline cannot be established nor 25% increase compared with nadir
PD (progressive disease)	At least 25% increase in SPD compared with nadir and/or unequivocal progression of non-index lesions and/or appearance of new lesions (at any single time point)	At least 25% increase in tumor burden compared with nadir (at any single time point) in two consecutive observations at least 4 weeks apart

Table 13.9 Major differences between WHO, RECICT 1.0, and SWOG criteria

Response	WHO	RECIST 1.0	SWOG
CR (complete response)	Complete disappearance of all targeted lesions	Disappearance of all target lesions (up to 5 measurable liver lesions)	Complete disappearance of all measurable and evaluable disease; no evidence of non-evaluable disease, including normalization of markers and other abnormal laboratory values for at least 3–6 weeks. Complete disappearance of all targeted lesions including normalization of markers and other abnormal laboratory values for at least 3–6 weeks
PR (partial response)	At least 50% decrease in tumor size	30% decrease of the sum of the greatest diameter of target lesions	Sum of products of all lesions decreased by ≥50% for at least 3–6 weeks; no new lesions; no progression of evaluated lesions
SD (stable disease)	Meets neither PR nor PD criteria	Meets neither PR nor PD criteria	Sum of products of lesions decreased by <50% or increased by <50% or 10 cm^2 for at least 3–6 weeks
PD (progressive disease)	>25% increase of at least one lesion or a new lesion	20% increase of the sum of the greatest diameter of target lesions	50% increase or an increase of 10 cm^2 (whichever is smaller) in the sum of products of all measurable lesions over the smallest sum observed; clear worsening of any evaluable disease; appearance of a new lesion

References

1. Zubrod CG, Schneiderman SM, Frei E III, et al. Appraisal of methods for the study of chemotherapy of cancer in man: comparative therapeutic trial of nitrogen mustard and triethylene thio-phosphamide. J Chronic Dis. 1960;11:7–33.
2. World Health Organization. WHO handbook for reporting results of cancer treatment. Geneva: World Health Organization; 1979.
3. Miller AB, Hoogstraten B, Staquet M, et al. Reporting results of cancer treatment. Cancer. 1981;47:207–14.
4. Therasse P, Arbuck SG, Eisenhauer EA, et al. New guidelines to evaluate the response to treatment in solid tumors. European organization for research and treatment of cancer, national cancer institute of the United States, National Cancer Institute of Canada. J Natl Cancer Inst. 2000;92:205–16.
5. Forner A, Ayuso C, Varela M, et al. Evaluation of tumor response after loco-regional therapies in hepatocellular carcinoma: are response evaluation criteria in solid tumors reliable? Cancer. 2009;115:616–23.
6. Eisenhauer EA, Therasse P, Bogaerts J, et al. New response evaluation criteria in solid tumors: revised RECIST guideline (version 1.1). Eur J Cancer. 2009;45:228–47.
7. Lencioni R, Llovet JM. Modified RECIST (mRECIST) assessment for hepato-cellular carcinoma. Semin Liver Dis. 2010;30:52–60.
8. Wahl RL, Jacene H, Kasamon Y, et al. From RECIST to PERCIST: evolving considerations for PET response criteria in solid tumors. J Nucl Med. 2009;50:S122–50.
9. Subbiah V, Chuang HH, Gambhire D, et al. Defining clinical response criteria and early response criteria for precision oncology: current state-of-the-art and future perspectives. Diagnostics (Basel). 2017;7(1):10.
10. Choi H, Charnsangavej C, Faria SC, et al. Correlation of computed tomography and positron emission tomography in patients with metastatic gastrointestinal stromal tumor treated at a single institution with imatinib mesylate: proposal of new computed tomography response criteria. J Clin Oncol. 2007;25:1753–17597.
11. Bruix J, Sherman M, Llovet JM, et al. Clinical management of hepatocellular carcinoma. Conclusions of the barcelona-2000 EASL conference. European association for the study of the liver. J Hepatol. 2001;35:421–30.
12. Hamaoka T, Madewell JE, Podoloff DA, et al. Bone imaging in metastatic breast cancer. J Clin Oncol. 2004;22:2942–53.

13. Green S, Weiss GR. Southwest oncology group standard response criteria, endpoint definitions and toxicity criteria. Invest New Drugs. 1992;10:239–53.

14. Macdonald DR, Cascino TL, Schold SC Jr, et al. Response criteria for phase II studies of supratentorial malignant glioma. J Clin Oncol. 1990;8:1277–80.

15. Wen PY, Macdonald DR, Reardon DA, et al. Updated response assessment criteria for high-grade gliomas: response assessment in neuro-oncology working group. J Clin Oncol. 2010;28:1963–72.

16. Young H, Baum R, Cremerius U, et al. European Organization for Research and Treatment of Cancer (EORTC) Pet Study Group Measurement of clinical and subclinical tumor response using [18F]-fluorodeoxyglucose and positron emission tomography: review and 1999 EORTC recommendations. Eur J Cancer. 1999;35:1773–82.

17. Kudo M, Kubo S, Takayasu K, et al. Liver Cancer Study Group of Japan Response evaluation criteria in cancer of the liver (RECICL) proposed by the Liver Cancer Study Group of Japan (2009 revised version). Hepatol Res. 2010;40:686–92.

18. Vassiliou V, Andreopoulos D. Assessment of therapeutic response in patients with metastatic skeletal disease: suggested modifications for the MDA response classification criteria. Br J Cancer. 2010;103(6):925–6.

19. Limouris GS, Toubanakis N, Shukla SK, et al. Prostate osseous metastases: evaluation of the combined application of disodium pamidronate/^{89}Sr-chloride/^{186}Re-HEDP. In: Bergmann H, Kroiss A, Sinzinger H, editors. Radioactive isotopes in clinical medicine and research XXII. Basel: © Birkhäuser Verlag; 1997.

20. Van der Veldt AA, Meijerink MR, van den Eertwegh AJ, et al. Choi response criteria for early prediction of clinical outcome in patients with metastatic renal cell cancer treated with sunitinib. Br J Cancer. 2010;102:803–9.

21. Stacchiotti S, Negri T, Palassini E, et al. Sunitinib malate and figitumumab in solitary fibrous tumor: patterns and molecular bases of tumor response. Mol Cancer Ther. 2010;9:1286–97.

22. Faivre S, Zappa M, Vilgrain V, et al. Changes in tumor density in patients with advanced hepatocellular carcinoma treated with sunitinib. Clin Cancer Res. 2011;17:4504–12.

23. Kudo M, Han KH, Kokudo N, et al. Liver cancer working group report. Jpn J Clin Oncol. 2010;40:i19–27.

24. Hoos A, Parmiani G, Hege K, et al. A clinical development paradigm for cancer vaccines and related biologics. J Immunother. 2007;30(1):1–15.

25. Wolchok JD, Hoos A, O'Day S, et al. Guidelines for the evaluation of immune therapy activity in solid tumors: immune-related response criteria. Clin Cancer Res. 2009;15:7412–20.

26. Hoos A, Eggermont AM, Janetzki S, et al. Improved endpoints for cancer immunotherapy trials. J Natl Cancer Inst. 2010;102:1388–97.

^{111}In-Octreotide Infusions for the Treatment of Bronchopulmonary Neuroendocrine Neoplasms

Georgios S. Limouris and Athanasios G. Zafeirakis

14.1 Introduction

According to Talal Hilal [1], although bronchopulmonary neoplasms are considered to be potentially curable by surgical resection, some patients present with locally advanced or metastatic disease with or without hormone-related syndromes that may prove to be more challenging in management. Furthermore, large-scale clinical trials are limited for this specific patient population due to the overall rarity of the malignancy.

Neuroendocrine tumors (NETs) are a relative rare and heterogeneous tumor type of neoplasms comprising about 2% of all malignancies, with a prevalence of approximately 200,000 cases in the United States, with no concrete therapeutic algorithm, thus called "orphan" disease [2]. The term "neuroendocrine" is applied to widely dispersed cells with "neuro" and "endocrine." The "neuro" property is based on the identification of dense-core granules (DCGs) [3] that are similar to DCGs present in serotonergic neurons, which store monoamines. (However, unlike neurons, neuroendocrine cells do not contain synapses.) The "endocrine" property refers to the synthesis

and secretion of these monoamines [4]. The GI track and lungs (Fig. 14.1) are the most common primary tumor sites [5]. In 1963, Williams and Sandler classified NETs, according to the embryonic divisions of the digestive tract as foregut [esophagus; thymus; respiratory tract (bronchopulmonary tree); stomach; duodenum, up to the ampulla of Vater; liver; biliary-gallbladder; pancreas and spleen], midgut [(duodenum-distal half of second, third, and fourth parts) jejunum,

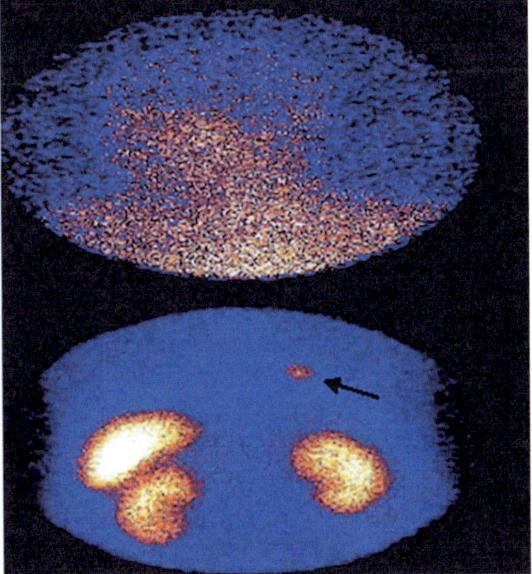

Fig. 14.1 OctreoScan® scintigraphy: Posterior view of a BNN (arrow) after 111 MBq ^{111}In-Octreotide i.v. 7 h post injection. Normal intense radiotracer uptake in kidneys and spleen (visual score II)

G. S. Limouris (✉)
Nuclear Medicine, Medical School, National and Kapodistrian University of Athens, Athens, Greece
e-mail: glimouris@med.uoa.gr

A. G. Zafeirakis
Nuclear Medicine Department, Army Share Fund Hospital of Athens, Athens, Greece

© Springer Nature Switzerland AG 2021
G. S. Limouris (ed.), *Liver Intra-arterial PRRT with ^{111}In-Octreotide*,
https://doi.org/10.1007/978-3-030-70773-6_14

ileum, cecum, appendix, proximal colon (ascending colon-hepatic flexure), transverse colon (proximal two-thirds)], and hindgut (the distal third of the transverse colon and the splenic flexure, the descending colon, sigmoid colon, and rectum) [6].

According to the WHO classification, lung NETs can be categorized in four subtypes as the following: well differentiated (low grade with long-life-expectancy typical carcinoids [TCs], intermediate grade with a more aggressive clinical course atypical carcinoids [ACs]) and poorly differentiated with dismal prognosis (high-grade large-cell neuroendocrine carcinomas (LCNECs) and small-cell lung carcinomas (SCLCs)) [7]. In 2004, according to Travis, the WHO divided neoplasms of the lung and thymus into three grades based on mitotic index and necrosis (Table 14.1) [8].

The incidence of these tumors is increasing, but disease awareness remains low among thoracic specialists, who are often involved in the diagnosis and early treatment for these patients. An accurate and timely diagnosis can ensure the implementation of an appropriate treatment and has a substantial impact on prognosis. However, lung NET classification and diagnosis, particularly regarding TCs/ACs, are adversely affected by several factors, including a variable natural history and nonspecific symptoms.

TCs/ACs, but there is a lack of precision-consensus between lung NET management and guidelines regarding optimal treatment approaches in the unresectable/metastatic setting on account of the limited availability of high-level clinical evidence [9]. As a result, a multidisciplinary approach for the management of lung NETs is required to ensure a consistent and optimal level of care (Table 14.2) [10].

Table 14.1 NETs 2004: WHO classification for the lung and thymus

Grade	Mitotic count per 10 HPFs	Necrosis
G1	<2	0
G2	2–10	In foci (+)
G3	>10	Present (+++)

HPFs high-power fields

Table 14.2 Multidisciplinary team approach to reviewing lung- and liver-metastasized patients

Nuclear medicine physician	Hepatic surgeon
Interventional radiologist	Medical oncologist
Radiation physicist	Pathologist
Lung surgeon	Anesthesiologist
Gastroenterologist	Dedicated nursing staff

Table 14.3 BPNN patients response to therapy with ^{111}In-Octreotide

Patient no.	Response evolution	PFS	OS
1.	SD ≫ PD ≫ D (5 i.a. and 4 i.v. infusions)	29	32
2.	PR (5 i.a. and 4 i.v. infusions)	>40	>40
3.	PR (9 i.a. infusions)	>84	>84
4.	SD ≫ PD ≫ D (5 i.a. and 4 i.v. infusions)	8	16
5.	PD ≫ D (5 i.a. and 4 i.v. infusions)	0	12
6.	PD ≫ D (5 i.a. and 4 i.v. infusions)	0	11
7.	SD ≫ PD ≫ D (5 i.a. and 4 i.v. infusions)	7	16

PR partial response, *SD* stable disease, *PD* progressive disease, *D* death, ≫ shifted to

Since historically limited clinical data are available regarding lung NETs, we aimed to evaluate and compare the effectiveness of PRRT with high doses using ^{111}In-Octreotide, in patients with inoperable BPNNs associated with liver metastases and positive for somatostatin receptors, discussing and analyzing the recent ergography developments. We report on the effectiveness of PRRT in seven patients [one with surgically excised primary tumor site (Table 14.3, patient no. 3) and in six with inoperable bronchial carcinoids (verified by OctreoScan® (Figs. 14.1, 14.2, and 14.3), confirmed by biopsy)]. *All of them had liver metastases*, treated with ^{111}In-Octrotide. We compared the dosimetric outcome with that obtained from the ergography, where ^{177}Lu-DOTA-TATE is used. After centesis of the dorsal vein hand system or the antecubital vein, the dose per session administered monthly to each patient ranged from 4.070 to 5.920 GBq. The same activity was

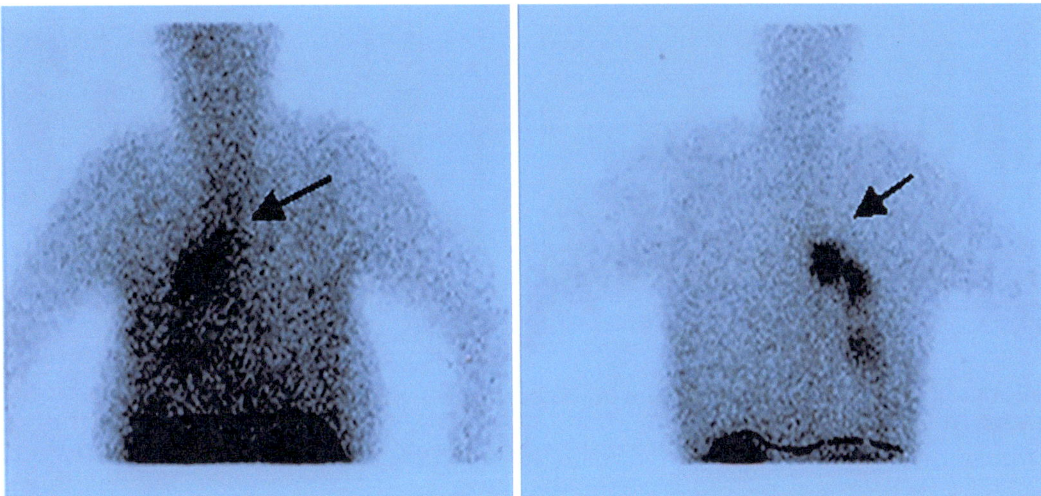

Fig. 14.2 OctreoScan® scintigraphy of a BPNN (arrow, post/ant view) after 185 MBq ^{111}In-Octreotide, i.v. 7 h post injection. Normally intense radiotracer uptake in liver and spleen (visual score II–III)

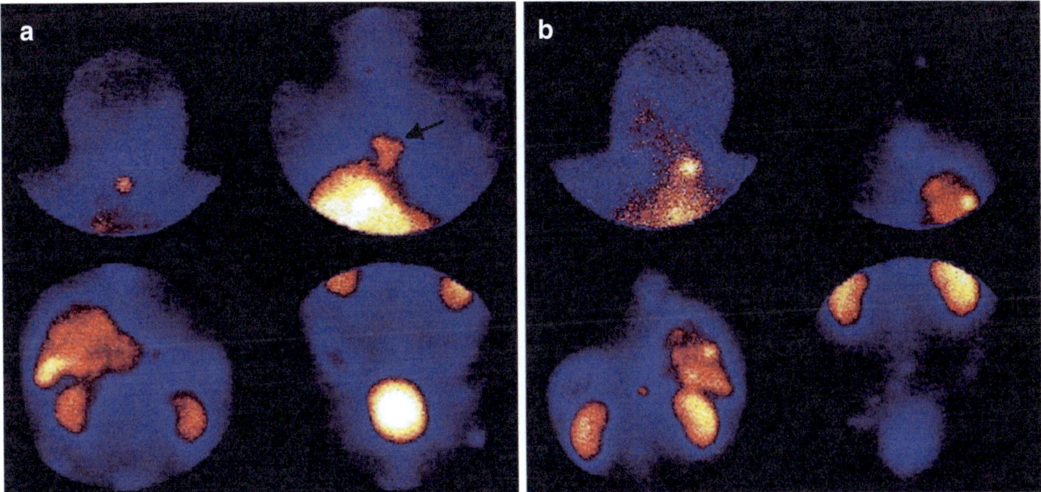

Fig. 14.3 OctreoScan® scintigraphy of a BPNN (before surgery) of the right lung-middle lobe-medial segment (arrow) with multiple metastases in liver and bone (sixth cervical and tenth thoracic vertebra) after 185 MBq ^{111}In-Octreotide, i.v. 7 h-post injection (visual score III); (**a**: anterior view, **b**: posterior view); normally intense radiotracer uptake in liver and spleen

infused intra-arterially, after catheterization of the hepatic artery. Repetitions did not exceed the nine sessions with treatment intervals of 5–8 weeks. Absorbed doses delivered to the primary BPNN, its liver metastases, kidneys, and red marrow were calculated according to OLINDA 1.1 program, and response assessment was classified, based on RECIST criteria. CT/MRI scans were performed before, during, and after the end of treatment, and monthly ultrasound images were used for liver follow-up measurements. Toxicity (WHO criteria) was measured using blood and urine tests of renal, hepatic, and bone marrow function.

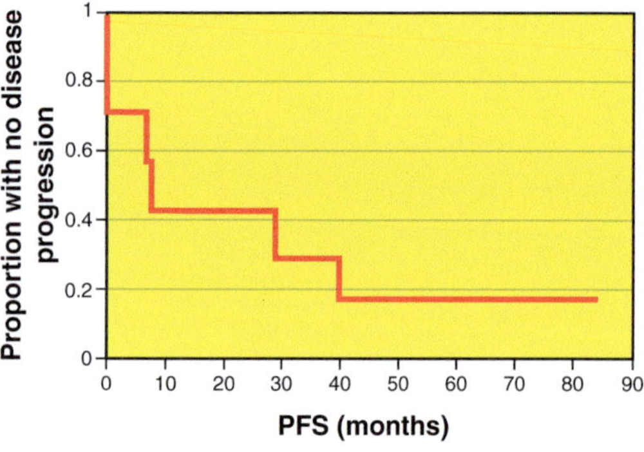

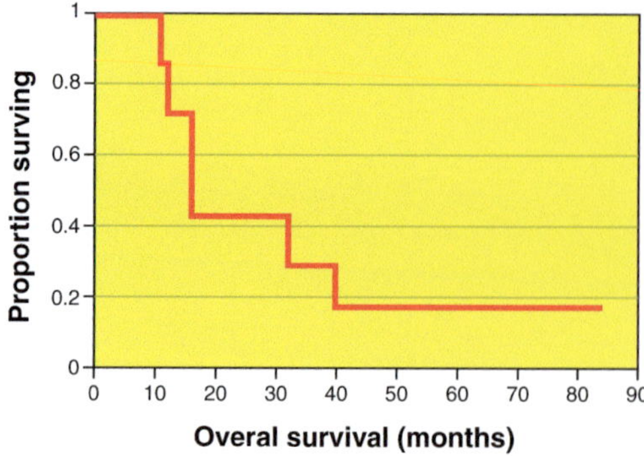

Fig. 14.4 Kaplan-Meier curves for progression-free (left) and overall survival (OS) of the seven BPNN patients' study, treated with ^{111}In-Octreotide

14.2 ^{111}In-Octreotide Treatment Results

Liver metastatic load: None of the seven treated patients resulted in complete response or partial response; disease stabilization was assessed in all seven cases. *Bronchopulmonary neuroendocrine (BPN) neoplasms load* (Table 14.3): Five out of the aforementioned seven cases resulted in disease stabilization, whereas two did not respond at all and died within 1 year after the initialization of the therapeutic scheme due to pulmonary aggravation (Table 14.3, Fig. 14.4). According to the therapy response results, the 12-month progression free ratio was found to be 3/7 (42.9%) while the 12-month overall survival ratio was 6/7 (85.7%).

On CT, the bronchial carcinoid tumor masses progressed dramatically, whereas the liver metastases showed a mean target diameter shrinkage ranging from 33 to 45%. Grade II to III erythro-, leuko-, and thrombocytopenia occurred in all seven cases. Dosimetric calculations (Table 14.4) were found as follows: (a) liver tumor 15.2 mGy/MBq, (b) liver 0.14 mGy/MBq, (c) kidneys 0.41 mGy/MBq, (d) spleen 1.4 mGy/MBq, (e) bronchial carcinoid 0.08 mGy/MBq, and (f) bone marrow 0.055 mGy/MBq. The average absorbed dose per session to a tumor for a spherical mass of 10 g was estimated to be 15 mGy/MBq. Remarkably, even though no significant bronchial tumor absorbed-dose difference is observed between intra-arterial (i.a.) and intravenous (i.v.) infusion, there is a threefold difference between the i.a. and i.v. of the liver metastatic absorbed-dose ratio.

Table 14.4 Tumor absorbed-dose comparison between i.v. and i.a. administration of ^{111}In-Octreotide

Organ	Intra-arterial infusion	Intravenous infusion
Liver dose	0.14 (mGy/MBq)	0.40 (mGy/MBq)
Kidney dose	0.41 (mGy/MBq)	0.51 (mGy/MBq)
Liver metastatic tumor dose	15.20 (mGy/MBq)	11.20 (mGy/MBq)
Bronchial carcinoid	0.08 (mGy/MBq)	0.07 up to 0.09 (mGy/MBq)
Spleen dose	1.40 (mGy/MBq)	1.56 (mGy/MBq)
Bone marrow dose	0.0035 (mGy/MBq)	0.022 (mGy/MBq)
Tumor/liver dose **ratio**	108.57[a]	28.00
Tumor/kidney dose **ratio**	37.07	21.96

[a]The average absorbed dose per session to a tumor for a spherical mass of 10 g was estimated to be 10.8 mGy/MBq, depending on the histotype of the tumor

14.3 Discussion

This prospective single-center analysis provides efficacy results including a clearly limited progression-free survival and overall survival of PRRT in a patient cohort with advanced well-differentiated pulmonary NETs after failing standard treatment with chemotherapy. Despite the small patient number ($n = 7$), these findings can act as a pilot study, as they forward the feature of the persistent antiproliferative activity of ^{111}In-Octreotide Auger and internal conversion electron emission in this specific NET entity at an advanced stage. However, this sort of electron emission achieves a rather insignificant disease control in almost all patients, intravenously treated, and a short-term stabilization with a median progressive free survival (PFS) of approximately 24 months, thus rendering ^{111}In-Octreotide not promising for an objective outcome in that context of lacking established treatment alternatives.

Chemotherapy: Effective treatment options for patients with functionally uncontrolled carcinoid syndrome or tumor progression in metastatic pulmonary NET of well-differentiated histology are very limited. The goals of medical therapy are to slow down tumor growth and control hormone-related symptoms in patients with functional tumors. Previous investigations with various chemotherapy agents, either as mono- or combined therapy, were generally discouraging. According to Ekeblad et al. [11], satisfactory results have been observed after treatment of 13 patients (10 typical and 3 atypical carcinoids) with oral temozolomide achieving PR in 4 (31%) patients and disease stabilization in 8 (62%) patients. Targeted treatments with tyrosine-kinase inhibitor such as sunitinib (Sutent®) or inhibitor of mammalian target of rapamycin

(mTOR) everolimus (Afinitor®) were also associated with limited efficacy in patients with non-pancreatic NET by Kulke et al. [12], Yao et al. [13], Duran et al. [14], and Pavel et al. [15]. In a recent trial by Yao et al. [16] on patients with nonfunctional neuroendocrine tumors of lung or gastrointestinal origin (RADIANT4), everolimus could prolong the PFS in 203 patients including 63 patients with pulmonary NET to less than 15 months. Particular efficacy in pulmonary NET, however, has only been reported by Fazio et al. [17], in an earlier study on 33 patients, and showed a statistically insignificant trend toward longer PFS (13.6 months) under everolimus compared to 11 patients who received placebo (5.6 months).

PRRT: Data supporting the efficacy of PRRT with radiolabelled somatostatin analogs in bronchopulmonary NETs with ^{111}In-Octreotide are restricted and cannot be considered as promising (Table 14.3, Figs. 14.3 and 14.4), particularly when compared with those obtained after the use of ^{177}Lu-DOTATATE (Table 14.5). Furthermore, it should not be ignored that these patients have already undergone chemo- and radiotherapy or a combination of these; also, the speculation that both chemotherapy and/or radiotherapy interact and activate proteins of the ATP-binding-cassette

Table 14.5 Experteers on PRRT in bronchopulmonary NETs

Author	Year/type	Radiopeptide	n	orr (%)	PFS (months)	OS (months)
Waldherr et al.	2001/ps	^{90}Y-DOTATOC	7	29	nr	nr
Waldherr et al.	2002/ps	^{90}Y-DOTATOC	3	0	nr	nr
van Essen et al.	2006/rs	^{177}Lu-DOTATATE	3	0	nr	5
van Essen et al.	2007/rs	^{177}Lu-DOTATATE	9	67	31	nr
Imhof et al.	2011/rs	^{90}Y-DOTATOC	84	29	nr	40
Filice et al.	2012/rs	^{90}Y-DOTATOC and ^{177}Lu-DOTATATE	13	62	nr	nr
Limouris et al.	2012/ps	^{111}In-Octreotide	7	71.4	24	30r
Mariniello et al.	2016/rs	^{90}Y-DOTATOC	45	18	32	46
		^{177}Lu-DOTATATE	48	29	40	110
		^{90}Y/^{177}Lu-DOTA-TOC/TATE	21	38	46	61
Ianniello et al.	2016/rs	^{177}Lu-DOTATATE	34	33	20	nr
Sabet et al.	2017/rs	^{177}Lu-DOTATATE	22	27	27	42
Brabander et al.	2017/ps	^{177}Lu-DOTATATE	23	30	20	52
Garske-Román et al.	2018/ps	^{177}Lu-DOTATATE	6	17	(5/6)20, (1/6)12	nr
van der Zwan et al.	2019/pr	^{177}Lu-DOTATATE	13	15.5	8.0	26.2

rs retrospective study, *ps* prospective study, *orr* objective response rate, *PFS* progression-free survival, *os* mean overall survival, *nr* non-referred

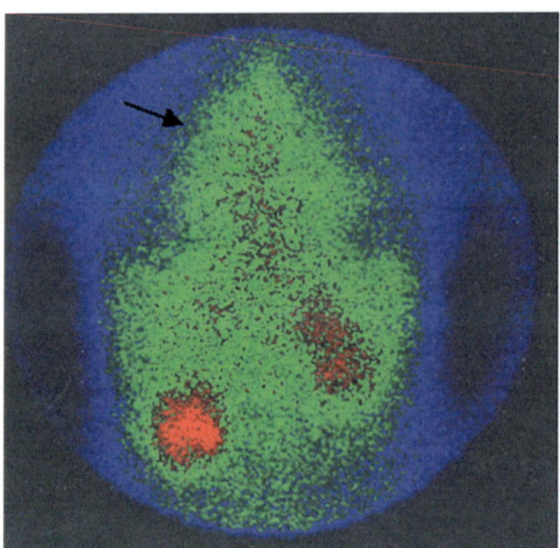

Fig. 14.5 OctreoScan® scintigraphy of a BPNN after 185 MBq ^{111}In-Octreotide i.v. 7 h post injection (anterior view); visual score II for lung tumor (arrow) and normal liver

(ABC) transporter family, accelerating the drug washout, outside the tumor

Cell should be taken into account; this probably leads to a lower amount of absorbed radiation/gram tumor tissue, thus reducing the chance of tumor remission, explaining this dismal response to PRRT treatment schemes. Additionally, the reduced density and affinity of somatostatin receptors play a negative role concerning the poor somatostatin receptors expressed in high-grade bronchial carcinomas and SCLCs (Fig. 14.5) compared with low-grade bronchial carcinoids, the former featuring a more aggressive behavior [18]. In the limited cohort of the present study, including seven patients suffering from bronchial carcinoids treated with ^{111}In-Octreotide, objective response was observed in five (71.4%) with a median PFS of 24 months [19]. On the contrary according to the relevant international literature, the outcome after ^{177}Lu-DOTATATE implementation is worth to notice. In 2001, Waldherr et al. [20] in a prospective phase II study on seven BPNN treated with ^{90}Y-DOTATOC reported an objective response rate of (2/7) 29%; PFS and OS were not referred. In 2002, the same authors [21] in another prospective study on three BPNN treated with ^{90}Y-DOTATOC reported a SD in all three patients;

PFS and OS were also not referred. In a large study of Imhof et al. [22] on more than 1000 patients with NET of different origins treated with ^{90}Y-DOTATOC, 84 patients with bronchopulmonary NETs had a median OS of 40 months (95% CI, 31–50) with no PFS data available. In a retrospective study on 59 patients by Filice et al. [23], with advanced NET, 13 patients with pulmonary NET were treated with ^{90}Y-DOTATOC and/or ^{177}Lu-DOTATOC. The reported objective response rate was 62% according to somatostatin receptor imaging; no further information regarding the characteristics and survival outcome of this subgroup was mentioned. In 23 patients with BPN neoplasms treated with ^{177}Lu-DOTATATE, Brabander et al. [24] reported a PR in 7 (30%), a SD in 7 (30%), and a PD in 6 (26%) patients, whereas the remaining 2 cases could not be evaluated; additionally, for these BPN neoplasms, the authors found a mean PFS of 20 months and a median OS of 52 months. In a study of van Essen et al. [25] on three patients with small-cell lung cancer (SCLC) treated with ^{177}Lu-Octreotate, all three died within 5 months after starting PRRT therapy, because of tumor progression. One year later, in the same group [26] on nine BPNN patients, five had partial remission, one had minor response, two had stable disease (SD), and one had progressive disease (PD) with a median time to progression of 31 months. The authors pointed out that regarding the atypical and typical pulmonary NETs no difference to the treatment outcome was observed. In a recent research of Sabet et al. [27], the considerable efficacy of ^{177}Lu-Octreotate in pulmonary NET is indicated and reported on 22 BPNN patients, with a partial response in 6 patients (27.3%), a median PFS of 27, and an overall survival of 42 months, respectively. In a recent prospective study of Garske-Román et al. [28], on six BNN NETs, median PFS was 20 months in five patients and 12 months in one patient, whereas OS was not tabulated.

A study restricted to patients with pulmonary NET describing the outcome in a heterogeneous cohort treated with ^{177}Lu-DOTATATE, ^{90}Y-DOTATOC, or the combination of both compounds over more than a decade is that of Mariniello et al. [29]. In this large cohort of patients with advanced bronchopulmonary NETs and followed up for a median of 45.1 months (range 2–191 months), PRRT proved to be promising in prolonging survival and delaying disease progression. Despite the potential selection biases, considering the risk-benefit ratio, ^{177}Lu-DOTATATE seemed superior to ^{90}Y-DOTATOC. They indicated that the use of PRRT in earlier stages of the disease could provide a more favorable outcome. In a similar study of Ianniello et al. [30] on 34 consecutive patients with advanced bronchial carcinoids treated also with ^{177}Lu-DOTATATE, 6% CR, 27% PR, and 47% SD were reported with a median PFS of 20 months; overall survival was not referred. Finally, in a recent prospective study of van de Zwan et al., on 13 patients, an objective response rate of 15.5%, a median PFS of 8 months, and a median overall survival of 26.2 months were reported [31].

14.4 Conclusion

In unresectable metastatic *liver* lesions, positive for somatostatin receptors, originated from BPNNs, repeated high doses of ^{111}In-Octreotide, tandem i.a. and i.v. infused, resulted in a stable disease in all affected secondaries, whereas the inoperable *pulmonary* primaries progressed dramatically. The dosimetric calculations proved the poor absorbed dose, predicting the disappointing results. Systematic PRRT for *bronchial carcinoids* with intravenously injected ^{111}In-Octreotide does not seem to have clinical effects in bronchial carcinoids and is not recommended to be performed.

References

1. Hilal T. Current understanding and approach to well differentiated lung neuroendocrine tumors: an update on classification and management. Ther Adv Med Oncol. 2017;9(3):189–99.
2. Basu B, Sirohi B, Corrie P. Systemic therapy for neuroendocrine tumours of gastroenteropancreatic origin. Endocr Relat Cancer. 2010;17(1):75–90.
3. Scalettar BA, Jacobs C, Fulwiler A, et al. Hindered submicron mobility and long-term storage of presynaptic dense-core granules revealed by single-particle tracking. Dev Neurobiol. 2012;72(9):1181–95.
4. Oronsky B, Ma PC, Morgensztern B, et al. Nothing but NET; a review of neuroendocrine tumors and carcinomas. Neoplasia. 2017;19:991–1002.
5. Anaizi A, Rizvi-Toner A, Valestin J, et al. Large cell neuroendocrine carcinoma of the lung presenting as pseudoachalasia: a case report. J Med Case Rep. 2015;9:56.
6. Williams E, Sandler M. The classification of carcinoid tumours. Lancet. 1963;281(7275):238–9.
7. Axiotis CA. The neuroendocrine lung. In: Volsi VL, Asa SL, editors. Endocrine pathology. New York: Churchill Livingstone; 2002. p. 261–96.
8. Travis WD. The concept of pulmonary neuroendocrine tumours. In: Travis WD, Brambilla E, Muller-Hermelink HK, Harris CC, editors. Pathology and genetics of tumours of the lung, pleura, thymus and heart. Lyon: IARC Press; 2004.
9. Hendifar AE, Marchevsky AM, Tuli R. Neuroendocrine tumours of the lung; current challenges and advances in the diagnosis and management of well-differentiated disease. J Thorac Oncol. 2017;12(3):425–36.
10. Limouris GS, Chatziioannou A, Kontogeorgakos D, et al. Selective hepatic arterial infusion of In-111-DTPA-Phe1-octreotide in neuro-endocrine liver metastases. Eur J Nucl Med Mol Imaging. 2008;35:1827–37.
11. Ekeblad S, Sundin A, Janson ET, et al. Temozolomide as monotherapy is effective in treatment of advanced malignant neuroendocrine tumours. Clin Cancer Res. 2007;13:2986–299.
12. Kulke MH, Lenz HJ, Meropol NJ, et al. Activity of sunitinib in patients with advanced neuroendocrine tumors. J Clin Oncol. 2008;26:3403–10.
13. Yao JC, Phan AT, Chang DZ, et al. Efficacy of RAD001 (everolimus) and octreotide LAR in advanced low- to intermediate-grade neuroendocrine tumors: results of a phase II study. J Clin Oncol. 2008;26:4311–8.
14. Duran I, Kortmansky J, Singh D, et al. A phase II clinical and pharmacodynamic study of temsirolimus in advanced neuroendocrine carcinomas. Br J Cancer. 2006;95:1148–54.
15. Pavel ME, Hainsworth JD, Baudin E, et al. Everolimus plus octreotide long-acting repeatable for the treatment of advanced neuroendocrine tumours associated with carcinoid syndrome (RADIANT-2): a randomised, placebo-controlled, phase 3 study. Lancet. 2011;378:2005–12.
16. Yao JC, Fazio N, Singh S, et al. RAD001 in Advanced Neuroendocrine Tumours, Fourth Trial (RADIANT-4) Study Group. Everolimus for the treatment of advanced, non-functional neuroendocrine tumours of the lung or gastrointestinal tract (RADIANT-4): a randomised, placebo-controlled, phase 3 study. Lancet. 2016;387(10022):968–77.
17. Fazio N, Granberg D, Grossman A, et al. Everolimus plus octreotide long-acting repeatable in patients with advanced lung neuroendocrine tumors: analy-

sis of the phase 3, randomized, placebo-controlled RADIANT-2 study. Chest. 2013;143:955–62.

18. Papotti M, Groce S, Macri D, et al. Correlative immuno-histochemical and reverse transcriptase polymerase chain reaction analysis of somatostatin receptor type 2 in neuroendocrine tumors of the lung. Diagn Mol Pathol. 2000;9:47–57.

19. Limouris GS, Karfis I, Paphiti MI, et al. The drawback to treat neuroendocrine bronchial tumors with high doses of radiolabelled somatostatin analogs. Eur J Nucl Med Mol Imaging. 2012;39(Suppl 2):457. [abstr].

20. Waldherr C, Pless M, Maecke HR, Haldemann A, Mueller-Brand J. The clinical value of [^{90}Y-DOTA]-D-Phe^{1}Tyr^{3}octreotide (^{90}Y-DOTATOC) in the treatment of neuroendocrine tumours: a clinical phase II study. Ann Oncol. 2001;12:941–5.

21. Waldherr C, Pless M, Maecke HR, et al. Tumor response and clinical benefit in neuroendocrine tumors after 7.4 GBq 90Y-DOTATOC. J Nucl Med. 2002;43(5):610–6.

22. Imhof A, Brunner P, Marincek N, et al. Response, survival, and long-term toxicity after therapy with the radiolabelled somatostatin analogue [90Y-DOTA]-TOC in metastasized neuroendocrine cancers. J Clin Oncol. 2011;29(17):2416–23.

23. Filice A, Fraternali A, Frasoldati A, et al. Radiolabeled somatostatin analogues therapy in advanced neuroendocrine tumors: a single centre experience. J Oncol. 2012;2012:320198. https://doi.org/10.1155/2012/320198.

24. Brabander T, van der Zwan WA, Teunissen JJM, et al. Long-term efficacy, survival, and safety of [^{177}Lu-DOTA^0, Tyr^3] octreotate in patients with gastroenteropancreatic and bronchial neuroendocrine tumors. Clin Cancer Res. 2017;23(16):4617–24.

25. Van Essen M, Krenning EP, Kooij PP, et al. Effects of therapy with peptide receptor radionuclide therapy with [^{177}Lu-DOTA^0, Tyr^3] octreotate in patients with paraganglioma, meningioma, small cell lung carcinoma, and melanoma. J Nucl Med. 2006;47:1599–606.

26. Van Essen M, Krenning EP, Bakker WH, et al. Peptide receptor radionuclide therapy with ^{177}Lu-octreotate in patients with foregut carcinoid tumours of bronchial, gastric and thymic origin. Eur J Nucl Med Mol Imaging. 2007;34(8):1219–27.

27. Sabet A, Haug AR, Eiden C, et al. Efficacy of peptide receptor radio-nuclide therapy with 177Lu-octreotate in metastatic pulmonary neuroendocrine tumors: a dual-centre analysis. Am J Nucl Med Mol Imaging. 2017;7(2):74–83.

28. Garske-Román U, Sandström M, Fröss-Baron K, et al. Prospective observational study of 177Lu-DOTA-octreotate therapy in 200 patients with advanced metastasized neuroendocrine tumours (NETs): feasibility and impact of a dosimetry-guided study protocol on outcome and toxicity. Eur J Nucl Med Mol Imaging. 2018;45:970–88.

29. Mariniello A, Bodei L, Tinelli C, et al. Long-term results of PRRT in advanced bronchopulmonary carcinoid. Eur J Nucl Med Mol Imaging. 2016;43(3):441–52.

30. Ianniello A, Sansovini M, Severi S, et al. Peptide receptor radionuclide therapy with (177) Lu-DOTATATE in advanced bronchial carcinoids: prognostic role of thyroid transcription factor 1 and (18)F-FDG PET. Eur J Nucl Med Mol Imaging. 2016;43(6):1040–6.

31. van der Zwan WA, Brabander T, Kam BLR, et al. Salvage peptide receptor radionuclide therapy with [177Lu-DOTA, Tyr3] octreotate in patients with bronchial and gastroenteropancreatic neuroendocrine tumours. Eur J Nucl Med Mol Imaging. 2019;46(3):704–17.

^{111}In-Octreotide Infusions for the Treatment of Colorectal Carcinoma

Georgios S. Limouris and Athanasios G. Zafeirakis

15.1 Introduction

The rate of detection of colorectal neuroendocrine neoplasms (NENs) is increasing, due to the widespread use of colonoscopy, including an established screening tool, and the followed biopsy of the removed lesions [1]. Colorectal cancer is a hindgut tumor which according to the statement of the authors of the recent ENETS consensus has to be treated not individually but as two different malignancies, i.e., the NEN of the rectum and the NEN of the colon [2].

Rectal NENs are usually small in size lesions (most <1 cm), and their histological malignancy is low to moderate (G1, G2), whereas NENs of the colon are often of larger dimension, aggressive, poorly differentiated, and more malignant (G3). Colonic NENs account for 7.8% and rectal NENs for 13.7% of all neuroendocrine neoplasms [3]. The most common site for colonic tumors is the caecum, and this location is more frequent in females [3]. The mean age at disease onset is 70 years [4, 5]. Rectal tumors are the third largest group of gastrointestinal NENs, accounting 1% of all rectal tumors. According to

Japanese and Korean data, rectal NENs are more common in the male population [6] with highest incidence in Asian and African patients [6, 7]. The mean age of patients with rectal NENs is 56 years. Statistically, rectal NENs record 4.2 cases per 1,000,000 citizens [6, 7]. Rectal NENs are usually single lesions. If neuroendocrine lesions are found in the rectum [8], complete colonoscopy is recommended.

According to the WHO classification of 2010, rectal NETs can be separated into three categories based on both Ki-67 index and mitotic count, as follows: low grade (G1) = <2 mitoses/10 high-power fields (HPFs) and ≤2% Ki-67 index; intermediate grade (G2) = 2–20 mitoses/10 HPFs or 3–20% Ki-67 index; or high grade (G3) = >20 mitoses/10 HPFs or >20% Ki-67 index [8, 9] (Table 15.1).

Surgery consists the only curative option for rectal NETs, but as in the bronchopulmonary NENs, there is a lack of precision-consensus between for both colonic and rectal NET management and guidelines regarding optimal treatment approaches in the unresectable/metastatic setting on account of the limited availability of high-level clinical evidence. As a result, a multidisciplinary approach for the management of colorectal NETs is required to ensure a consistent and optimal level of care (Table 15.2) [10]. Lesions ≤10 mm without invasion of the muscularis propria and without depression or ulceration seen macroscopically

G. S. Limouris (✉)
Nuclear Medicine, Medical School, National and Kapodistrian University of Athens, Athens, Greece
e-mail: glimouris@med.uoa.gr

A. G. Zafeirakis
Nuclear Medicine Department, Army Share Fund Hospital of Athens, Athens, Greece

© Springer Nature Switzerland AG 2021
G. S. Limouris (ed.), *Liver Intra-arterial PRRT with ^{111}In-Octreotide*,
https://doi.org/10.1007/978-3-030-70773-6_15

Table 15.1 NETs 2010: WHO classification for rectal NETs

Differentiation	Grade	Mitoses per 10 HPFs	Ki-67 index
Well differentiated	Low grade (G1)	<2	<3%
Well differentiated	Intermediate grade (G2)	2–20	3–20%
Poorly differentiated	High grade (G3)	>20	>20%

HPFs high-power fields

Table 15.2 Multidisciplinary team approach to reviewing colorectal and liver-metastasized patients

Nuclear medicine physician	Hepatic surgeon
Interventional radiologist	Medical oncologist
Radiation physicist	Pathologist
Colorectal surgeon	Anesthesiologist
Gastroenterologist	Dedicated nursing staff

Table 15.3 Colorectal patients' response to therapy with ^{111}In-Octreotide

Patients' no.	Age/ sex	Response evolution	PFS (months)	O S (months)
1	76/f	PR	54	61
2	63/m	PD	5	27
3	62/f	PR	78	>96
4	59/f	PR	60	60
5	56/f	PR	30	69
6	63/f	PR	49	71
7	79/f	PD	7	17
8	55/f	PR	33	41
9	52/m	PR	36	48
10	49/f	SD	29	35
11	68/m	PR	42	46

PR partial response, *SD* stable disease, *PD* progressive disease, *D* death

could be locally resected safely [11]. Rectal NETs between 10 and 20 mm have sparked more controversy and can be managed with endoscopy or surgery depending on the stage. Alternatively, larger lesions >20 mm should be managed like rectal adenocarcinoma with low anterior resection or, in rare cases, abdomino-perineal resection [8].

We report on the effectiveness of PRRT in 11 colorectal, liver metastasized patients [3 males, 8 females (Table 15.3)] discussing and analyzing the recent ergography developments. Indication for PRRT was decided in an interdisciplinary tumor board. Planar and SPECT scans were performed for all therapy cycles to calculate tumor and critical organ doses, followed by quantitative dosimetry. Accordingly, absorbed doses delivered to liver metastases, kidneys, and red marrow were calculated according to OLINDA 1.1 program, and response assessment was classified, based on RECIST 1.1 criteria. Response to salvage PRRT was assessed by CT/MRI scans performed before, during, and after the end of treatment and monthly ultrasound images for liver follow-up measurements. Toxicity (WHO criteria) was measured using blood and urine tests of renal, hepatic, and bone marrow function. Progression-free survival

(PFS) analysis was performed with the Kaplan-Meier survival plot. High doses [4070–5920 MBq (110–160 mCi)] of ^{111}In-Octreotide were intra-arterially infused, after catheterization of the hepatic artery of these 11 patients with surgically removed ascendant colonic (2 cases), descendant colonic (4 cases), sigmoid (3 cases), cecum (1 case), and rectal (1 case) NENs, associated with liver metastases, positive for somatostatin receptors [verified by OctreoScan® (Figs. 15.1 and 15.2) and confirmed by biopsy].

15.2 ^{111}In-Octreotide Treatment Results

Liver metastatic load: None of the 11 treated patients resulted in complete response, and partial response was assessed in 8 cases. Table 15.3: One out of the aforementioned 11 cases resulted in disease stabilization, whereas 2 did not respond at all and died within about 1 year after the initialization of the therapeutic scheme (patients 2 and 7) due to disease aggravation (Fig. 15.3). The 36-month PFS ratio was 6/11 (54.54%), and the ratio for OS was 8/11 (72.72%).

In both U/S and CT, liver-metastasized tumor lesions showed a mean target diameter shrinkage ranging from 33 to 45%. A Grade II to III erythro-, leuko-, and thrombocytopenia occurred in all PD cases. Dosimetric calculations

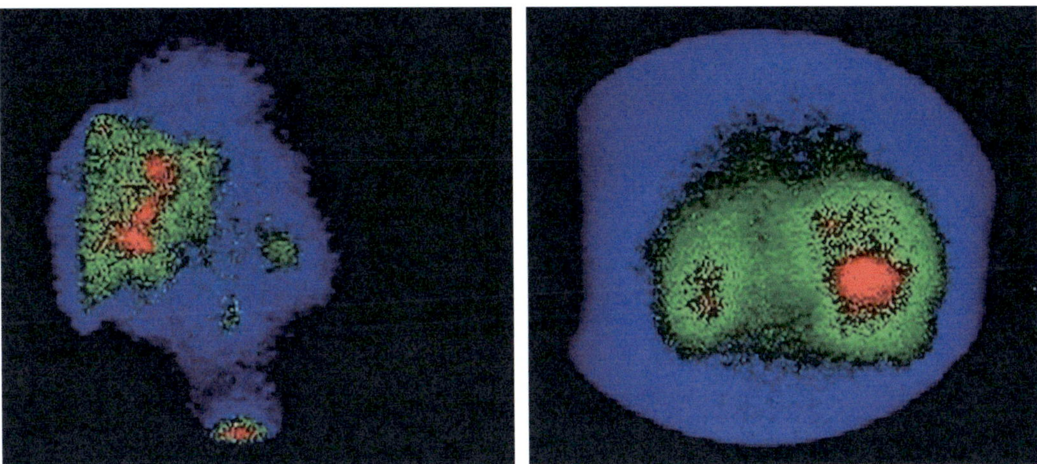

Fig. 15.1 OctreoScan® scintigraphy (anterior/posterior view) of a colorectal carcinoma after 185 MBq ¹¹¹In-Octreotide, i.v. 7 h post injection. Overintense radiotracer uptake in liver and spleen (visual score IV)

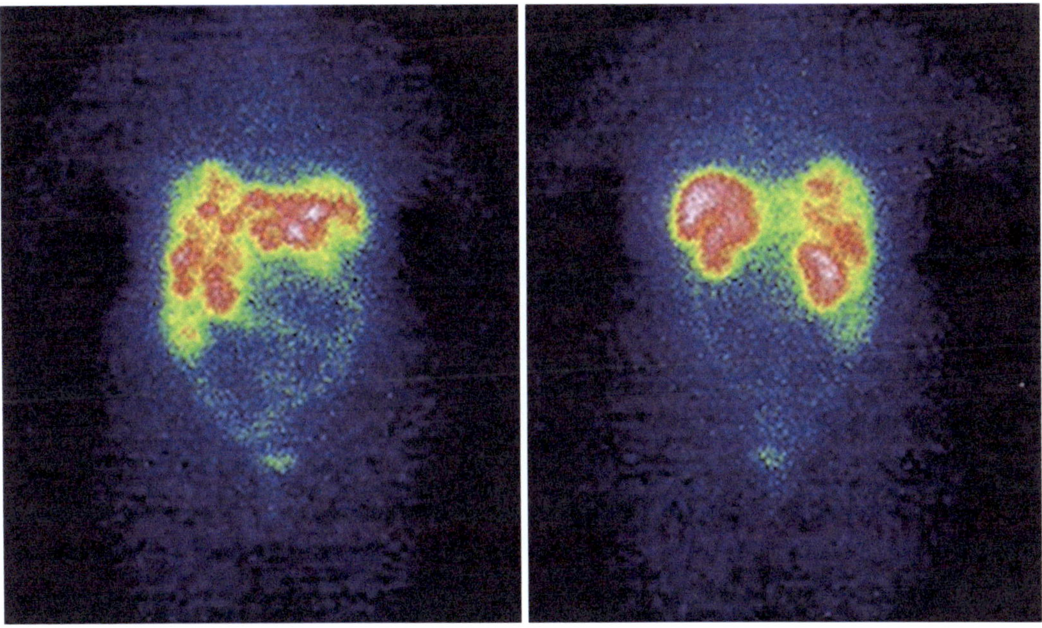

Fig. 15.2 OctreoScan® scintigraphy of a BPNN after 185 MBq ¹¹¹In-Octreotide, i.v. 7 h post injection (left: anterior view; right, posterior view). Overintense radiotracer uptake in the liver and spleen (visual score IV)

(Table 15.4) were found as follows: (a) liver tumor 15.2 mGy/MBq, (b) liver 0.14 mGy/MBq, (c) kidneys 0.41 mGy/MBq, (d) spleen 1.4 mGy/MBq, and (e) bone marrow 0.0035 mGy/MBq. Remarkably, a threefold tumor-/liver-absorbed dose difference is observed between intra-arterial (i.a.) and intravenous (i. v.) one.

15.3   Discussion

In the limited cohort of the present study of 11 patients suffering from liver-metastasized colorectal NENs treated with ¹¹¹In-Octreotide with surgically removed primaries, an objective response was observed in 8 (72.72%) patients

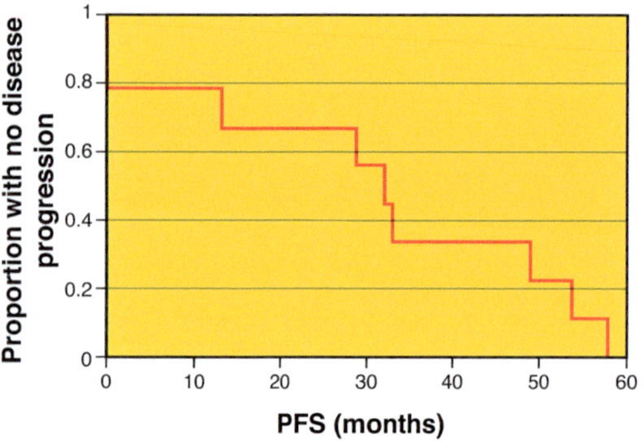
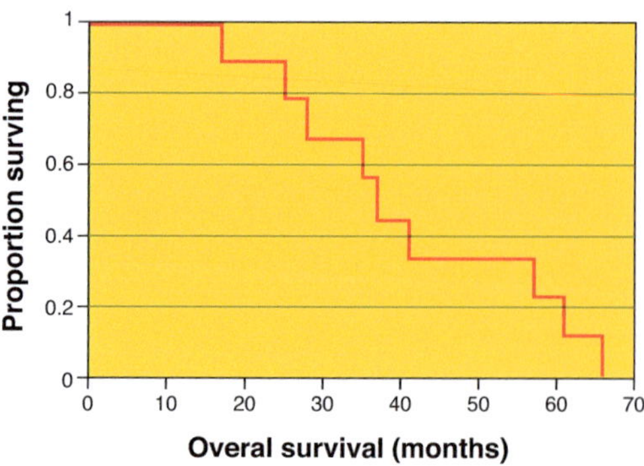

Fig. 15.3 Kaplan-Meier curves for progression-free (left) and overall survival (OS) of the 11 colorectal patients' study, treated with ^{111}In-Octreotide

Table 15.4 Tumor-absorbed dose comparison between i.v. and i.a. administration of ^{111}In-Octreotide

	Intra-arterial infusion	Intravenous infusion
Liver dose	0.14 (mGy/MBq)	0.40 (mGy/MBq)
Kidney dose	0.41 (mGy/MBq)	0.51 (mGy/MBq)
Tumor dose	15.20 (mGy/MBq)	11.20 (mGy/MBq)
Spleen dose	1.40 (mGy/MBq)	1.56 (mGy/MBq)
Bone marrow dose	0.0035 (mGy/MBq)	0.022 (mGy/MBq)
Tumor/liver dose ratio	108.57[a]	28.00
Tumor/kidney dose ratio	37.07	21.96

[a]The average absorbed dose per session to a tumor for a spherical mass of 10 g was estimated to be 10.8 mGy/MBq, depending on the histotype of the tumor

with a median PFS of 36 months. This single-center analysis provides efficacy results including a clearly limited progression-free survival and overall survival as well. Despite the small patient number ($n = 11$), these findings can act as a first class forwarding the feature of the persistent antiproliferative activity of ^{111}In-Octrerotide Auger and internal conversion electron emission in this specific NET entity at an advanced stage.

Few data are available internationally concerning the effectiveness of targeted therapy with radioisotope-labeled somatostatin analogues in patients with colorectal NENs (Table 15.5), and

according to Kwekkeboom et al., the observed survival following PRRT is shorter than in midgut tumors [12]. The relevant international references report on [90]Y- and ^{177}Lu-labeled peptides but not with [111]In.

In a retrospective study of Lung et al., in 2017, 6 out of 26 patients with metastatic G3 advanced NETs, originated from the rectum, were treated with ^{177}Lu-DOTATE [13]. The authors reported an OS of 18 months and a median time to death (TNTD) of 12 months with a poor prognosis and limited treatment options (usually based on chemotherapy). In a recent prospective study of Garske-Román et al. on 11 rectal NETs, median PFS and OS were 34 (17–35) and 50 months, respectively, in 8 out of 11 patients, in whom the absorbed dose to the kidneys reached 23 Gy; in the rest three, in whom it did not, PFS and OS were 12 (3–12) and 12 (11–33) months, accordingly [14]. In another similar retrospective review study of Kong et al. on 27 patients with rectal NETs, treated with ^{177}Lu-DOTATATE, 10 patients died with a median OS of 81 months and a median PFS of 29 months. The authors reported a PR in 19 (70%) patients and a SD in 7 (26%) [15].

15.4 Conclusion

In unresectable metastatic liver lesions positive for somatostatin receptors, colorectal originated, repeated, intra-arterially infused, high doses of

Table 15.5 Experts on PRRT in colorectal NETs

Author	Year	Radiopeptide	Origin	n	orr (%)	PFS (months)	OS (months)
Lung et al.	2017	^{177}Lu-DOTATATE	Rectal	6	nr	nr	18
Garske-Román et al.	2018	^{177}Lu-DOTATATE	Rectal	11	5	34 (8/11) 12 (3/11)	50 (8/11) 12 (3/11)
Kong G et al.	2019	^{177}Lu-DOTATATE	Colorectal	27	70	29	81
Limouris et al.	Present study	^{111}In-Octreotide	Total	11	71.4	36	48
			desc	4		45.5	53.5
			sigm	3		61	68
			asc	2		44	82.5
			rect	1		5	27
			cecum	1		36	48

orr objective response rate, *dcr* disease control rate, *PFS* progression-free survival, *os* overall survival, *nr* non-referred, *desc* descending colon, *sigm* sigmoid, *r* rectum

^{111}In-Octreotide resulted in an 11 NET patient cohort an overall response rate of 72.72%. The Auger and internal conversion electron emission of ^{111}In-Octreotide seems to be a promising therapeutic tool to confront liver-metastasized hindgut tumors, especially in those secondaries not exceeding the 20 mm in diameter, having the same successful outcome observed in GEP-NET cases.

References

1. Bogacka B, Marlicz W, Białek A,˙ et al. Trends in colorectal neuroendocrine tumors: a 10 years review. Gut. 2009;58:A296.
2. Ramage JK, De Herder WW, Delle Fave G, et al. Vienna Consensus Conference participants. ENETS consensus guidelines update for colorectal neuroendocrine neoplasms. Neuroendocrinology. 2016;103(2):139–43.
3. Modlin IM, Lye KD, Kidd M. A 5-decade analysis of 13,715 carcinoid tumors. Cancer. 2003;97:934–59.
4. Modlin I, Kidd M, Latich I, et al. Current status of gastrointestinal carcinoids. Gastroenterology. 2005;128:1717–51.
5. Rydzewska G, Cichocki A, Ćwikła JB, et al. Gastroduodenal neuro-endocrine neoplasms including gastrinoma—management guidelines (recommended by the Polish Network of Neuroendocrine Tumours). Endokrynol Pol. 2013;64(6):444–58.
6. Maggard MA, O'Connell JB, Ko CY. Updated population-based review of carcinoid tumours. Ann Surg. 2004;240:117–22.
7. Matsui K, Iwase T, Kitagawa M. Small, polypoid-appearing carcinoid tumors of the rectum: clinicopathologic study of 16 cases and effectiveness of endoscopic treatment. Am J Gastroenterol. 1993;88:1949–53.
8. Caplin M, Sundin A, Nillson O, et al. ENETS Consensus guidelines for the management of patients with digestive neuroendocrine neoplasms: colorectal neuroendocrine neoplasms. Neuroendocrinology. 2012;95:88–97.
9. Anthony LB, Strosberg JR, Klimstra DS, et al. The NANETS consensus guidelines for the diagnosis and management of gastrointestinal neuroendocrine tumors (nets): well-differentiated nets of the distal colon and rectum. Pancreas. 2010;39:767–74.
10. Limouris GS, Chatziioannou A, Kontogeorgakos D, et al. Selective hepatic arterial infusion of In-111-DTPA-Phe1-octreotide in neuro-endocrine liver metastases. Eur J Nucl Med Mol Imaging. 2008;35:1827–37.
11. Kobayashi K, Katsumata T, Yoshizawa S, et al. Indications of endoscopic polypectomy for rectal carcinoid tumors and clinical usefulness of endoscopic ultrasonography. Dis Colon Rectum. 2005;48:285–91.
12. Kwekkeboom DJ, de Herder WW, van Eijck CHJ, et al. Peptide receptor radionuclide therapy in patients with gastroenteropancreatic neuroendocrine tumors. Semin Nucl Med. 2010;40(2):78–88.
13. Lung MS, Hofman M, Kong G. Outcomes of peptide receptor radionuclide therapy (PRRT) in metastatic grade 3 neuroendocrine tumors (NETs). J Clin Oncol. 2017;2017:35. (15 suppl. Abstract e15694).
14. Garske-Román U, Sandström M, Fröss-Baron K, et al. Prospective observational study of 177Lu-DOTA-octreotate therapy in 200 patients with advanced metastasized neuroendocrine tumours (NETs): feasibility and impact of a dosimetry-guided study protocol on outcome and toxicity. Eur J Nucl Med Mol Imaging. 2018;45:970–88.
15. Kong G, Grozinsky-Glasberg S, Hofman MS, et al. Highly favorable outcomes with peptide receptor radionuclide therapy (PRRT) for metastatic rectal neuroendocrine neoplasia (NEN). Eur J Nucl Med Mol Imaging. 2019;46(3):718–27.

¹¹¹In-Octreotide Infusions for the Treatment of Paraganglioma

Georgios S. Limouris, Valery Krylov, Michael B. Dolgushin, and Athanasios G. Zafeirakis

16.1 Introduction

Paragangliomas are rare, non-epithelial NETs [1], which derive from paraganglial system, and are classified as (a) sympathetic, almost always producing catecholamines, and (b) parasympathetic, usually not releasing catecholamines [2].

They are metastatic in about 10% of cases. Paragangliomas are known to express high levels of somatostatin receptors (sst), especially subtype sst2. However, according to Saveanu et al. [3], Reubi et al. [4], and Binderup et al. [5], some paragangliomas have cytoplasmic localization of sst2 receptor rather than a membrane, and it has been suggested that this might account for not only the failure of sst2 agonists in controlling catechol-amine secretion and tumor proliferation but also failure of ¹¹¹In-Octreotide imaging to detect some of them. ¹¹¹In-Octreotide shows a modest sst2 binding, having a good sensitivity (up to 90%) for head and neck paragangliomas [6] and according to Charrier et al. [7] a mediocre sensitivity as low as 20% as far as the abdominal ones. Nowadays, for their diagnosis, a new generation of somatostatin analogs with superior sst2 binding affinity has been developed for use with PET/CT imaging such as ⁶⁸Ga-DOTATOC, ⁶⁸Ga-DOTANOC, and ⁶⁸Ga-DOTATATE [8, 9] (Table 16.1).

According to WHO, paragangliomas are classified into two groups, based on their clinical and biological behavior: those arising from the parasympathetic system, primary located in the head and neck and less frequently in the thorax and pelvis, and those from the sympathetic one (Table 16.2).

16.1.1 Parasympathetic (Head and Neck) Paragangliomas

Accounting approximately a 20% of all paragangliomas [10–12] are generally nonfunctioning subcategorized according to their anatomical sites of origin as carotid body paragangliomas, jugulo-tympanic paragangliomas (Fig. 16.1), vagal paragangliomas, and laryngeal paragangliomas [13]. As a whole, less than 5% of head and neck paragangliomas metastasize. Hereditary cases of head and neck paragangliomas could be multiple and

G. S. Limouris (✉)
Nuclear Medicine, Medical School, National and Kapodistrian University of Athens, Athens, Greece
e-mail: glimouris@med.uoa.gr

V. Krylov
Nuclear Medicine Department, "A. Tsyb Research Center", Obninsk, Russia

M. B. Dolgushin
N.N. Blokhin Russian Oncological Research Center, Moscow, Russia

A. G. Zafeirakis
Nuclear Medicine Department, Army Share Fund Hospital of Athens, Athens, Greece

© Springer Nature Switzerland AG 2021
G. S. Limouris (ed.), *Liver Intra-arterial PRRT with ¹¹¹In-Octreotide*,
https://doi.org/10.1007/978-3-030-70773-6_16

Table 16.1 Affinity profiles (IC50) of somatostatin receptor subtypes for imaging and therapy

Sst and its analogs	sst1	sst2	sst3	sst4	sst5
Somatostatin-28	5.2	2.7	7.7	5.6	4.0
[111]In-Octreotide	>10,000	22	182	>1000	237
68Ga-DOTATOC	>10,000	2.5	613	>1000	73
68Ga-DOTANOC	>10,000	1.9	40	260	7.2
68Ga-DOTATATE	>10,000	0.2	>1000	300	377

IC50 is expressed in nanomoles (the lower the values, the higher the receptor affinity)

Table 16.2 WHO classification for paragangliomas

	Sympathetic	Parasympathetic
Location/ frequency	Below the diaphragm/85%	Head-neck/20%
Function	+++	+
Norepinephrine levels	+++	+
Dopamine levels	+++	+
Metastatic tension	High risk	Seldom (<5%)

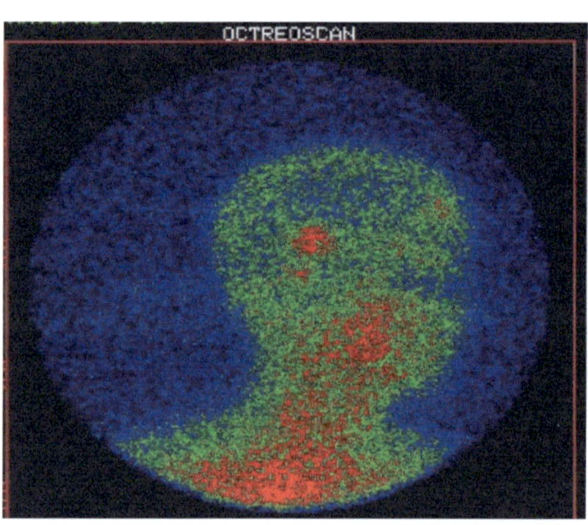

Fig. 16.1 OctreoScan® scintigraphy (right lateral view) of a petrous-bone paraganglioma, after 185 MBq ^{111}In-Octreotide, i.v. 7 h post injection (visual score II to III)

occur in association with sympathetic ones. The germline mutation, most commonly noted in one of the succinate dehydrogenase genes (SDHx), can be screened by immunohistochemical staining for SDHB protein. Paragangliomas associated with SDHB mutations have a high risk of metastasis. Thus, even in the absence of family history, genetic testing should be recommended for at least the most common genes in all patients, depending on local resources [14].

16.1.2 Sympathetic Paragangliomas

Approximately 85% of sympathetic paragangliomas arise below the diaphragm. Sympathetic paraganglioma could be found in retroperitoneum around the adrenal/renal area, around the organ of Zuckerkandl or in the urinary bladder [15]. The other sympathetic paragangliomas are noted in the thorax, heart, and other locations [16–18]. Sympathetic paragangliomas are more likely to be functioning when compared to head and neck paragangliomas [19]. Patients with sympathetic paragangliomas usually have elevated norepinephrine only or both norepinephrine and dopamine. Sympathetic paragangliomas have high risk of metastases and even higher (even up to 50%) in those with SDHB mutation [20].

16.1.3 Treatment Stratification

Although most paragangliomas are benign, factors such as genetic background, tumor size, tumor location, and high methoxy-tyramine levels are associated with higher rate of metastatic disease. Their proximity to cranial nerves and vasculature may result in considerable morbidity due to compression or infiltration of the adjacent structures, necessitating balanced decisions between a wait-and-see policy and active treatment [21]. Surgery is the only curative treatment. Treatment options for patients with metastatic disease are limited. Paragangliomas have a strong genetic background, with at least one-third of all cases linked with germline mutations in 11 susceptibility genes. As genetic testing becomes more widely available, the diagnosis assessment of paragangliomas will be made earlier due to

Table 16.3 Multidisciplinary team approach for the paraganglioma patient's management

Nuclear medicine physician	Hepatic surgeon
Interventional radiologist	Medical oncologist
Radiation physicist	Pathologist
Colorectal surgeon	Anesthesiologist
Gastroenterologist	Dedicated nursing staff

routine screening of at-risk patients. As a result, a multidisciplinary approach for the management of paragangliomas is required to ensure a consistent and optimal level of care and treatment (Table 16.3).

For both sympathetic and parasympathetic PGLs, surgery is the treatment of choice, in cases where it can be performed. Further options of therapeutic schemes include systematic treatment with agents as gemcitabine, cisplatin or sunitinib, and radiotherapy (external-beam radiotherapy or stereotactic surgery). However, surgery and radiotherapy can cause severe side effects: the former hemostatic complications and nerve damage, particularly when tumor is in tight proximity with cranial nerves, and the latter vascular complications and peripheral nerve damage as well. In the international library, limited clinical data are available focused on radiopeptide schemes as treating option to confront paragangliomas. By the present, we describe and discuss the challenges of treating these rare tumors with ^{111}In-octreotide in high doses, using established protocols, performed in our institution for other NET histotypes.

We report on the effectiveness of PRRT in three paraganglioma patients [one with surgically excised primary in the lower part of the sigmoid colon associated with liver metastases and two inoperable cases (one at the petrous portion of the right temporal bone of the skull and the second situated in the lower half of the mediastinum)], verified by Octreo-Scan® (Figs. 16.1 and 16.2) and biochemically and radiologically confirmed. The dose per session administered monthly to each patient ranged from 4.070 to 5.920 GBq. Repetitions for the inoperable cases did not exceed the nine sessions and for liver secondaries the twelve, with treatment intervals of 5–8 weeks.

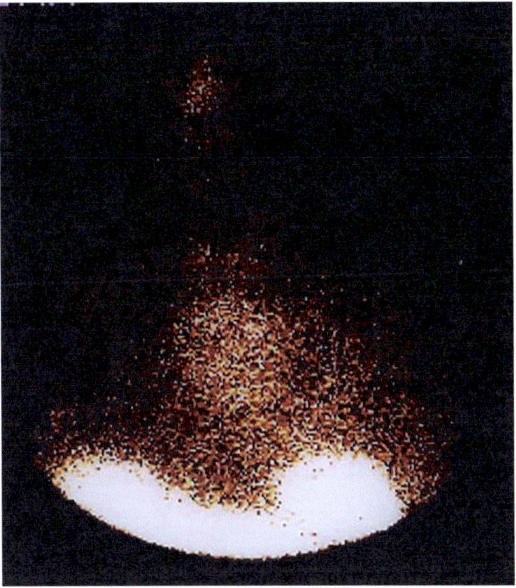

Fig. 16.2 OctreoScan® scintigraphy (anterior view) of an inoperable paraganglioma of the lower half of mediastinum, after 185 MBq ^{111}In-Octreotide, i.v. 7 h-post injection (visual score II to III)

Patients with inoperable PGLs were infused intravenously, after centesis of the dorsal vein hand system or the antecubital vein, whereas for the liver secondaries, ^{111}In-Octreotide was infused intra-arterially, after catheterization of the hepatic artery. Absorbed doses delivered to the primaries, to the liver metastases, kidneys, and red marrow were calculated according to OLINDA/EXM program, and response assessment was classified, based on RECIST criteria 1.1. CT/MRI scans were performed before, during, and after the end of treatment and monthly ultrasound images for the follow-up of the liver lesions.

16.2 ^{111}In-Octreotide Treatment Results

Liver metastatic load: None of the three treated patients resulted in complete response; partial response was assessed in one, whereas disease stabilization in two. *Petrous bone and mesothorax primary neoplasms load:* The aforementioned two cases resulted in initially disease stabilization for a short term, whereas on the

Table 16.4 Patients response to therapy with ^{111}In-octreotide

Patient's no./infusion way	Tumor origin	Response evolution	PFS	OS
1. Intravenously	Inoperable, mediastinum	SD ≫ PD ≫ D	25	29
2. Intravenously	Inoperable, petrous bone	SD ≫ PD ≫ D	19	26
3. Intra-arterially	Surgically excised, sigmoid	PR	108	120

PD partial response, *SD* stable disease, *PD* progressive disease, *D* death, ≫ shifted to

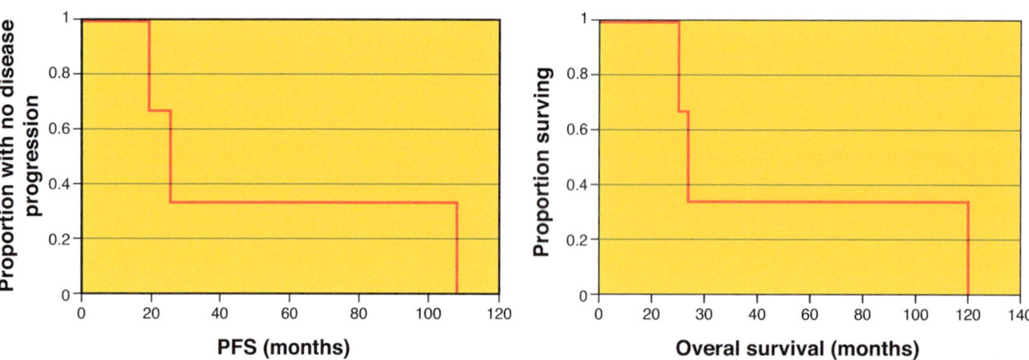

Fig. 16.3 Kaplan-Meier curves for PFS and OS of the three paraganglioma patients' study, treated with ^{111}In-Octreotide

progress of the therapy, they did not respond at all and died within 26–29 months after the initialization of the therapy due to aggravation and complications of the tumors (Table 16.4). According to the therapy response results, the 24-month PFS ratio was found to be 2/3 (66.6%) while the 24-month OS was 3/3 (100%) (Fig. 16.3). On CT, the mesothorax and petrous bone tumor masses progressed dramatically, whereas the liver metastases showed a mean target diameter shrinkage ranging from 33 to 45%. Grade I to II erythro-, leuko-, and thrombocytopenia occurred in all three cases. Dosimetric calculations for both the intra-arterial and intravenous infusions are tabulated in Table 16.5. Remarkably, an over than threefold higher tumor absorbed dose in favor of the intra-arterial one was noticed.

16.3 Discussion

This single-center analysis provides results including the respective progression-free survival and overall survival rates of PRRT in three patients with advanced paragangliomas of different primary origins after failing standard treatment. Despite the tiny patient number ($n = 3$), the treatment results forward the feature of the persistent anti-proliferative activity of ^{111}In-Octreotide Auger and internal conversion electron emission in this specific NET rare entity at an advanced stage. However, this sort of electron emission achieves a rather insignificant disease control in the case of inoperable mediastinum and petrous paraganglioma patients, intravenously treated, a short-term stabilization, and a median progression-free survival (PFS) of 19–25 months, thus rendering ^{111}In-Octrerotide not promising for an objective outcome in that context of lacking established treatment alternatives. On the contrary, concerning the intra-arterially treated hepatic metastases originating from the surgically excised colorectal paraganglioma, a long-term partial response was achieved with a PFS of 108 months.

According to the worldwide ergography, few studies report on the effect of PRRT in the management of patients suffering from metastatic or unresectable paragangliomas and no one on the

Table 16.5 Tumor-absorbed dose comparison between i.v. and i.a. administration of ^{111}In-Octreotide

Organs	Intra-arterial infusion	Intravenous infusion
Liver dose	0.14 (mGy/MBq)	0.40 (mGy/MBq)
Kidney dose	0.41 (mGy/MBq)	0.51 (mGy/MBq)
Tumor dose	15.20 (mGy/MBq)	11.20 (mGy/MBq)
Spleen dose	1.40 (mGy/MBq)	1.56 (mGy/MBq)
Bone marrow dose	0.0035 (mGy/MBq)	0.022 (mGy/MBq)
Tumor/liver dose ratio	108.57[a]	28.00
Tumor/kidney dose ratio	37.07	21.96

[a]The average absorbed dose per session to a tumor for a spherical mass of 10 g was estimated to be 10.8 mGy/MBq, depending on the histotype of the tumor

response and efficacy of Auger and internal conversion indium's electron emission. As in the majority of NETs, surgery consists the treatment of choice to confront this rare neuroendocrine histotype; however, even after radical operation, patients lurk the risk of recurrence and the development of metastases, even after many years. Fortunately, the low toxicity of the neoplasm and the usually settled long-term follow-up create good conditions for an efficient disease control. However, the real challenge for clinicians is the treatment of inoperable or metastatic tumors. Furthermore, the functioning cases, the elevated risk for severe cardiovascular disease, and the risk of malignancy add additional doctors' dilemmas [22–27].

We studied the PRRT results after ^{111}In-Octreotide administration in three patients suffering from paragangliomas. Comparing the internal references of several experteer reports on PRRT (Table 16.6), not with ^{111}In-octreotide (an Auger and internal conversion emitter) but with ^{90}Y-DOTATATE/DOTATOC or ^{177}Lu-DOTATATE (β-emitters), an objective response was observed in one of three (33.3%) patients of the treated cases, with a median PFS of 25 and median OS of 29 months. The outcome of this three-patient cohort gives a disease stabilization in two patients

and a partial response in one. In 2006, in a ^{177}Lu-DOTATATE study by van Essen et al. [28], including 12 PGL patients during a median of 13 (range 4–30) months follow-up, an ORR of 16.7% and a SD of 58.3% were reported. PD was 25%, whereas PFS and OS were not tabulated. In a ^{90}Y DOTATOC study by Imhof et al. [29], in a cohort of 28 paragangliomas, a median OS of 82 months was reported; ORR and PFS were not clearly discriminated. The same year, Zovato et al. [30] achieved in a cohort of four paragangliomas, treated with ^{177}Lu DOTATATE, a median PFS in a range of 15–25 months with a 50% ORR; median OS was not referred. Cecchin et al. [31] in a paraganglioma case study reported a PR (100%) with a median PFS of 16 months; median OS was not referred. Pinato et al. [32], in a study of five paraganglioma-treated cases implementing ^{177}Lu DOTATATE, reported a median PFS and a mean OS of 17 and 53 months, respectively; median OS was not achieved. In a paraganglioma case study of Ashwathanarayana et al., in 2017 [33], a 100% objective response was observed with a mean PFS of about 5 months and a mean OS of 11 months. In a study of Kong et al. [34], 20 patients with paragangliomas, treated with ^{177}Lu-DOTATATE, reached a median PFS of 39 months, whereas the median OS was not reached. The authors reported a PR in 19 (70%) patients and a SD in 7 (26%). In a study by Nastos et al. [35] in 15 paraganglioma cases treated with ^{131}I-mIBG as well as with ^{177}Lu DOTATATE, the median PFS was 20.6 and 38.5 months, respectively. The authors achieved a median OS of 41.8 months for ^{131}I-mIBG and 60.8 months for ^{177}Lu DOTATATE; ORR was not clearly discriminated and tabulated. In a recent prospective study of Garske-Román et al. [36] on 11 rectal NETs, median PFS and OS were 34 (17–35) and 50 months, respectively, in 8 out of 11 patients, in whom the absorbed dose to the kidneys reached 23 Gy; in the rest three, in whom it did not, PFS and OS were 12 (3–12) and 12 (11–33) months accordingly. Yavad et al. [37] evaluated in a recent study the role of combined capecitabine and ^{177}Lu-DOTATATE in malignant PGL patients. He observed in a cohort of 25 cases a 28% objective response with a median PFS of

Table 16.6 Experts on PRRT paraganglioma treatment

Author	Year	Radiopeptide	n	orr (%)	Median PFS (months)	Median OS (months)
van Essen et al.	2006	^{177}Lu-DOTATATE	12	16.7	nr	nr
Imhof et al.	2011	[90]Y DOTATOC	28	a	a	82
Zovato et al.	2011	^{177}Lu-DOTATATE	4	50	>15.8–25	nr
Cecchin et al.	2011	^{177}Lu-DOTATATE	1	100	16	nr
Pinato et al.	2016	^{177}Lu-DOTATATE	5	20	17	nr
Ashwathanarayana et al.	2017	^{177}Lu-DOTATATE	1	100	~5	11
Kong et al.	2017	^{177}Lu-DOTATATE	20	a	30	nr
Nastos et al.	2017	[131]I MIBG ^{90}Y/^{177}Lu-DOTATATE	15	a	20.6 38.5	41.2 60.8
Garske-Román et al.	2018	^{177}Lu-DOTATATE	3	0	14	37
Yadav et al.	2019	^{177}Lu-DOTATATE	25	28	32	nr
Vyakaranam et al.	2019	^{177}Lu-DOTATATE	13	7.7	16.7	37.3
Kolasinska-Cwikła et al.	2019	^{90}Y-DOTATATE	13	8	35	68
Limouris et al.	This study	^{111}In-Octreotide	3	100	25	29

rs retrospective study, *ps* prospective study, *orr* objective response rate, *PFS* progression-free survival, *os* overall survival, *nr* non-referred

[a]not clearly reported nor discriminated and tabulated

32 months; median OS was not referred. Vyakaranam et al. [38] in a recent study in 13 paraganglioma patients, treated with ^{177}Lu-DOTATATE, reported a PR in 1 out of 13 (7.7%) patients, a median OS of 37.3 months, and a median PFS of 21.6 months.

Finally, in a prospective open-label, single-center, phase II study of 13 patients with unresectable advanced paraganglioma treated with ^{90}Y DOTATATE by Kolasinska-Cwikła et al. [39], a median PFS of 35 and a median OS of 68 months were observed.

In our three patients' cohort, the equivocal and almost expected disappointing response to ^{111}In-Octreotide intravenous infusions in PGL primaries was also predicted and expected during each PRRT cycle by scintigraphy, including both whole-body scans and SPECT/CT. Furthermore, the visual rating (score) of the tumor radiotracer uptake ranges between II and III, never reaching the visual score IV of the hepatic secondaries.

16.4 Conclusion

In unresectable metastatic liver lesions positive for somatostatin receptors, originated from PGLs, repeated, intra-arterial high doses of ^{111}In-Octreotide resulted in a partial response in all the affected liver lesions. As far as both primaries, i.e., that of the inoperable petrous bone and the other of the mesothorax, after a short-term disease stabilization, progressed dramatically. The dosimetric calculations proved the poor absorbed dose, predicting the disappointing results. Systematic PRRT in primary PGLs with intravenously injected ^{111}In-Octreotide does not seem to have clinical effects in PGLs due to the over 20 mm tumor size and has no meaning to perform. On the contrary, liver secondaries not exceeding the 20 mm in diameter, intra-arterially treated, show the same successful results observed in GEP-NET histotype (Chap. 7).

References

1. Rindi G, Klimstra DS, Abedi-Ardekani B, et al. A common classification framework for neuroendocrine neoplasms: an International Agency for Research on Cancer (IARC) and World Health Organization (WHO) expert consensus proposal. Mod Pathol. 2018;31(12):1770–86.
2. Hayashi T, Mete O. Head and neck paragangliomas: what does the pathologist need to know? Diagn Histopathol. 2014;20:316–25.
3. Saveanu A, Muresan M, de Micco C, et al. Expression of somatostatin receptors, dopamine D2 receptors,

noradrenaline transporters, and vesicular monoamine transporters in 52 pheochromocytomas and paragangliomas. Endocr Relat Cancer. 2011;18:287–300.

4. Reubi JC, Waser B, Liu Q, Laissue JA, et al. Subcellular distribution of somatostatin sst2A receptors in human tumors of the nervous and neuroendocrine systems: membranous versus intracellular location. J Clin Endocrinol Metab. 2008;85:3882–91.

5. Binderup T, Knigge U, Mellon Mogensen A, et al. Quantitative gene expression of somatostatin receptors and noradrenaline transporter underlying scintigraphic results in patients with neuroendocrine tumors. Neuroendocrinology. 2008;87:223–32.

6. Koopmans KP, Jager PL, Kema IP, et al. 111In-octreotide is superior to 123I-metaiodobenzylgianidine for scintigraphic detection of head and neck paragangliomas. J Nucl Med. 2008;49:1232–7.

7. Charrier N, Deveze A, Fakhry N, et al. Comparison of [111In] pentetreotide-SPECT and [18F]FDOPA-PET in the localization of extra-adrenal paragangliomas: the case for a patient-tailored use of nuclear imaging modalities. Clin Endocrinol. 2011;74:21–9.

8. Reubi JC, Schar JC, Waser B, et al. Affinity profiles for human somatostatin receptor subtypes SST1-SST5 of somatostatin radiotracers selected for scintigraphic and radiotherapeutic use. Eur J Nucl Med. 2000;27:273–82.

9. Wild D, Schmitt JS, Ginj M, et al. DOTA-NOC, a high-affinity ligand of somatostatin receptor subtypes 2, 3 and 5 for labelling with various radiometals. Eur J Nucl Med Mol Imaging. 2003;30:1338–47.

10. Sajid MS, Hamilton G, Baker DM, Joint Vascular Research Group. A multicenter review of carotid body tumour management. Eur J Vasc Endovasc Surg. 2007;34:127–30.

11. Chan JKC, Kimura N, Capella C, et al. Chapter 10: Paraganglion tumours. In: El-Nigger AK, Chan JKC, Grandis JF, Takata T, Slootweg PJ, editors. WHO classification of head and neck tumours. 4th ed. Lyon: IARC; 2017.

12. Blumenfeld J, Cohen N, Anwar M, et al. Hypertension and a tumor of the glomus jugular region. Evidence for epinephrine biosynthesis. Am J Hypertens. 1993;6:382–7.

13. Piccini V, Rapizzi E, Bacca A, et al. Head and neck paragangliomas: genetic spectrum and clinical variability in 79 consecutive patients. Endocr Relat Cancer. 2012;19:149–55.

14. Lam KY, Lo CY, Wat NMS, et al. The clinicopathological features and importance of p53, Rb and mdm2 expression in pheochromocytomas and paragangliomas. J Clin Pathol. 2001;54:443–8.

15. Lam KY, Chan ACL. Paraganglioma of urinary bladder: an immunohistochemical study and report of an unusual association with intestinal carcinoid. Aust N Z J Surg. 1993;63:740–5.

16. Garg A, Mishra D, Bansal M, et al. Right atrial paraganglioma: an extremely rare primary cardiac neoplasm mimicking myxoma. J Cardiovasc Ultrasound. 2016;24:334–6.

17. Michałowska I, Ćwikła J, Prejbisz A, et al. Mediastinal paragangliomas related to SDHx gene mutations. Kardiochir Torakochirurgia Pol. 2016;13:276–82.

18. Soomro NH, Zahid AB, Zafar AA. Non-functional paraganglioma of the mediastinum. J Pak Med Assoc. 2016;66:609–11.

19. Blanchet EM, Martucci V, Pacak K. Pheochromocytoma and paraganglioma: current functional and future molecular imaging. Front Oncol. 2012;1:58.

20. Assadipour Y, Sadowski SM, Alimchandani M, et al. SDHB mutation status and tumor size but not tumor grade are important predictors of clinical outcome in pheochromocytoma and abdominal paraganglioma. Surgery. 2017;161:230–9.

21. Coresmitt EP, Romijn JA. Clinical management of paragangliomas. Eur J Endocrinol. 2014;171(6):232–43.

22. Berends AMA, Buitenwerf E, de Krijger R, et al. Incidence of pheochromocytoma and sympathetic paraganglioma in the Netherlands: a nationwide study and systematic review. Eur J Intern Med. 2018;51:68–73.

23. Lenders JW, Duh QY, Eisenhofer G. Pheochromocytoma and paraganglioma: an endocrine society clinical practice guideline. J Clin Endocrinol Metab. 2014;99:1915–42.

24. Jimenez C, Rohren E, Habra MA, et al. Current and future treatments for malignant pheochromocytoma and sympathetic paraganglioma. Curr Oncol Rep. 2013;15:356–71.

25. Fishbein L, Orlowski R, Cohen D. Pheochromocytoma/paraganglioma; review of perioperative management of blood pressure and update on genetic mutations associated with pheochromocytoma. J Clin Hypertens (Greenwich). 2013;15:428–34.

26. Elston MS, Meyer-Rochow GY, et al. Increased SSTR2A and SSTR3 expression in succinate dehydrogenase-deficient pheochromocytomas and paragangliomas. Hum Pathol. 2015;46:390–6.

27. Lenders JWM, Eisenhofer G. Update on modern management of pheochromocytoma and paraganglioma. Endocrinol Metab. 2017;32:152–61.

28. van Essen M, Krenning EP, Kooij PP, et al. Effects of therapy with [177Lu-DOTA0, Tyr3]-octreotate in patients with paraganglioma, meningioma, small cell lung carcinoma, and melanoma. J Nucl Med. 2006;47(10):1599–606.

29. Imhof A, Brunner P, Marincek N, et al. Response, survival, and long-term toxicity after therapy with the radiolabeled somatostatin analogue [^{90}YDOTA]-TOC in metastasized neuroendocrine cancers. J Clin Oncol. 2011;29(17):2416–23.

30. Zovato S, Kumanova A, Demattè S, et al. Peptide receptor radionuclide therapy (PRRT) with 177Lu-DOTATATE in individuals with neck or mediastinal paraganglioma (PGL). Horm Metab Res. 2012;44(5):411–4.

31. Cecchin D, Schiavi F, Fanti S, et al. Peptide receptor radionuclide therapy in a case of multiple spinal canal and cranial paragangliomas. J Clin Oncol. 2011;29(7):e171–4.

32. Pinato DJ, Black JR, Ramaswami R, et al. Peptide receptor radionuclide therapy for metastatic paragangliomas. Med Oncol. 2016;33(5):47.

33. Ashwathanarayana AG, Biswal CK, Sood A, et al. Imaging guided use of combined 177Lu-DOTATATE and capecitabine therapy in metastatic mediastinal paraganglioma. J Nucl Med Technol. 2017;45(4):314–6.

34. Kong G, Grozinsky-Glasberg S, Hofman MS, et al. Efficacy of peptide receptor radionuclide therapy for functional metastatic paraganglioma and pheochromocytoma. J Clin Endocrinol Metab. 2017;102(9):3278–87.

35. Nastos K, Cheung VT, Toumpanakis C, et al. Peptide Receptor Radionuclide Treatment and (131)I-MIBG in the management of patients with metastatic/progressive pheochromocytomas and paragangliomas. J Surg Oncol. 2017;115(4):425–34.

36. Garske-Román U, Sandström M, Fröss Baron K, et al. Prospective observational study of ^{177}Lu-DOTA-octreotate therapy in 200 patients with advanced metastasized neuroendocrine tumours (NETs): feasibility and impact of a dosimetry-guided study protocol on outcome and toxicity. Eur J Nucl Med Mol Imaging. 2018;45(6):970–88.

37. Yadav MP, Ballal S, Bal C. Concomitant ^{177}Lu-DOTATATE and capecitabine therapy in malignant paragangliomas. EJNMMI Res. 2019;9:13. https://doi.org/10.1186/s13550-019-0484-y.

38. Vyakaranam AR, Crona J, Norlén O. Favorable outcome in patients with pheochromocytoma and paraganglioma treated with 177Lu-DOTATATE. Cancers. 2019;11(7):909. https://doi.org/10.3390/cancers11070909.

39. Kolasinska-Cwikła A, Peczkowska M, Cwikła JB. A clinical efficacy of PRRT in patients with advanced, nonresectable, paraganglioma-pheochromocytoma, related to SDHx gene mutation. J Clin Med. 2019;8:952. https://doi.org/10.3390/jcm8070952www.mdpi.com/journal/jcm.

Georgios S. Limouris, Valery Krylov,
Michael B. Dolgushin,
and Athanasios G. Zafeirakis

17.1 Introduction

Neuroendocrine tumors (NETs) comprise a heterogeneous group of malignancies that arise from neuroendocrine cells throughout the body, most commonly originating from the lung and the gastrointestinal tract.

In the case of brain tumors (Fig. 17.1) a high incidence of sst receptors has been reported in meningiomas, gliomas, and well-differentiated astrocytomas and neuroendocrine secondaries [1–5]. These tumors express a high density of somatostatin receptors compared to the surrounding tissue that allow them to be readily visualized by in vivo receptor imaging methods using labelled somatostatin analogs such as octreotide [4, 6].

NETs were called "carcinoid" 100 years ago and considered as benign neoplasms. Currently, WHO characterized them as malignant, elimi-

nated in 2000, the "carcinoid" label, whereas in 2010 classified them [7–10], including both Ki-67 index and mitotic count, as the following: Low Grade (G1) =<2 mitoses/10 high power fields (HPFs) and $\leq$2% Ki-67 index; Intermediate Grade (G2) = 2–20 mitoses/10 HPFs or 3–20% Ki-67 index; and High Grade (G3) =>20 mitoses/10 HPFs or >20% Ki-67 index [11, 12] (Table 17.1).

The incidence of NETs is increasing, and it is therefore attracting interest and attention. Generally, the majority of metastases occur in the liver (Fig. 17.2), lungs, and bone. Other sites are rarer, and brain metastases are very rare, so an

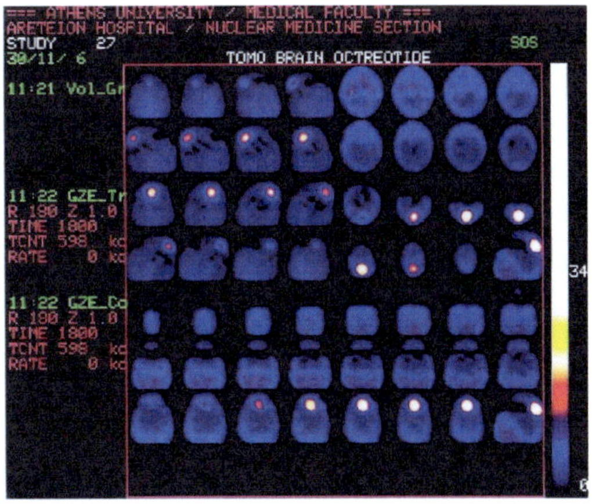

Fig. 17.1 OctreoScan® brain tomo-scintigraphy of a radiologically confirmed meningioma after 111 MBq ^{111}In-Octreotide i.v. 7 h post-injection. Intense radiotracer uptake to the right of the mid-line of the parietooccipital area (visual score IV)

G. S. Limouris (✉)
Nuclear Medicine, Medical School, National and Kapodistrian University of Athens, Athens, Greece
e-mail: glimouris@med.uoa.gr

V. Krylov
Nuclear Medicine Department, "A. Tsyb Research Center", Obninsk, Russia

M. B. Dolgushin
N.N. Blokhin Russian Oncological Research Center, Moscow, Russia

A. G. Zafeirakis
Nuclear Medicine Department, Army Share Fund Hospital of Athens, Athens, Greece

© Springer Nature Switzerland AG 2021
G. S. Limouris (ed.), *Liver Intra-arterial PRRT with ^{111}In-Octreotide*,
https://doi.org/10.1007/978-3-030-70773-6_17

accurate and timely diagnosis can ensure the implementation of appropriate treatment and have a substantial impact on prognosis.

With a worldwide incidence of 45,000 cases [13], meningiomas are the most common non-glial primary intracranial tumors where surgery consists a promising curative option; however, after complete tumor resection Galldiks et al.

Table 17.1 NETs 2010—WHO classification for rectal NETs

Grade	Mitoses per 10 HPFs	Ki-67 index
G1	<2	≤2%
G2	2–10	3–20%
G3	>10	>20%

HPFs high power fields

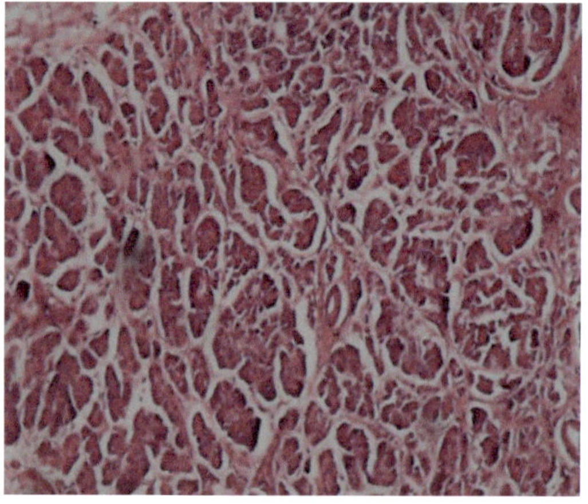

Fig. 17.2 Histological section of a low-grade pancreatic NET metastasized to the liver (Hematoxylin Eosin ×10)

[14] and Goldbrunner et al. [15] reported that a 5-year recurrence rate is estimated to 5%, 40%, and 80% in grades I (benign), II (atypical), and III (anaplastic) of the tumor, respectively. At this step very few treatment options are available. According to Kaley et al. [16] and Guedj et al. [13], the progression-free survival of aggressive recurrent meningiomas decreases below 30% at 6 months, while the median overall survival accounts to 3 years for patients with grade III. Surgery remains the only curative option for treatment of meningioma, whereas external beam radiotherapy offers another curative option in meningioma manipulation [15, 17, 18]. Accordingly, a multidisciplinary approach to the management of brain tumors, positive for soma-tostatin receptors, is required to ensure a consistent and optimal level of care (Table 17.2) [19].

Even after complete surgical removal, meningiomas recur in about 10–32% of the cases within 10 years. As a sequence, among the tumor histo-type treated, we evaluated the effectiveness of high doses of ^{111}In-Octreotide infusions following selective catheterization of the internal

Table 17.2 Multidisciplinary team approach to reviewing lung and liver metastasized patients

Nuclear medicine physician	Hepatic surgeon
Interventional radiologist	Medical oncologist
Radiation physicist	Pathologist
Neurosurgeon	Anesthesiologist
Gastroenterologist	Dedicated nursing staff

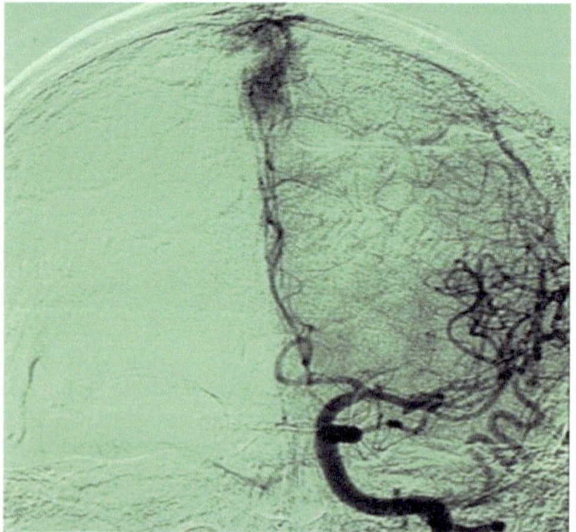
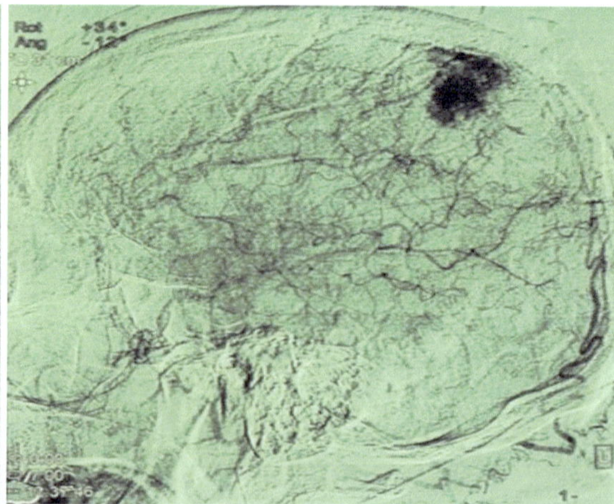

Fig. 17.3 Selective catheterization of the right carotid artery and followed angiography of the meningioma remnant

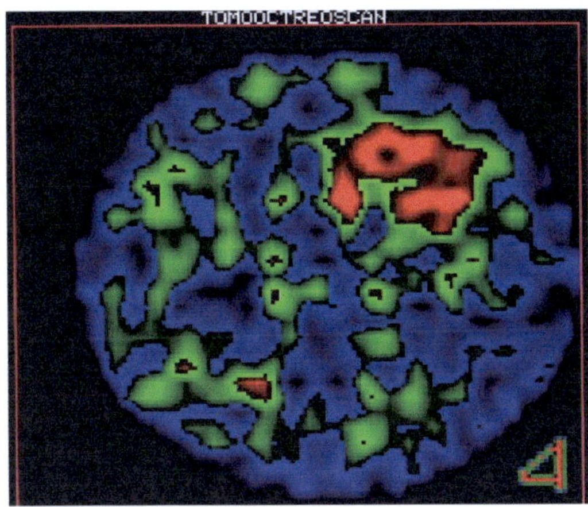

Fig. 17.4 Diagnostic OctreoScan® brain tomoscintigraphy of a radiologically confirmed meningioma after 111 MBq ^{111}In-Octreotide i.v. 7 h post-injection. Intense radiotracer uptake to the right of the midline of the parieto-occipital area (visual score IV) at the level of the tumor remnant

carotid artery (Fig. 17.3), in a recurrent WHO grade II brain meningioma residuals and sst receptor (OctreoScan)-positive, due to the effect of ^{111}In Auger electron emission (Fig. 17.4).

17.2 ^{111}In-Octreotide Treatment Results

A 76-year-old male patient (Table 17.3) had a median Karnofsky performance status 90 at inclusion; the high diagnostic probability of meningioma was based on typical radiologic patterns in CT/MR imaging and positive ^{111}In-Octreotide uptake. The patient had been treated by surgery and radiotherapy.

The average dose per session administered was 5.4 ± 1.7 GBq GBq. Repetitions did not exceed threefold. Response assessment was classified according to the modified Response Evaluating Criteria in Solid Tumors (RECIST). CT/MRI scans were performed as baseline before, during, and after the end of treatment. Toxicity (WHO criteria) was measured using blood and urine tests of renal and bone marrow function.

Brain meningioma load (Table 17.3): A complete and partial response could be not achieved to the treated patient, whereas disease stabilization was observed.

Table 17.3 Patient response to therapy with ^{111}In-Octreotide

Patients	Response evolution	PFS	O S
Meningioma	SD ≫ PD ≫ D	29	43

Table 17.4 Tumor-absorbed dose comparison between i.v. and i.a. administration of ^{111}In-Octreotide

	Intra-arterial infusion	Intravenous infusion
Liver dose	0.14 (mGy/MBq)	0.40 (mGy/MBq)
Kidney dose	0.41 (mGy/MBq)	0.51 (mGy/MBq)
Tumor dose	15.20 (mGy/MBq)	11.20 (mGy/MBq)
Spleen dose	1.40 (mGy/MBq)	1.56 (mGy/MBq)
Bone marrow dose	0.0035 (mGy/MBq)	0.022 (mGy/MBq)
Tumor/liver dose ratio	108.57[a]	28.00
Tumor/kidney dose ratio	37.07	21.96

[a]The average absorbed dose per session to a tumor for a spherical mass of 10 g was estimated to be 10.8 mGy/MBq, depending on the histotype of the tumor

A 43-month overall survival time was estimated with a 29-month PFS. Grade 1 erythro-, leuko-, and thrombo-cytopenia was noticed.

On CT the brain tumor mass progressed dramatically. Dosimetric calculations for the intra-arterial infusions are tabulated in Table 17.4 and compared with intra-venous data obtained from cases, rarely intravenously treated.

17.3 Discussion

With a PFS of 29 and 43 months OS in our study (Table 17.5), ^{111}In-Octreotide may represent a promising PRRT option for meningioma cases, antra-arterially treated. PRRT, intravenously performed not with ^{111}In-Octreotide but with β-emitters, i.e., ^{90}Y-DOTATOC or ^{177}Lu-DOTATATE, consists a promising tool for the confrontation not only for low-grade meningiomas but also for high-grade tumors. In a study of Bartolomei et al. [20] on 29 meningioma patients intravenously infused with ^{90}Y-DOTATOC, a SD was observed in 19/29 and a PD in 10/29 cases, accordingly. The authors report a median PFS (from beginning of PRRT)

Table 17.5 Experts on PRRT in brain NETs

Author	Year	Radiopeptide	Origin	ptsno	orr (%)	PFS (months)	OS (months)	CR, PR%	SD%	PD%
van Essen et al.	2006	^{177}Lu-DOTATATE	Meningioma	5	0	nr	nr	0	2 (40)	3 (60)
Bartolomei et al.	2009	^{90}Y-DOTATOC	Meningioma	29	0	13–61	nr	0	19 (65.5)	10 (34.5)
Kreissl et al.	2012	^{177}Lu-DOTATATE and E B R T	Meningioma	10	20	nr	18	1.1	8	0
Minutoli et al.	2014	^{111}In-Octreotide ^{90}Y-DOTATOC ^{177}Lu-DOTATATE	Meningioma	8	25	nr	nr	0.2	5	1
Gerster-Gilliéron et al.	2015	^{90}Y-DOTATOC	Meningioma	15	nr	24	49.7	0.0	13 (86.7)	2 (13.3)
Marincek et al.	2015	^{90}Y-DOTATOC ^{177}Lu-DOTATATE	Meningioma	34	nr	(8/11) 34 (3/11) 12	50 (8/11), 12 (3/11)	0	23	11
Limouris et al.	This study	^{111}In-Octreotide		1	nr	29	43	0	1 (100)	0

rv review study, *rs* retrospective study, *ps* prospective study, *orr* objective response rate, *dcr* disease control rate, *PFS* progression-free survival, *os* overall survival, *nr* non-referred, *E B R T* external beam radiotherapy, *pts no* patients' number of 61 months for the low-grade group and 13 months for the high-grade cases. According to the results of Kreissel et al. [21], a combination of PRRT using ^{177}Lu-labeled somatostatin analogs with fractionated external-beam radiotherapy is feasible and well tolerated. The authors had an orr of 20% a SD in 80% and an OS of 18 months. Minutoli et al. [22] reported that ^{111}In-labeled somatostatin analogs might be used instead of β-emitting radionuclides in cases with a higher risk of renal toxicity. The authors report a PR for two patients, a SD for five, and a PD for one. According to Guedj and Graillon [13] with a worldwide incidence of 45,000 cases, meningioma is the most common non-glial primary intracranial tumor where many of them present with aggressive features and poor outcomes. In a study of Kaley et al. [16], the PFS of recurrent cases decreases below 30% at 6 months, whereas the median OS is 3 years for grade III.

Peptide receptor radionuclide therapy (PRRT) has gained popularity and an increasing role in positive for somatostatin receptor (SSTR) tumors, confirmed after scintigraphy with ^{111}In-Octreotide or preferably with Gallium-68 DOTATOC. Besides NETs that are the leading example of tumors with SSTR overexpression, meningiomas belong to non-neuroendocrine malignancies overexpressing SSTR too and might serve as a potent option in the meningioma-therapy armamentariums. According to Graillon T et al. [23], meningiomas overexpress SSTR2 in a 67% of cases, confirmed scintigraphically with 68Ga-DOTA-peptides that showed highly elevated uptake [24, 25].

Based on a plethora of studies [26–30], over a hundred meningioma patients were treated with PRRT. Although half of them were pre-treated with external radiotherapy, patients showed safe as well an excellent clinical tolerance. In their report Guedj and Graillon [13] notice that these studies are limited by mixing various types of meningiomas, different PRRT schedules, and follow-up imaging studies. In addition, the growth rate before treatment is not always documented, limiting the interpretation of the PFS, particularly in grade I and "low" grade II menin-

gioma patients. Regarding oncologic endpoints, these promising studies have described disease stabilization for grades I and less aggressive grades II meningiomas in most cases, with a 6-month PFS ranging from 57 to 100%. By contrast, no clear benefit can be seen for more aggressive grade II and III meningiomas, so far. Van Essen et al. [26] report that in a small cohort of four patients treated with [^{177}Lu-DOTA0, Tyr3] octreotate, one of four patients with progressive meningioma had SD and three had PD. One patient with stable meningioma at the beginning of therapy had SD. The authors emphasized that PRRT can be effective only if uptake in tumor deposits on somatostatin receptor scintigraphy with ^{111}In-Octreotide (OctreoScan; Mallinckrodt) is equal to or higher than liver uptake. In a study by Backhaus et al. [27], in a case of a 54-year-old male patient with atypical (WHO grade II) meningioma who underwent one cycle of peptide receptor radionuclide therapy, the post-therapeutic whole-body ^{177}Lu-DOTATATE scintigraphy revealed thoracic uptake arising from previously undetected pulmonic meningioma metastases. The case highlights the importance of consideration of rare/untypical metastatic sides and the value of radiotracer whole-body imaging in identifying these. According to Sabet et al. [28] a patient with anaplastic meningioma and lung metastases resistant to conventional treatment underwent radiopeptide therapy with ^{177}Lu-DOTA-octreotate. The treatment resulted in significant improvement in patient's quality of life and inhibition of tumor progression. The authors noticed that this case may eventually help to establish the value of radiopeptide therapy in patients with this rare condition. In a study of Gerster-Gilliéron et al. [29] reporting on a cohort of 15 recurrent and progressive meningiomas treated with ^{90}Y-DOTATOC in two sessions of 7.4 GBq/m^2 each, a median PFS of 24 months and a mean OS of at least 49.7 months were achieved. Marincek et al. [30], in 34 patients with progressive meningiomas treated with ^{90}Y-DOTATOC and ^{177}Lu-DOTATOC, achieved a SD in 23 patients who showed a mean PFS ranging from 12 months (in 3/11 patients) to 34 months (in 8/11 patients) from the initialization of the PRRT treatment; the mean OS was 12 months in 3/11 patients and 50 months in 8/11 patients.

As regards dosimetry, according to Cremonesi et al. [31], two main options can be proposed in order to increase the absorbed dose while preserving at risk organs: either to treat with standard activity, i.e., 7.4 GBq/cycle but with variable number of cycles until the biological effective dose limits of the kidney and bone marrow are reached [32] or to treat with four fixed cycles with variable activity per cycle to reach the dose limits [33]. The authors underline the need for the PRRT schedule to be tailored to each situation taking into account the extent of disease, the growth rate, the grade, and SST expression and receptor affinity.

17.4 Conclusions

Prospective randomized trials, with a longer follow-up and a larger number of patients, are required to confirm the efficiency of PRRT in meningiomas. In recurrent WHO grade II tumor residuals, positive for somatostatin receptors, repeated, high doses of ^{111}In-Octreotide fallowing selective catheterization of the internal carotid artery showed an effective therapeutic outcome, i.e., a promising disease control. Given the locoregional modality character of the administration technique plus the extremely short range of [111]In Auger and internal conversion electron emission, no nephro-, liver, or myelo-toxicity has so far been observed. This approach in intra-arterially treating meningiomas and generally brain tumors, i.e., oligodendrogliomas positive for sstr2, represents an attractive strategy for the treatment of recurring or progressive symptomatic meningioma, which should be further evaluated.

References

1. Reubi JC, Maurer R, Klijn JGM, et al. High incidence of somatostatin receptors in human meningiomas: biochemical characterization. J Clin Endocrinol Metab. 1986;63:433–8.

2. Reubi JC, Lang W, Maurer R, et al. Distribution and biochemical characterization of somatostatin receptors in tumors of the human central nervous system. Cancer Res. 1987;47:5758–64.

3. Reubi JC, Horisberger U, Laissue J. High density of somatostatin receptors in veins surrounding human cancer tissue: role in tumor-host interaction. Int J Cancer. 1994;56:681–8.

4. Reubi JC, Waser B, Lamberts SWJ, et al. Somatostatin (SRIH) messenger ribonucleic acid expression in human neuroendocrine and brain tumors using in situ hybridization histochemistry: comparison with SRIH receptor content. J Clin Endocrinol Metab. 1993;76:642–7.

5. Hildebrandt G, Scheidauer K, Luyken C, et al. High sensitivity of the in vivo detection of somatostatin receptors by Indium (DTPA-Octreotide) scintigraphy in meningioma patients. Acta Neurochir. 1994;126:63–71.

6. Reubi JC. Neuropeptide receptors in health and disease: the molecular basis for in vivo imaging. J Nucl Med. 1995;36:1825–35.

7. Klimstra DS, Modlin IR, Coppola D, et al. The pathologic classification of neuroendocrine tumors: a review of nomenclature, grading, and staging systems. Pancreas. 2010;39(6):707–12.

8. Öberg K, Castellano D. Current knowledge on diagnosis and staging of neuroendocrine tumors. Cancer Metastasis Rev. 2011;30(1):3–7.

9. Liu T-C, Hamilton N, Hawkins W, et al. Comparison of WHO classifications (2004, 2010), the Hochwald grading system, and AJCC and ENETS staging systems in predicting prognosis in locoregional well-differentiated pancreatic neuro-endocrine tumors. Am J Surg Pathol. 2013;37(6):853–9.

10. Yamaguchi T, Fujimori T, Tomita S, et al. Clinical validation of the gastrointestinal NET grading system: Ki67 index criteria of the WHO 2010 classification is appropriate to predict metastasis or recurrence. Diagn Pathol. 2013;8(1):65.

11. Caplin M, Sundin A, Nillson O, et al. ENETS Consensus guidelines for the management of patients with digestive neuroendocrine neoplasms: colorectal neuroendocrine neoplasms. Neuroendocrinology. 2012;95:88–97.

12. Anthony LB, Strosberg JR, Klimstra DS, et al. The NANETS consensus guidelines for the diagnosis and management of gastrointestinal neuroendocrine tumors (nets): well-differentiated nets of the distal colon and rectum. Pancreas. 2010;39:767–74.

13. Guedj E, Graillon T, et al. Treatment of aggressive recurrent meningiomas: spinning towards peptide receptor radionuclide therapy. Eur J Nucl Med Mol Imaging. 2019;46(3):537–8.

14. Galldiks N, Albert NL, Sommerauer M, et al. PET imaging in patients with meningioma-report of the RANO/PET Group. Neuro Oncol. 2017;19:1576–87.

15. Goldbrunner R, Minniti G, Preusser M, et al. EANO guidelines for the diagnosis and treatment of meningiomas. Lancet Oncol. 2016;17:e383–91.

16. Kaley T, Barani I, Chamberlain M, et al. Historical benchmarks for medical therapy trials in surgery- and radiation-refractory meningioma: a RANO review. Neuro Oncol. 2014;16:829–40.

17. Simpson D. The recurrence of intracranial meningiomas after surgical treatment. J Neurol Neurosurg Psychiatry. 1957;20:22–39.

18. Aizer AA, Bi WL, Kandola MS, et al. Extent of resection and overall survival for patients with atypical and malignant meningioma. Cancer. 2015;121:4376–81.

19. Limouris GS, Chatziioannou A, Kontogeorgakos D, et al. Selective hepatic arterial infusion of In-111-DTPA-Phe1-octreotide in neuro-endocrine liver metastases. Eur J Nucl Med Mol Imaging. 2008;35:1827–37.

20. Bartolomei M, Bodei L, De Cicco C, et al. Peptide receptor radionuclide therapy with (90)Y-DOTATOC in recurrent meningioma. Eur J Nucl Med Mol Imaging. 2009;36:1407–16.

21. Kreissl MC, Hänscheid H, Löhr M, et al. Combination of peptide receptor radionuclide therapy with fractionated external beam radiotherapy for treatment of advanced symptomatic meningioma. Radiat Oncol. 2012;7:99–108.

22. Minutoli F, Amato E, Sindoni A, et al. Peptide receptor radionuclide therapy in patients with inoperable meningiomas: our experience and review of the literature. Cancer Biother Radiopharm. 2014;29(5):193–9.

23. Graillon T, Romano D, Defilles C, et al. Octreotide therapy in meningiomas: in vitro study, clinical correlation, and literature review. J Neurosurg. 2017;127:660–9.

24. Soto-Montenegro ML, Peña-Zalbidea S, Mateos-Pérez JM, et al. Meningiomas: a comparative study of 68Ga-DOTATOC, 68Ga-DOTANOC and 68Ga-DOTATATE for molecular imaging in mice. PLoS One. 2014;9:e111624.

25. Sommerauer M, Burkhardt JK, Frontzek K, et al. 68Gallium DOTATATE PET in meningioma: a reliable predictor of tumor growth rate? Neuro Oncol. 2016;18:1021–7.

26. van Essen M, Krenning EP, Kooij PP, et al. Effects of therapy with [177Lu-DOTA0, Tyr3]octreotate in patients with paraganglioma, meningioma, small cell lung carcinoma, and melanoma. J Nucl Med. 2006;47:1599–606.

27. Backhaus P, Huss S, Kösek V, et al. Lung metastases of intracranial atypical meningioma diagnosed on posttherapeutic imaging after ¹⁷⁷Lu-DOTATATE therapy. Clin Nucl Med. 2018;43:e184–5.

28. Sabet A, Ahmadzadehfar H, Herrlinger U, et al. Successful radiopeptide targeting of metastatic anaplastic meningioma: case report. Radiat Oncol. 2011;6:94.

29. Gerster-Gilliéron K, Forrer F, Maecke H, et al. 90Y-DOTATOC as a therapeutic option for complex recurrent or progressive meningiomas. J Nucl Med. 2015;56:1748–51.

30. Marincek N, Radojewski P, Dumont RA, et al. Somatostatin receptor-targeted radiopeptide therapy with ⁹⁰Y-DOTATOC and ¹⁷⁷Lu-DOTATOC in progressive meningioma: long-term results of a phase II clinical trial. J Nucl Med. 2015;56:171–6.

31. Cremonesi M, Ferrari ME, Bodei L, et al. Correlation of dose with toxicity and tumour response to. Eur J Nucl Med Mol Imaging. 2018;45(13):2426–41.

32. Strigari L, Benassi M, Chiesa C, et al. Dosimetry in nuclear medicine therapy: radiobiology application and results. Q J Nucl Med Mol Imaging. 2011;55:205–21.

33. Sandström M, Garske-Román U, Granberg D, et al. Individualized dosimetry of kidney and bone marrow in patients undergoing 177Lu-DOTA-octreotate treatment. J Nucl Med. 2013;54:33–41.

Georgios P. Fragulidis, Athanasios G. Zafeirakis, and Georgios S. Limouris

18.1 Introduction

Neuroendocrine tumors (NETs) of the gastrointestinal tract are often metastatic, taken into account that nearly 10% of all tumor liver metastases are of neuroendocrine origin [1]. Despite the introduction of new chemotherapeutics and immunological agents, surgery remains the most efficient approach to metastatic disease and offers practically the longest benefits. Surgical removal of hepatic cancerous load has been shown to improve survival. Unfortunately, there is a lack of prospective randomized data on the treatment of liver metastases in neuroendocrine tumors where worldwide reports are mostly based on single institution experience and comparisons are made with limited number of cases. Survival, progression-free survival, and progression improvements can justify an aggressive approach. Although the indication for surgical treatment is usually a logic approach to the tumor load, the safety of a comprehensive debulking risk or of cytoreductive surgery needs to be evaluated to standardize this intervention. However, since the time of our first clinical experience, we have observed a worldwide trend toward the nonsurgical treatment of neuroendocrine metastases in the liver, mainly by TAE, TACE, radiofrequency ablation, etc. [2].

In addition to the abovementioned, over the last 15 years, there has been significant scientific advancement in the field of radiopeptide therapies. Standardization of practice and indications has made this procedure routine in experienced centers. Among them the "Aretaieion" University Hospital has mainly focused on intra-arterial radionuclide infusions under the tight collaboration of the Nuclear Medicine Division (Prof Dr. med GS Limouris), the Hemodynamic Unit (Prof Dr. med L Vlahos, Prof Dr. med A Chatziioannou), and the 2nd Surgery Clinic (Prof Dr. med D Voros, Prof Dr. med GP Fragulidis); this collaboration has led to the establishment of a "specific manipulation protocol" on the course of the infusion, the "Aretaieion Protocol," reported in details previously [3–14].

G. P. Fragulidis (✉)
2nd Department of Surgery, School of Medicine, "Aretaieion" Hospital, National and Kapodistrian University of Athens, Athens, Greece
e-mail: gfragulidis@aretaieio.uoa.gr

A. G. Zafeirakis
Nuclear Medicine Department, Army Share Fund Hospital of Athens, Athens, Greece

G. S. Limouris
Medical School, Nuclear Medicine, National and Kapodistrian University of Athens, Athens, Greece

18.2 Neuroendocrine Liver Metastases and Surgical Intervention

In the last two decades, there are many reports on patients undergoing surgery for neuroendocrine liver secondaries, a strenuous outcome of the

© Springer Nature Switzerland AG 2021
G. S. Limouris (ed.), *Liver Intra-arterial PRRT with ^{111}In-Octreotide*,
https://doi.org/10.1007/978-3-030-70773-6_18

Table 18.1 Surgical strategies in liver neuroendocrine secondaries

Strategy	Curative	Palliative	Cytoreductive	Debulking
Definition	Complete removal of tumor tissue with significant peritumoral margin of excision	If at least 90% of liver metastases are resectable with limited extrahepatic tumor mass	If less than 70% of liver is tumor infiltrated with inoperable extrahepatic disease	Debulking is the reduction of as much of the bulk
Remarks	Nearby lymph nodes may also be removed	–	–	–

increasing acceptance of the aggressive surgical strategy, and its associated benefits for the management of liver metastases [15]. A first-class example was some 30 years ago from the Mayo Clinic's review, reporting on patients treated with carcinoid tumors, between 1970 and 1989, having undergone less than 10% surgical intervention due to liver metastases ($n = 37$) [16]. Yet earlier, in 1986, in a paper of Galland and Blumgart, it was reported that only 2 candidates were found, among 30 NET cases for liver surgical exeresis [17]. In 2002, Sarmiento et al. [18] in a review paper on liver neuroendocrine metastases, running from 1973 to 1999, only 57 patients underwent partial hepatectomy vs over 170 NET patients undergoing surgical resection from 1977 to 1998, reported in another Mayo Clinic study [19]. More recently, another study comparing liver resection vs intra-arterially infused cases for NETs at 9 institutions reported that more than 300 cases underwent surgery [20]. However, it is important to note that due to the lack of cases, even in large institutions and due to the nonrandomized uncontrolled nature of these studies, biases might occur. Following up the aforementioned ergography starting from 1996 with Ahlman et al. [15], a continuing growing of NET cases is observed which among others increases the surgeons' experience and their evaluation resulted in many curative resections to be defined differently. We see that in some papers, the curative intention is defined only for an achieved Ro[1]

resection, while others classify the resection as complete without reference to the margin status or characterize a curative procedure when all visible gross disease has been removed [23].

Based on the experience achieved upon our patients, and focused on neuroendocrine liver secondaries, surgical excision of neuroendocrine liver lesions is the best option for curing and alleviating symptoms, despite the availability of a plethora of treatment options (Table 18.1).

ual tumor. The R classification takes into account clinical and pathological findings. A reliable classification requires the pathological examination of resection margins. The R classification has considerable clinical significance, particularly being a strong predictor of prognosis. A plethora of general and specific procedures for performing pathological R classification on resection specimens of different organs has been described. New methods in R classification comprise imprint cytology, cytological examination of ascites, and examination of bone marrow biopsy [21]. A **resection margin** or **surgical margin** is the margin of apparently non-tumorous tissue around a tumor that has been surgically removed, called "resected," in surgical oncology. The resection is an attempt to remove a cancer tumor so that no portion of the malignant growth extends past the edges or margin of the removed tumor and surrounding tissue. These are retained after the surgery and examined microscopically by pathologists to see if the margin is indeed free from tumor cells. If cancerous cells are found at the edges, the operation is much less likely to achieve the desired results [22].

Margins are classified by the pathologist as:

- R0—no cancer cells seen microscopically at the resection margin
- R1—cancer cells present microscopically at the resection margin (microscopic positive margin)
- R2—gross examination by the naked eye shows tumor tissue present at the resection margin (macroscopic positive margin)

---

[1]The R classification, adopted in 1987 by the UICC, denotes absence or presence of residual tumor after treatment. Residual tumor may be localized in the area of the primary tumor and/or as distant metastases. **R0** corresponds to resection for cure or complete remission, **R1** to microscopic residual tumor, and **R2** to macroscopic resid-

18.3   Exeresis of Liver Neuroendocrine Metastases as a Curative Approach

In surgical oncology, curative resection is defined as the complete removal of tumor tissue with a significant margin of excision described on pathological examination (hepatic and extrahepatic anatomical status). Principally, liver resection in metastatic disease has been widely accepted as a potentially curative modality in patients with colorectal cancer [19, 24, 25]. With improvements in the safety of major liver resection and an operative mortality rate of approximately 5% in most series, liver excision gained popularity as a possible "cure" of metastatic disease from neuroendocrine tumors.

18.3.1   Ergography on Curative Liver Excision of Neuroendocrine Liver Metastases

Surgical removal for neuroendocrine liver metastases is a standard methodology against all other forms of liver-targeted system therapies. Unfortunately, due to the relatively low incidence of the neuroendocrine disease, complicated with the biological heterogeneity between the primaries and the liver secondaries, there is a lack of prospective randomized studies that might provide a first-level evidence. The worldwide ergography is based on encouraging results almost basically from large retrospective studies and the authors' experience; it includes radical surgery resection of the primary tumor, proceeding to a second approach for the potentially resectable advanced neuroendocrine secondaries that were metastasized to the liver. It is estimated that since patients with untreated liver metastases have a 5-year survival of approximately 20–40% [26, 27], aggressive surgery for the liver secondaries appears the goal of prolonging survival [19, 26–34]. Due to the tardy nature of the disease, overall survival after liver lesion resection can be considered as satisfactory. This is obvious even for stage 4 disease and despite high post-curative 5-year recurrence rates of more than 40–70% in

most cases. Overall survival ranges from 46 to 86% at 5 years and 35 to 79% at 10 years [19, 26, 27, 30, 31, 33, 35–37]. Patients who were in a good clinic-laboratory disease status after removing the liver metastases had a significantly better overall median survival and 5 years survival than patients with inoperable liver disease [27, 31, 32, 38]. According to Mayo et al. [20] and Reddy et al. [39], the median survival time ranges from 52 to 123 months for patients who have received a neuroendocrine liver metastasis resection. Based on the results of Ahlman et al. [15] and Grazi et al. [31], a curative neuroendocrine liver metastasis resection is achieved in a range of 22–84%. Sarmiento et al. [19] achieved a major hepatectomy (one or more lobes) in 91 patients (54%) and reported a morbidity of 14% and an operative mortality of 1.2%., but the recurrence rate was 84% at 5 years. Mayo et al. [40] reported the largest and only multi-institutional experience of surgical management of neuroendocrine liver metastases where in a cohort of 339 patients a 77.6% underwent resection, a 19.5% resection and ablation, and a 2.9% ablation, achieving a curative resection (R0 status) in 53.7% of the patients and 5- and 10-year survival rates of 74% and 51%, respectively. According to Clary [41] differences in survival data need to be scholastically interpreted as the resectability criteria are not the same which must be taken into account when comparing recent series with older studies. As stated by Glazer et al. [42] and Hibi et al. [43], the biological behavior of NETs and their metastases is variable, emphasizing that patients with NETs originated from lungs have the worst predictions compared to other primary sites, a statement not verified in our patient cohort (Chap. 14). To note, NET patients with liver secondaries from a colon primer appear to have a longer relapse-free survival [42]. Apart from the tumor site, other preoperative factors for a poor prognosis are the nonfunctioning primaries, the multiple and/or bilobar liver metastases, and the invasion extension of more than 75% of the liver parenchyma [26, 30, 44].

Besides the distinguishing feature of the neuroendocrine tumors to metastasize is the potential for unregulated endocrine activity. This unregulated endocrine activity complicates the therapy but serves as one of the main reasons for the role of palliative surgery. Even if a curative excision is not feasible, either due to extrahepatic disease or extensive intrahepatic secondaries, a role for the operation remains, although less well defined. The goals of palliative surgery aim to alleviate mass symptoms and the symptoms of hormonal hypersecretion, to slow down tumor cell growth, prolong survival, and ultimately achieve long-term quality of life. Some authors [45], as we did, have developed surgical treatment to resect more than 90% of the bulk of the tumor; this is an incomplete resection of the tumor attempting to slow down the symptoms. The debulking operation is defined as a surgical resection of residual disease beyond the criteria of cytoreductive surgery. According to the Mayo Clinic group, palliative resection is justified if at least 90% of liver metastases are resectable and extrahepatic tumor mass is limited [46], referred separately in the consensus report of the European Neuroendocrine Tumor Society [47]. According to Frilling et al., cytoreductive liver resections should be considered if there are no inoperable extrahepatic diseases and less than 70% of the liver is affected by the tumor [23]. As Lee et al. stated [1] in the palliative situation where symptomatic control of quality of life rather than survival is the primary goal, the benefit-risk balance must be clearly determined to justify surgery, because liver resection is not without significant morbidity and mortality. Furthermore, when cytoreductive surgery can increase survival, the use of surgical intervention in a patient population that can survive many years of symptomatic disease is doubly justified and is a "sine qua non."

18.4 Resectability of Neuroendocrine Liver Metastases

The definition of "resectability" is determined by many circumstances, including patient, disease, and technical factors. The principle lies in the technical ability to leave a liver remnant with adequate function, lowering in parallel the perioperative morbidity and mortality with long-term

survival outcomes and quality of life. On the other hand, a rapidly progressing intrahepatic or an extensive extrahepatic disease consists significant comorbidities, thus contraindications for hepatectomy. Fortunately, the growth pattern of liver neuroendocrine secondaries allows an aggressive surgical approach, as the lesions displace rather than envelop the intrahepatic vessels and the lesions are often discrete. For large dominant tumors with sluggish growth, resection of the dominant tumor is suggested for cytoreductive purposes to alleviate the symptoms [48]. Abdalla et al. [49–51] in their studies report that after liver excision, a 20–25% of residual functional healthy liver parenchyma is sufficient, permitting an acceptable liver function; most surgeons will not recommend surgery if the estimated volume of functional residual liver is either less than 20–25% of the total liver or less than 0.5% of the total body weight. In addition, the use of indocyanine green clearance (ICG) in our institution as an objective adjunct in liver function assessment is also performed for patients with "borderline seriousness" [52–55]. Such selected cases have the safer option of inducing hypertrophy in the remaining functional liver by portal embolization to reduce the risk of postoperative liver failure, rarely observed in NETs.

In cases where neuroendocrine liver metastases are numerous or large, surgical resectability is a major concern. Once it has been established that a curative or cytoreductive resection is indicated, resectability is determined from two factors: anatomical feasibility and volumetric tolerance. A multidisciplinary approach, involving a liver surgeon, a dedicated hepatobiliary radiologist, and a medical oncologist, is mandatory, so the decision should be confirmed.

18.5 Width of Resection Margins in Neuroendocrine Liver Metastases

The optimal excised margins consist another important issue regarding the resection of liver metastases, because there is no definite consensus or evidence about the width of clear margins for NETs due to the plethora of parenchymal transection techniques in different centers [56]. Most of the experience and data reported come from colorectal carcinoma and are extrapolated to NET liver metastases. In general, a positive resection margin inclines to marginal recurrence and is a main independent predictor of poor survival [57–59]. Additionally, some centers have shown improved results with margins of more than 1 cm, since micro-metastases can be detected within peritumoral tissue remnants of 1 cm or less [60–63] decreasing patients' median survival; in contrast other authors report that the width of the resection margin does not affect survival as long as it is negative [64–66].

18.6 Hepatic Lymphadenectomy in Neuroendocrine Liver Metastases

The management and the role as well of hepatic lymphadenectomy in neuroendocrine liver metastases is not well established [67] since most of the experience and data are extrapolated from colorectal liver metastatic cases with nodal involvement of the hepatoduodenal ligament [68–70]. A Mayo Clinic report identified metastatic hepatoduodenal lymph nodes as an independent predictor of survival with an over threefold increase in 5-year survival rates in node-negative patients after hepatectomy for colorectal metastases [68]. In a French study, a 3-year survival of 38% is reported after hepatic lymphadenectomy [71]. Even though these data suggest that regional lymphadenectomy is important in all patients undergoing curative hepatectomy for malignant tumors, there is little information about neuroendocrine liver metastases and no consensus on whether the colorectal metastatic experience is to be extrapolated to liver neuroendocrine tumor cases.

18.7 Role of Prophylactic Cholecystectomy

In the most recent Nordic guidelines of 2010 [72] prophylactic cholecystectomy was not recommended, contending that (a) the somatostatin-induced gallstone are normally asymptomatic, (b) in the co-existance of cholecystitis peptide receptor radionuclide therapy (PRRT) is not over-burdened and (c) even the risk of complications in cholecystectomy is low (3%) it has not to be ignored. However, prophylactic cholecystectomy should be recommended when considering surgery for advanced neuroendocrine tumors [47]. The reason is that, somatostatin treatment in neuroendocrine tumors can induce gallstone disease in up to 50% of cases. Morbidity of the cholecystectomy is negligible [73, 74].

18.8 Palliative Liver Resection for NET Liver Metastases

Neuroendocrine tumor behavior and biological properties justify the use of cytoreductive therapy. In most NETs, the tumors have a long doubling time, especially in gastrointestinal neuroendocrine tumors, where hepatic and regional lymph node metastases are the predominant site of spread. In most metastatic NETs, metastases are restricted to the liver, which are susceptible to (chemo) embolization and tumor volume correlated with the level of endocrine symptoms. It is crucial to know that the primary tumors are often resectable despite extensive metastases [48]. Metastatic patients with gastrointestinal neuroendocrine tumors clearly have a better survival compared to patients with metastatic adenocarcinoma of the gastrointestinal tract [75, 76].

18.8.1 Results of Palliative Liver Resection for NET Liver Metastases

In the last 20 years, a plethora of retrospective, unfortunately not prospective, studies dealing with an efficient, yet aggressive, approach favoring cytoreductive liver resection, partial hepatectomy, and ablation report on prolonged survival and symptom relief in neuroendocrine liver metastatic patients [16, 27, 77–79]. Berger et al. [80] compared resection versus embolic treatment results in symptomatic metastatic NETs and found that cytoreductive surgery was superior (69% vs 59%) providing a better and longer relief of symptoms. Furthermore, the guidelines suggested by them are either not based or not widely accepted on a cohort that is rather heterogenous.

Based on the literature [19, 77, 78], excision of neuroendocrine liver metastatic lesions results in hormone-related symptom relief and low morbidity and mortality with symptom reduction ranging from 16 to 26 months. About 10 years ago, Que et al. [77] noticed that the recurrence of symptoms occurred earlier in patients undergoing palliative resection (11.3 months versus 20.4 months) compared to those with curative liver lesion exeresis. Using Karnofsky index, Knox et al. reported an improvement in quality of life lasting more than 4 years after surgery [79].

18.9 Liver Transplantation for Neuroendocrine Liver Metastases (NELM)

According to Mazzaferro et al., liver transplantation has a particular role in NELM and is proposed for certain candidates with a 5-year overall survival of up to 70% and 5-year relapse-free survival of up to 50% [81]. In a large meta-analysis of Lehnert et al., including 103 patients [82], the 5-year survival rate was 47%, with only 24% of patients showing no recurrence, whereas in another large series of liver transplants for NELM of Le Treut et al. including 85 cases, overall survival was 47% and recurrence-free survival 20% at 5 years [83, 84]. Mazzaferro et al. [81] proposed guidelines for the selection of liver transplant candidates, considering well-differentiated, low-grade endocrine tumors eligible candidates for liver transplantation, known as "Milan criteria." To notice according to European Neuroendocrine Tumor Society, patients with inoperable liver secondaries or **cases** with life-threatening hormonal imbalances, refractory to drug therapy, are also candidates for liver transplantation as a potential treatment option. Finally, patients most likely to benefit from liver transplantation are those who are less than 50 years old and free of extrahepatic tumors and have low expression of Ki-67 [85].

18.10 Surgery and Combined Therapies

According to the gathered experience, the most successful and effective combination with surgery is indisputably that with PRRT. Principally, tandem treatment schemes with other therapeutic modalities as chemotherapy or radiofrequency ablation (RFA) cannot be considered as well-established procedures. However, there are reports [86] showing that patients with carcinoid syndrome had a partial or complete symptom response and patients could potentially benefit from this combined ablative treatment [19]. In another paper [32] also it was shown that systemic chemotherapy or trans-arterial embolization combined with surgery and RFA resulted in 100% symptom control and improved 3-year survival (83% versus 31%).

18.11 Perioperative Care and Speculations

The surgical and anesthetic techniques as well as the perioperative care of these patients have improved greatly, leading to a significant reduction of the morbidity and mortality rates after hepatectomy. Regarding the perioperative morbidity and mortality rates for liver metastasectomy in neuroendocrine tumors, these are similar to those for colorectal carcinomas [77, 87] directly related to postoperative liver function, with the most important determinant the extent of liver resection [88]. Perioperative mortality in neuroendocrine liver metastasectomy ranges between 0 and 9% in patients without underlying hepatic dysfunction, whereas the overall morbidity rate ranges from 3 to 24% [87]. Thus, patients with severe morbidities should be screened by the anesthesia team to assess preoperative risk factors related to the American Society of Anesthesiologists (ASA) score [89].

Preoperative preparation with 150–500 µg somatostatin in the pre-induction phase in the operating room prevents hemodynamic instability intraoperatively [23]. Special preoperative preparation is required, i.e., for **insulinomas** to monitor regular glucose and **for gastrinomas** to introduce H2 receptor antagonists or H + -K + ATPase inhibitors [48]. Finally, the perioperative risk is in general not elevated in specific endocrinopathies, with the exception of **carcinoid heart disease**, where selected patients may require surgical repair of carcinoid heart disease prior to liver resection for symptomatic carcinoid syndrome to reduce the risk of massive bleeding from intrahepatic venous hypertension in case of right heart failure [90].

Patients with tumors near vascular structures or with multiple lesions located at different sites require large volume resections leaving small functional residual liver. The surgeon has to choose the best strategy having in mind to manage this challenge as (a) the parenchyma-preserving, segmental approach to resection, (b) the inclusion of concomitant wedges or thermal ablations for small tumors outside the delineated safe area of resection, and/or rarely (c) either preoperative portal vein embolization for extended hepatectomy or stepped resections to induce hypertrophy of the future liver remnant [91]. Furthermore, according to Glaser et al. [42] intra-abdominal fluid accumulation as an independent risk factor for perioperative mortality has not to be ignored.

18.12 Conclusion

The presence of liver secondaries is a distinguishing feature of neuroendocrine tumors and an anti-restrictive step in patient survival [92, 93]. Surgery plays a strong role in neuroendocrine liver tumors and should be the treatment of preference when patients are sane, and the disease clinicolaboratory factors allow it in both curative and palliative management. A multidisciplinary meeting among the specialties involved is suggested, has to be a "premise," and should be the platform for decision-making. In patients with curable lesions, curative excision should be the treatment of first choice. In cases where healing cannot be achieved by surgery alone, PRRT can be combined with surgery to achieve "healing." If curative intent cannot be achieved, **cytoreductive surgery should be performed** if at least 90% of tumor burden can be excised. If surgery and PRRT cannot reach this 90%, liver transplantation can be the ultimate consideration. According to Frilling et al. [23], neuroendocrine liver tumors are further classified in various patterns: type I as a single metastasis of any size, type II as an isolated metastatic mass with smaller deposits in both liver lobes, and type III as disseminated metastatic spread in both liver lobes always involved with virtually no normal liver parenchyma. By this classification, the authors found that the three categories of neuroendocrine liver metastases differ in biology and behavior and express the only significant independent predictors of survival [23]. This study suggests that although aggressive surgery is generally recommended, the individualization of the treatment strategy should be tailored to each patient, as the therapy response is not the expected one and some patients benefit more from the surgical intervention than others [20]; thus, a multidisciplinary team approach may be the platform for this decision-making process (Table 18.2). The experts participating in such a team may include nuclear physicians, interventional radiologists, medical oncologists, gastroenterologists, hepatobiliary surgeons, and pathologists. According to our observations, we suggest that in neuroendocrine liver metastases surgery should be maintained for patients with low-volume or for symptomatic high-volume disease also mentioned else-where [20]. Even though PRRT is currently indicated in patients with fully resected NENs, further adjuvant schemes should be investigated in clinical trials [94]. The analysis of such

Table 18.2 Multidisciplinary consultants' board

Nuclear medicine physician	Interventional radiologist
Hepatobiliary surgeon	Medical oncologist
Gastroenterologist	Pathologist
Radiation physicist	Dedicated nursing staff

data should also help to identify subgroups of patients at high risk of recurrence and to validate scoring systems to make predictions about the most likely to benefit [26]. Additionally, the development of histopathological and staging criteria should also improve the selection of appropriate patients for clinical trials.

References

1. Lee SY, Cheow PC, Teo JY, et al. Surgical treatment of neuroendocrine liver metastases. Int J Hepatol. 2012;2012:146590. https://doi.org/10.1155/2012/146590.
2. Tao L, Xiu D, Sadula A, Ye C, et al. Oncotarget. 2017;8(45):79785–92.
3. Limouris GS, Dimitropoulos N, Kontogeorgakos D, et al. Evaluation of the therapeutic response to In-111-DTPA octreotide-based targeted therapy in liver metastatic neuroendocrine tumors according to CT/MRI/US findings. Cancer Biother Radiopharm. 2005;20:215–7.
4. Kontogeorgakos D. Dosimetry during therapeutic applications with octreotide labeled with In-111. ND 22105; 2006. http://hdl.handle.net/10442/hedi/22105.
5. Kontogeorgakos D, Dimitriou P, Limouris GS, et al. Patient-specific dosimetry calculations using mathematic models of different atomic sizes during therapy with In-111-DTPA-DPhe1 Octreotide infusions after catheterization of the hepatic artery. J Nucl Med. 2006;47(9):1476–82.
6. Koutoulidis V. Intraarterial administration of 111 in labeled octreotide for the therapeutic treatment of neuroendocrine hepatic metastases. ND 24891; 2006. http://hdl.handle.net/10442/hedi/24891.
7. Kontogeorgakos D, Limouris GS, Kamenopoulou V, et al. Optimization of doses received by the hospital staff and the members of the family of patients undergoing 111In-DTPA-DPhe1-Octreotide therapy. Radiat Prot Dosim. 2007;125(1–4):403–6.
8. Limouris GS, Chatziioannou A, Kontogeorgakos D, et al. Selective hepatic arterial infusion of In-111-DTPA-Phe1-octreotide in neuroendocrine liver metastases. Eur J Nucl Med Mol Imaging. 2008;35(10):1827–37.
9. Vamvakas I, Lagopati N, Andreou M, et al. Patient specific computer automated dosimetry calculations during therapy with 111In Octreotide. Eur J Radiogr. 2009;1(4):180–3.
10. Papakonstantinou I, Lykoudis PM, Contis JC, et al. A case of hepatic flexure carcinoid with extended brain metastases. J BUON. 2011;16(4):779–80.
11. Limouris GS, Karfis I, Chatziioannou A, et al. Super-selective hepatic arterial infusions as established technique ('Aretaieion' protocol) of 177 Lu DOTA-TATE inoperable neuroendocrine liver metastases of gastro-entero-pancreatic tumors. Q J Nucl Med Mol Imaging. 2012;56:551–8.
12. Fragulidis GP, Derpapas MK, Vezakis A, et al. Non-functioning pancreatic-endocrine tumors: eleven-year experience in a single institute. J BUON. 2014;19(2):449–52.
13. Troumpoukis ND. Evaluation of the therapeutic response of hepatic metastases due to neuroendocrine tumors with In-111 Octreotide after super-selective catheterization of the hepatic artery. ND 37639; 2016. http://hdl.handle.net/10442/hedi/37639.
14. Karfis IL. Intra-arterial therapeutic approach of hepatic neuroendocrine character neoplasiae with 111indium-pentetreotide after temporary installation of a catheter—port system. ND 37597; 2016. http://hdl.handle.net/10442/hedi/39579.
15. Ahlman H, Westberg G, Wängberg B, et al. Treatment of liver metastases of carcinoid tumors. World J Surg. 1996;20(2):196–202.
16. McEntee GP, Nagorney DM, Kvols LK, et al. Cytoreductive hepatic surgery for neuroendocrine tumors. Surgery. 1990;108(6):1091–6.
17. Galland RB, Blumgart LH. Carcinoid syndrome. Surgical management. Br J Hosp Med. 1986;35(3):166–70.
18. Sarmiento JM, Farnell MB, Que FG, et al. Pancreaticoduodenectomy for islet cell tumors of the head of the pancreas: long-term survival analysis. World J Surg. 2002;26(10):1267–71.
19. Sarmiento JM, Heywood G, Rubin J, et al. Surgical treatment of neuroendocrine metastases to the liver: a plea for resection to increase survival. J Am Coll Surg. 2003;197(1):29–37.
20. Mayo SC, de Jong MC, Bloomston M, et al. Surgery versus intra-arterial therapy for neuroendocrine liver metastasis: a multicenter international analysis. Ann Surg Oncol. 2011;18(13):3657–65.
21. Hermanek P, Wittekind C, et al. Pathol Res Pract. 1994;190(2):115–23.
22. Emmadi R, Wiley EL. Evaluation of resection margins in breast conservation therapy: the pathology perspective-past, present, and future. Int J Surg Oncol. 2012;2012:180259. https://doi.org/10.1155/2012/180259.
23. Frilling A, Li J, Malamutmann E, Schmid KW, et al. Treatment of liver metastases from neuroendocrine tumours in relation to the extent of hepatic disease. Br J Surg. 2009;96(2):175–84.
24. Rosen CB, Nagorney DM, Taswell HF, et al. Perioperative blood transfusion and determinants of survival after liver resection for metastatic colorectal carcinoma. Ann Surg. 1992;216(4):493–505.
25. Scheele J, Stangl R, Altendorf-Hofmann A, et al. Indicators of prognosis after hepatic resection for colorectal secondaries. Surgery. 1991;110(1):13–29.
26. Chamberlain RS, Canes D, Brown KT, et al. Hepatic neuroendocrine metastases: does intervention alter outcomes? J Am Coll Surg. 2000;190(4):432–45.
27. Chen H, Hardacre JM, Uzar A, et al. Isolated liver metastases from neuroendocrine tumors:

does resection prolong survival? J Am Coll Surg. 1998;187(1):88–93.

28. Touzios JG, Kiely JM, Pitt SC, et al. Neuroendocrine hepatic metastases: does aggressive management improve survival? Ann Surg. 2005;241(5):776–85.

29. Norton JA, Warren RS, Kelly MG, et al. Aggressive surgery for metastatic liver neuroendocrine tumors. Surgery. 2003;134(6):1057–65.

30. Elias D, Lasser P, Ducreux M, et al. Liver resection (and associated extrahepatic resections) for metastatic well-differentiated endocrine tumors: a 15-year single center prospective study. Surgery. 2003;133(4):375–82.

31. Grazi GL, Cescon M, Pierangeli F, et al. Highly aggressive policy of hepatic resections for neuroendocrine liver metastases. Hepatogastroenterology. 2000;47(32):481–6.

32. Musunuru S, Chen H, Rajpal S, et al. Metastatic neuroendocrine hepatic tumors: resection improves survival. Arch Surg. 2006;141(10):1000–4.

33. Yao KA, Talamonti MS, Nemcek A, et al. Indications and results of liver resection and hepatic chemoembolization for metastatic gastrointestinal neuroendocrine tumors. Surgery. 2001;130(4):677–85.

34. Nave H, Mössinger E, Feist H, et al. Surgery as primary treatment in patients with liver metastases from carcinoid tumors: a retrospective, unicentric study over 13 years. Surgery. 2001;129(2):170–5.

35. Gomez D, Malik HZ, Al-Mukthar A, et al. Hepatic resection for metastatic gastrointestinal and pancreatic neuroendocrine tumours: outcome and prognostic predictors. HPB. 2007;9(5):345–51.

36. Dousset B, Saint-Marc O, Pitre J, et al. Metastatic endocrine tumors: medical treatment, surgical resection, or liver transplantation. World J Surg. 1996;20(7):908–15.

37. Coppa J, Pulvirenti A, Schiavo M, et al. Resection versus transplantation for liver metastases from neuroendocrine tumors. Transplant Proc. 2001;33(1–2):1537–9.

38. House MG, Cameron JL, Lillemoe KD, et al. Differences in survival for patients with resectable versus unresectable metastases from pancreatic islet cell cancer. J Gastrointest Surg. 2006;10(1):138–45.

39. Reddy SK, Clary BM. Neuroendocrine liver metastases. Surg Clin N Am. 2010;90(4):853–61.

40. Mayo SC, de Jong MC, Pulitano C, et al. Surgical management of hepatic neuroendocrine tumor metastasis: results from an international multi-institutional analysis. Ann Surg Oncol. 2010;17(12):3129–36.

41. Clary B. Treatment of isolated neuroendocrine liver metastases. J Gastrointest Surg. 2006;10(3):332–4.

42. Glazer ES, Tseng JF, Al-Refaie W, et al. Long-term survival after surgical management of neuroendocrine hepatic metastases. HPB. 2010;12(6):427–33.

43. Hibi T, Sano T, Sakamoto Y, et al. Surgery for hepatic neuroendocrine tumors: a single institutional experience in Japan. Jpn J Clin Oncol. 2007;37(2):102–7.

44. Azimuddin K, Chamberlain RS. The surgical management of pancreatic neuroendocrine tumors. Surg Clin N Am. 2001;81(3):511–25.

45. Wong RJ, DeCosse JJ. Cytoreductive surgery. Surg Gynecol Obstet. 1990;170(3):276–81.

46. Que FG, Sarmiento JM, Nagorney DM. Hepatic surgery for metastatic gastrointestinal neuroendocrine tumors. Cancer Control. 2002;9(1):67–79.

47. Falconi M, Bettini R, Boninsegna L, et al. Surgical strategy in the treatment of pancreatic neuroendocrine tumors. JOP. 2006;7(1):150–6.

48. Que FG, Sarmiento JM, Nagorney DM. Hepatic surgery for metastatic gastrointestinal neuroendocrine tumors. Adv Exp Med Biol. 2006;574:43–56.

49. Abdalla EK, Barnett CC, Doherty D, et al. Extended hepatectomy in patients with hepatobiliary malignancies with and without preoperative portal vein embolization. Arch Surg. 2002;137(6):675–81.

50. Abdalla EK, Denys A, Chevalier P, et al. Total and segmental liver volume variations: implications for liver surgery. Surgery. 2004;135(4):404–10.

51. Berge T, Linell F. Carcinoid tumours. Frequency in a defined population during a 12 year period. Acta Pathol Microbiol Scand A. 1976;84(4):322–30.

52. Fan ST. Liver functional reserve estimation: state of the art and relevance for local treatments—the Eastern perspective. J Hepato-Biliary-Pancreat Surg. 2009;17(4):380–4.

53. Manizate F, Hiotis SP, Labow D, et al. Liver functional reserve estimation: state of the art and relevance for local treatments—the Western perspective. J Hepato-Biliary-Pancreat Surg. 2010;17(4):385–8.

54. Makuuchi M, Kosuge T, Takayama T, et al. Surgery for small liver cancers. Semin Surg Oncol. 1993;9(4):298–304.

55. Kubota K, Makuuchi M, Kusaka K, et al. Measurement of liver volume and hepatic functional reserve as a guide to decision-making in resectional surgery for hepatic tumors. Hepatology. 1997;26(5):1176–81.

56. Bodingbauer M, Tamandl D, Schmid K, et al. Size of surgical margin does not influence recurrence rates after curative liver resection for colorectal cancer liver metastases. Br J Surg. 2007;94(9):1133–8.

57. DeMatteo RP, Palese C, Jarnagin WR, et al. Anatomic segmental hepatic resection is superior to wedge resection as an oncologic operation for colorectal liver metastases. J Gastrointest Surg. 2000;4(2):178–84.

58. Pawlik TM, Scoggins CR, Zorzi D, et al. Effect of surgical margin status on survival and site of recurrence after hepatic resection for colorectal metastases. Ann Surg. 2005;241(5):715–24.

59. Hamady ZZR, Cameron IC, Wyatt J, et al. Resection margin in patients undergoing hepatectomy for colorectal liver metastasis: a critical appraisal of the 1 cm rule. Eur J Surg Oncol. 2006;32(5):557–63.

60. Elias D, Bonnet S, Honoré C, et al. Comparison between the minimum margin defined on preoperative imaging and the final surgical margin after hepatectomy for cancer: how to manage it? Ann Surg Oncol. 2008;15(3):777–81.

61. Torzilli G, Del Fabbro D, Palmisano A, et al. Contrast-enhanced intraoperative ultrasonography during hepatectomies for colorectal cancer liver metastases. J Gastrointest Surg. 2005;9(8):1148–54.
62. Abdalla EK, Adam R, Bilchik AJ, et al. Improving resectability of hepatic colorectal metastases: expert consensus statement. Ann Surg Oncol. 2006;13(10):1271–80.
63. Wakai T, Shirai Y, Sakata J, et al. Appraisal of 1 cm hepatectomy margins for intrahepatic micrometastases in patients with colorectal carcinoma liver metastasis. Ann Surg Oncol. 2008;15(9):2472–81.
64. de Haas RJ, Wicherts DA, Flores E, et al. R1 resection by necessity for colorectal liver metastases: is it still a contraindication to surgery? Ann Surg. 2008;248(4):626–36.
65. Are C, Gonen M, Zazzali K, et al. The impact of margins on outcome after hepatic resection for colorectal metastasis. Ann Surg. 2007;246(2):295–300.
66. Shirabe K, Takenaka K, Gion T, et al. Analysis of prognostic risk factors in hepatic resection for metastatic colorectal carcinoma with special reference to the surgical margin. Br J Surg. 1997;84(8):1077–80.
67. Ercolani G, Grazi GL, Ravaioli M, et al. The role of lymphadenectomy for liver tumors: further considerations on the appropriateness of treatment strategy. Ann Surg. 2004;239(2):202–9.
68. Zakaria S, Donohue JH, Que FG, et al. Hepatic resection for colorectal metastases: value for risk scoring systems? Ann Surg. 2007;246(2):183–91.
69. Beckurts KTE, Hölscher AH, Thorban S, et al. Significance of lymph node involvement at the hepatic hilum in the resection of colorectal liver metastases. Br J Surg. 1997;84(8):1081–4.
70. Laurent C, Sa Cunha A, Rullier E, et al. Impact of microscopic hepatic lymph node involvement on survival after resection of colorectal liver metastasis. J Am Coll Surg. 2004;198(6):884–91.
71. Jaeck D, Nakano H, Bachellier P, et al. Significance of hepatic pedicle lymph node involvement in patients with colorectal liver metastases: a prospective study. Ann Surg Oncol. 2002;9(5):430–8.
72. Janson ET, Sørbye H, Welin S, et al. Nordic Guidelines 2010 for diagnosis and treatment of gastroenteropancreatic neuroendocrine tumours. Acta Oncol. 2010;49(6):740–56.
73. Sarmiento JM, Que FG. Hepatic surgery for metastases from neuroendocrine tumors. Surg Oncol Clin N Am. 2003;12(1):231–42.
74. Trendle MC, Moertel CG, Kvols LK. Incidence and morbidity of cholelithiasis in patients receiving chronic octreotide for metastatic carcinoid and malignant islet cell tumors. Cancer. 1997;79(4):830–4.
75. Moertel CG. Karnofsky memorial lecture. An odyssey in the land of small tumors. J Clin Oncol. 1987;5(10):1502–22.
76. Thompson GB, van Heerden JA, Grant CS, et al. Islet cell carcinomas of the pancreas: a twenty-year experience. Surgery. 1988;104(6):1011–7.
77. Que FG, Nagorney DM, Batts KP, et al. Hepatic resection for metastatic neuroendocrine carcinomas. Am J Surg. 1995;169(1):36–43.
78. Osborne DA, Zervos EE, Strosberg J, et al. Improved outcome with cytoreduction versus embolization for symptomatic hepatic metastases of carcinoid and neuroendocrine tumors. Ann Surg Oncol. 2006;13(4):572–81.
79. Knox CD, Feurer ID, Wise PE, et al. Survival and functional quality of life after resection for hepatic carcinoid metastasis. J Gastrointest Surg. 2004;8(6):653–9.
80. Berger LA, Osborne D. Treatment of pyogenic liver abscesses by percutaneous needle aspiration. Lancet. 1982;1(8264):132–4.
81. Mazzaferro V, Pulvirenti A, Coppa J. Neuroendocrine tumors metastatic to the liver: how to select patients for liver transplantation? J Hepatol. 2007;47(4):460–6.
82. Lehnert T. Liver transplantation for metastatic neuroendocrine carcinoma: an analysis of 103 patients. Transplantation. 1998;66(10):1307–12.
83. Le Treut YP, Grégoire E, Belghiti J, et al. Predictors of long-term survival after liver transplantation for metastatic endocrine tumors: an 85-case French multicentric report. Am J Transplant. 2008;8(6):1205–13.
84. Öberg K, Eriksson B. Endocrine tumours of the pancreas. Best Pract Res Clin Gastroenterol. 2005;19(5):753–81.
85. Steinmüller T, Kianmanesh R, Falconi M, et al. Consensus guidelines for the management of patients with liver metastases from digestive (neuro)endocrine tumors: foregut, midgut, hindgut, and unknown primary. Neuroendocrinology. 2007;87(1):47–62.
86. Eriksson J, Stålberg P, Nilsson A, et al. Surgery and radiofrequency ablation for treatment of liver metastases from midgut and foregut carcinoids and endocrine pancreatic tumors. World J Surg. 2008;32(5):930–8.
87. Jamison RL, Donohue JH, Nagorney DM, et al. Hepatic resection for metastatic colorectal cancer results in cure for some patients. Arch Surg. 1997;132(5):505–11.
88. Boleslawski E, Dharancy S, Truant S, et al. Surgical management of liver metastases from gastrointestinal endocrine tumors. Gastroenterol Clin Biol. 2010;34(4–5):274–82.
89. Doyle DJ, Garmon EH. American Society of Anesthesiologists Classification (ASA Class) [Updated 2019 Jan 19]. In: StatPearls [Internet]. Treasure Island: StatPearls Publishing; 2019. https://www.ncbi.nlm.nih.gov/books/NBK441940/.
90. McDonald ML, Nagorney DM, Connolly HM, et al. Carcinoid heart disease and carcinoid syndrome: successful surgical treatment. Ann Thorac Surg. 1999;67(2):537–9.

91. Hemming AW, Reed AI, Howard RJ, et al. Preoperative portal vein embolization for extended hepatectomy. Ann Surg. 2003;237(5):686–93.
92. Weber HC, Venzon DJ, Lin JT, et al. Determinants of metastatic rate and survival in patients with Zollinger-Ellison syndrome: a prospective long-term study. Gastroenterology. 1995;108(6):1637–49.
93. Hellman P, Lundström T, Öhrvall U, et al. Effect of surgery on the outcome of midgut carcinoid disease with lymph node and liver metastases. World J Surg. 2002;26(8):991–7.
94. Kulke MH, Siu LL, Tepper JE, et al. Future directions in the treatment of neuroendocrine tumors: consensus report of the National Cancer Institute Neuroendocrine Tumor Clinical Trials Planning Meeting. J Clin Oncol. 2011;29(7):934–43.

Cytoreductive Surgery in Peritoneal Neuroendocrine Neoplasm Metastases: The Adjuvant Endoperitoneal PRRT with ^{111}In-Octreotide Perspective

19

Ioannis Kyriazanos and Georgios S. Limouris

19.1 Introduction

Neuroendocrine neoplasms (NENs) are rather uncommon malignancies occurring with an annual incidence of two to four cases per 100,000 population. However, their incidence has been on the rise in the last four decades, presumably due to improvements in imaging and pathognomonic diagnostic techniques that enhance detection [1–3] (Fig. 19.1).

The prognosis of these tumors compares favorably with other forms of intra-abdominal malignancies, while prolonged survival is observed even in the presence of metastatic disease [4].

19.2 Metastatic NENs

Unfortunately, NENs carry a significant risk for metastatic development, documented in 20.8% at presentation and in an additional 38% of patients subsequent to initial diagnosis [5–7] (Fig. 19.2).

I. Kyriazanos (✉)
1st Surgery Clinic, Naval and Veterans Hospital of Athens, Athens, Greece

G. S. Limouris
Nuclear Medicine, Medical School, National and Kapodistrian University of Athens,
Athens, Greece

Several primary sites have official identification codes (ICD), significantly affecting prognosis [5]; such a practice is imperative in metastatic disease investigation for primary identification [5] (Fig. 19.3). Different metastatic potential among primary sites indicates differing biology and genetics as NENs have been recognized as a heterogeneous group of tumors [8]. The liver remains the most common site of metastasis in NENs with both a known and unknown primary tumor and with 80–90% of metastatic patients to initially present with liver involvement [9] (Fig. 19.4). This is also reported for disseminated metastatic disease, present in a large proportion of gastrointestinal NENs at diagnosis, with liver being the most common site, detected in 60–80% of cases at presentation.

Intra-abdominal extrahepatic metastases have been reported with an incidence varying from 5 to 29% for different primary tumors, with the colon being the commonest source of such a kind of metastasis. In odds ratio analyses, most prominent sources for extrahepatic intraperitoneal dissemination were the small bowel, colon, and hepatopancreatobiliary primary tumors (Fig. 19.5). Peritoneal metastases are generally recognized in about 25% of small bowel NENs and may also occur in midgut well-differentiated neuroendocrine tumors, albeit their influence on survival is ill-defined [10, 11].

© Springer Nature Switzerland AG 2021
G. S. Limouris (ed.), *Liver Intra-arterial PRRT with ^{111}In-Octreotide*,
https://doi.org/10.1007/978-3-030-70773-6_19

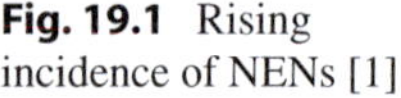

Fig. 19.1 Rising incidence of NENs [1]

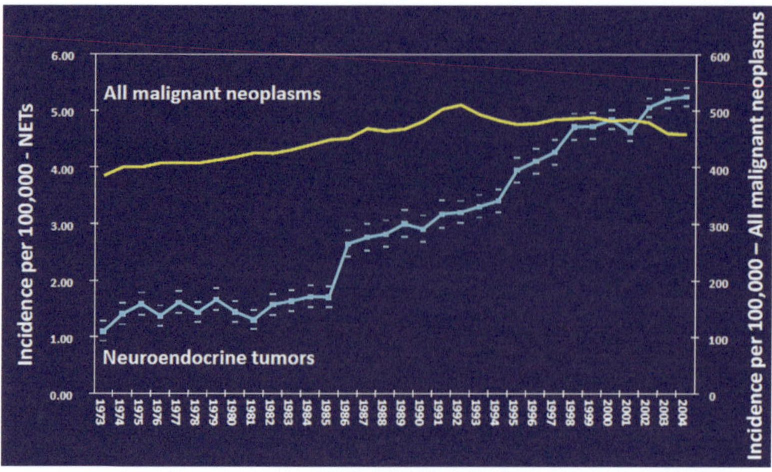

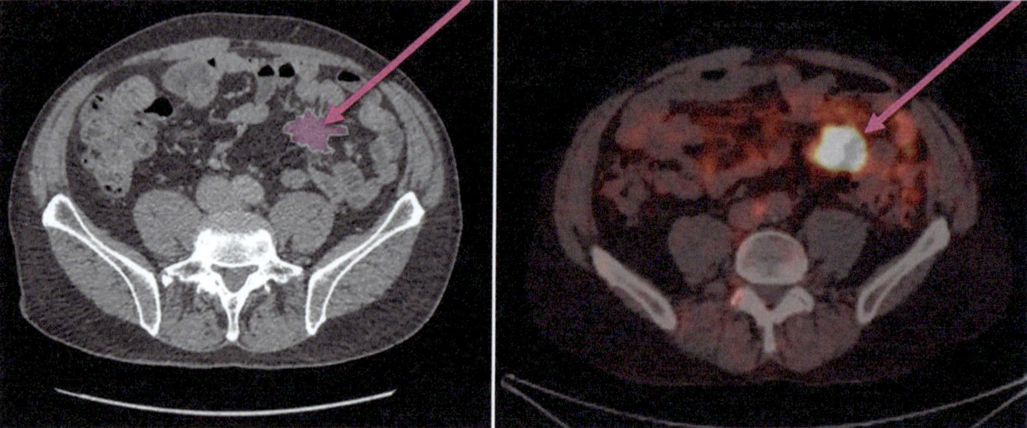

Fig. 19.2 Imaging in metastatic NET; CT (left) and PET/CT (right)

19.3 Peritoneal Carcinomatosis (PC) Due to NENs

Several gastrointestinal and gynecological malignancies have the potential to disseminate and grow in the peritoneal cavity. This condition is known as peritoneal carcinomatosis (PC), and it is often associated with disease progression and poor prognosis. The occurrence of PC from NENs is not a rare event even though there are insufficient data regarding its exact prevalence [12]. Based mainly on two reports from Vasseur et al. in 1996 and Elias et al. in 2005, an overall peritoneal dissemination prevalence ranging from 10 to 33% has been reported. The incidence of PC in patients with NENs is approximately 17% according to the French National Register and 17% among the 603 consecutive small intestinal NENs treated in Uppsala. The US National Cancer Institute's Surveillance, Epidemiology, and End Results (SEER) data in 2003 reported a 13.6% peritoneal metastases prevalence [7, 13–16].

19.4 Molecular Mechanism of Peritoneal Metastases

Tumor dissemination to the peritoneal cavity consists of a multistep process. Individual or clusters of tumor cells detach from primary site and gain freedom to access to the peritoneal cavity. Adhesion molecules play *an important role in this* process. For the formation of perito-

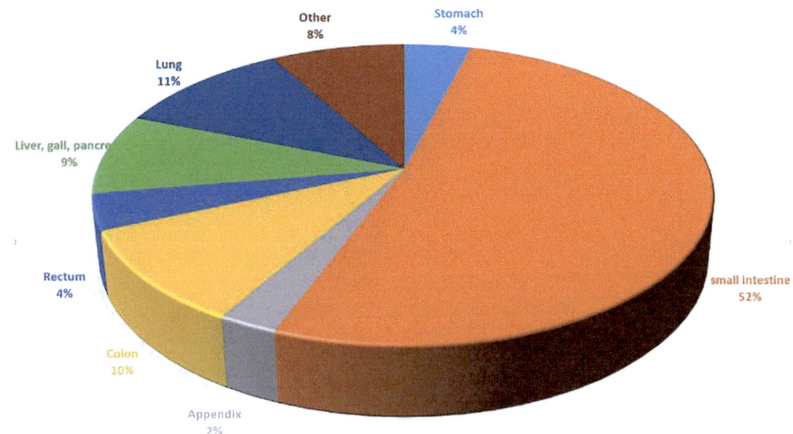

Fig. 19.3 Distribution of primary site in metastatic NENs [5]

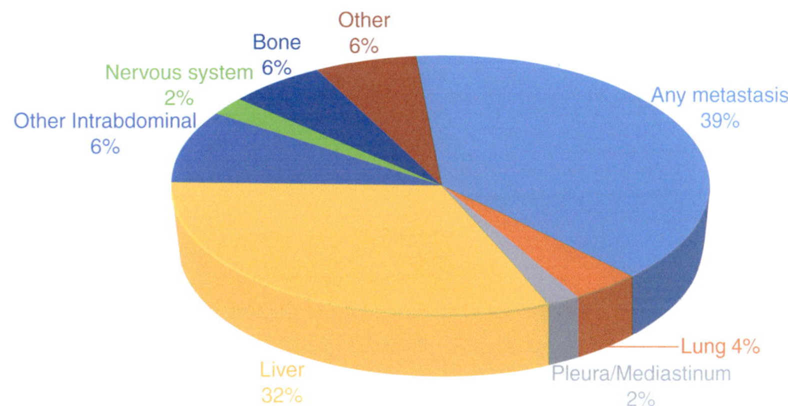

Fig. 19.4 Distribution of metastases in NENs [5]

neal metastases, attachment of peritoneal-free cancer cells to the peritoneum is necessary, and two different processes have so far been proposed: the trans-mesothelial process and the trans-lymphatic process. In brief, the multistep processes in the peritoneal dissemination can be summarized in the following steps: *process 1,* detachment of cancer cells from serosa with participation of E-cadherin, S100A4, and motility factors (AMF/AMFR, HGF/c-Met, Rho); *process 2,* adhesion to mesothelial cells (CD-44, CEA, ICAM, CA19-9); **process 3,** contraction of mesothelial cells (cytokines: interleukins, EGF, HGF, VEGF-C); **process 4,** adhesion molecules (integrins, CD44); **process 5,** invasion: motility factors, matrix metalloproteinases, urokinase, and UKPR; **process 6,** vascular neogenesis (VEGF, VEGFC, bFGF), lymph angiogenesis, and lymphatic dilatation (VEGF-C, VEGF-D); **process 7,** exposure of lymphatic stomata (cytokines: interleukins EGF,HGF,VEGF-C) or lymphatic orifices; and **process 8,** invasion through lymphatic stomatas and lymphangiogenesis (VEGF-C, VEGF-D) [17] (Fig. 19.6).

19.5 Distribution of Peritoneal Metastases Due to NENs

The peritoneal cavity contains less than 100 mL of serous fluid similar in composition to plasma ultrafiltrate. This fluid lubricates the visceral peritoneum and typically contains a few cells, including desquamated mesothelial cells, perito-

Fig. 19.5 Distribution of extra-hepatic intraperitoneal metastases in NENs [5]

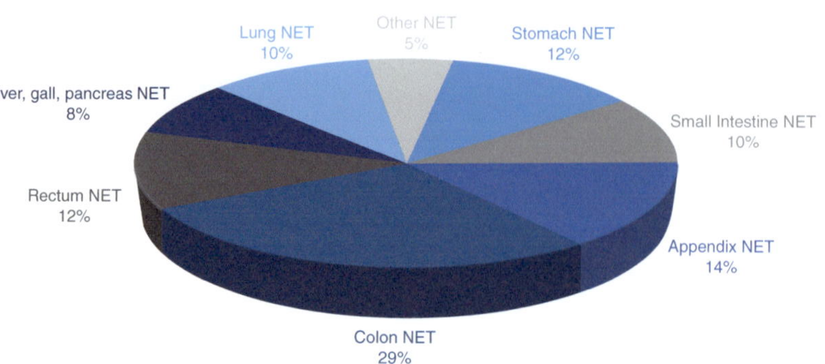

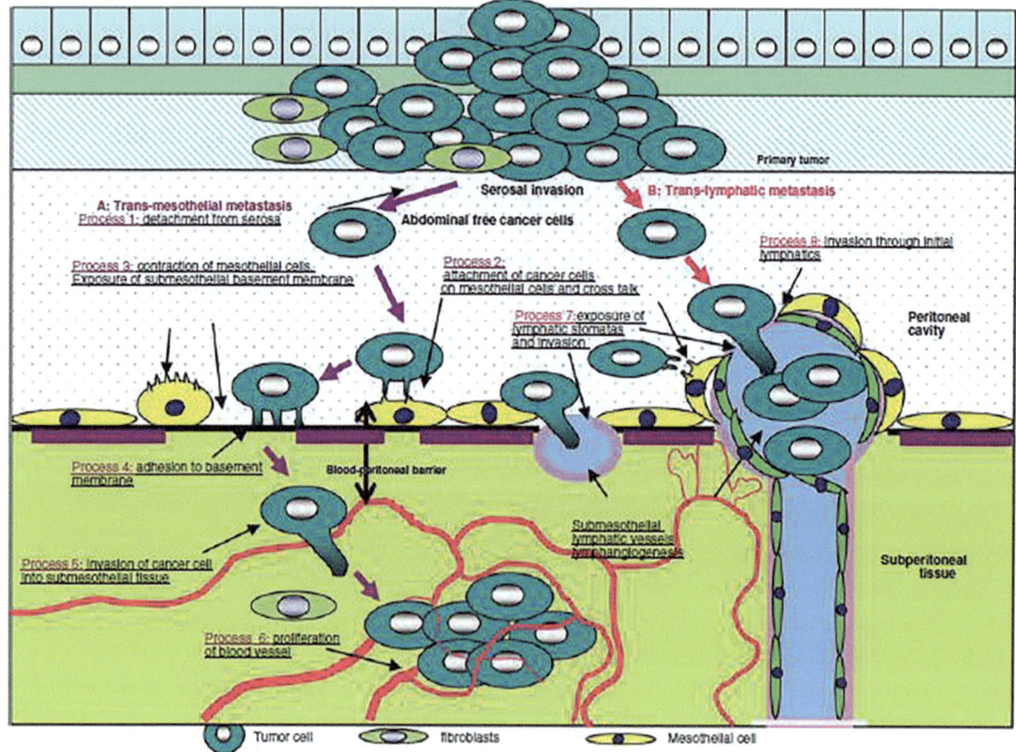

Fig. 19.6 Molecular mechanism of peritoneal metastases [17]

neal macrophages, mast cells, fibroblasts, lymphocytes, and other leukocytes.

Force of gravity drives pool of peritoneal fluid preferentially in pelvic cavity which follows a circular clockwise route, and through the paracolic gutters, it is directed to subphrenic regions to final reabsorption and recirculation [18] (Fig. 19.7).

The exfoliated cancer cells from the primary tumor are disseminated throughout the peritoneal cavity by this natural flow of the peritoneal fluid. A mechanism implicating gravity on biological fluids (i.e., ascites) is associated with it. Since, normally, there is only a small volume of the peritoneal fluid present, dissemination is predominantly limited to the organs in the vicinity of

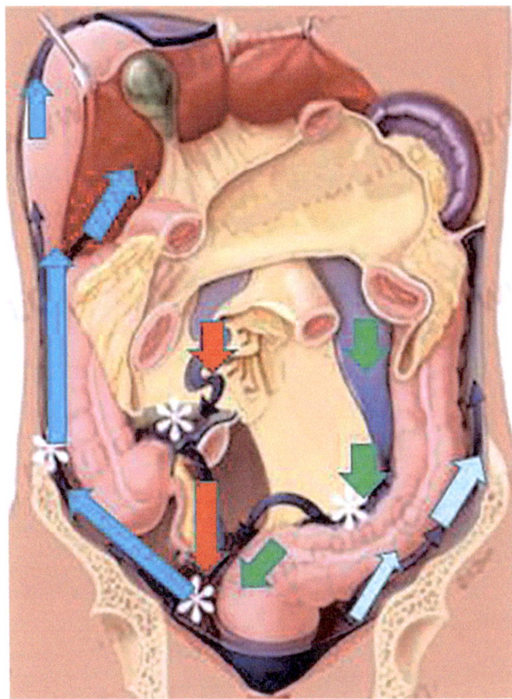

Fig. 19.7 Intraperitoneal fluid circulation [18]

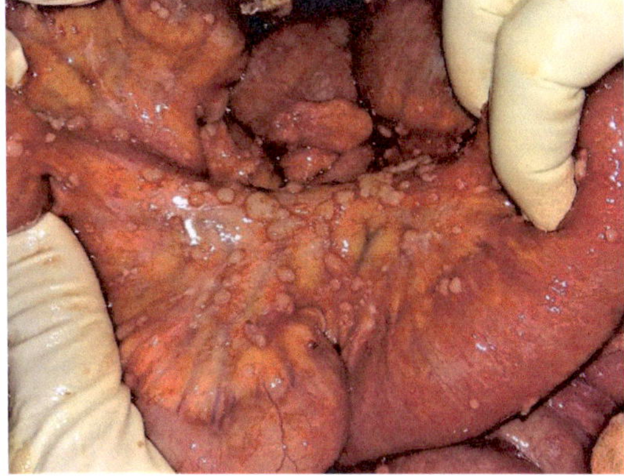

Fig. 19.8 Massive peritoneal metastases due to NEN in Douglas pouch (pelvic peritoneum)

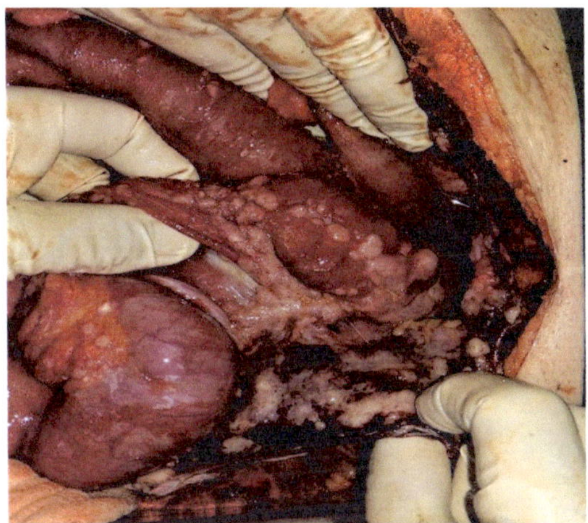

Fig. 19.9 Massive involvement in small bowel mesentery

the primary tumor. As the disease progresses, more and more ascites are produced, and this enables the spread of the cancer cells to more distant sites in the abdomen.

Free cancer cells float into the peritoneal space forming cell aggregation in spotted areas as a consequence of gravity and concentration in places of peritoneal fluid absorption. Reabsorption of peritoneal fluids takes place at the omentum and the diaphragmatic peritoneum. The most frequently affected locations are pelvis (Fig. 19.8), subphrenic areas, parietocolic grooves, and the Morrison's pouch [19].

In the absence of tumor fluid production, cancer cell motility is limited, implanting close to the primary site. Distant areas are affected when the fluid carrier is present, such as at the Treitz ligament and the lesser omentum; in the absence of fluid carriers, these sites are unaffected.

In general, in early stages, the mesenteric surfaces and serosa of the small intestine are spared; the presence of peristaltic motility inhibits cancer cell adhesion. In advanced carcinomatosis, small bowel wall or mesenteric involvement with partial or complete lumen obstruction is a common finding (Fig. 19.9). Conversely, fixed areas, such as the duodenum, ileocecal, and rectosigmoid passages, are frequently involved by PM [20]. One of the predominant sites of cancer metastasis is the omentum covering the bowel with "omental cake" formation (Fig. 19.10).

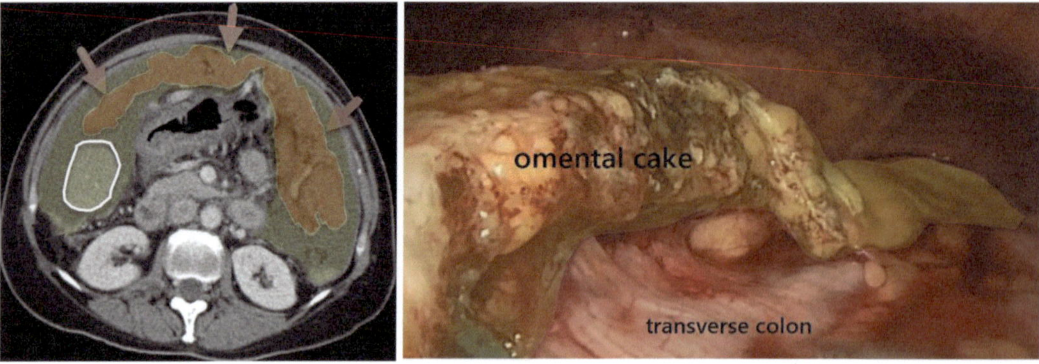

Fig. 19.10 Massive involvement of greater omentum from NENs peritoneal meta-stases; CT (left) and laparoscopic appearance of "omental cake" in ascitic environment

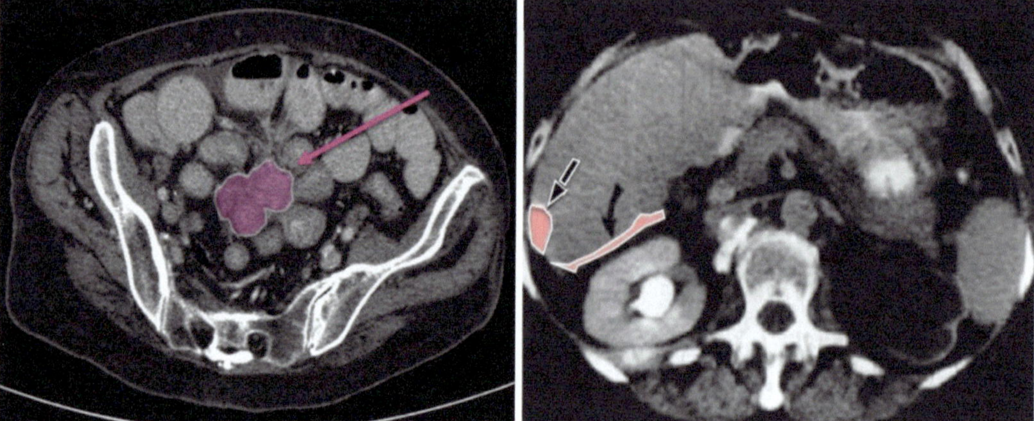

Fig. 19.11 CT imaging of peritoneal metastases due to NENs in small bowel mesentery and liver Glisson's capsule

19.6 Diagnostic Procedures for Peritoneal Carcinomatosis Due to NENs

Signs and symptoms of peritoneal disease are usually absent during initial stages of the disease. After their occurrence, symptoms are strong indicators for peritoneal carcinomatosis presence. Signs usually include omentum stranding to discrete nodules to omental caking, whereas in other abdominal locations, they can result in "Sister Mary Joseph nodule," nodularity in thin areas of the abdominal wall, such as a hernia or diastasis, and/or nodularity in the cul-de-sac. Once peritoneal disease is significant enough to block the infra-diaphragmatic lymphatics, ascites may be present at the time of diagnosis [21].

The clinical presentation of peritoneal carcinomatosis may include mild bloating and distention, which may be due to ascites, an enlarged omentum, gas-filled bowel, or a single lesion pressing on the rectum or stomach. Urinary urgency can occur with lesions pressing the bladder, or on the contrary, urinary retention can be related to ureter encasement. More obvious symptoms, such as pain due to peritoneal carcinomatosis, are largely dependent on the location of peritoneal nodules [22].

The preoperative exact localization (Fig. 19.11) of the lesion is of crucial importance.

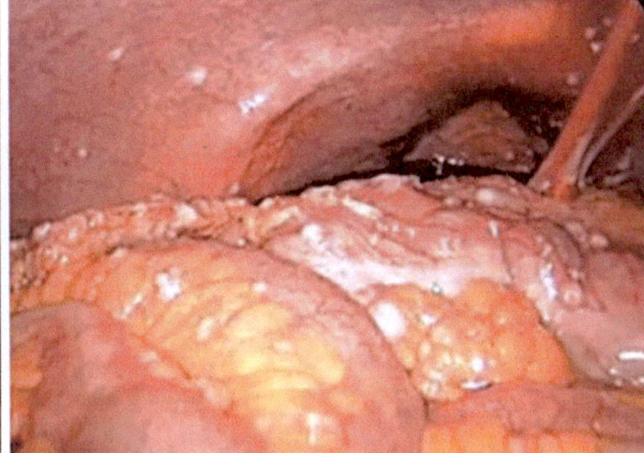

Fig. 19.12 Diagnostic laparoscopy able to improve detection of disseminated small nodules

Diagnostic procedures most commonly used for peritoneal metastasis identification, especially for large nodules >1 cm, include use of CT scan, MRI with conventional and diffusion-weighted (DWI) sequences, FDG-positron emission tomography (FDG-PET or PET/CT or PET/MRI), and laparoscopy. Specifically, for peritoneal disease arising from neuroendocrine neoplasms, and due to high levels of expression of somatostatin receptors (SSTRs) in the majority of NENs, these neoplasms can also be detected by somatostatin receptor scintigraphy (SRS; Octreoscan or Tektrotyd) or by positron emission tomography (PET; ^{68}Ga-DOTATOC PET/CT) [23]. Diagnostic laparoscopy (Fig. 19.12) is a safe and feasible tool, able to improve the selection of patients eligible for cytoreduction, avoiding at the same time a significant number of unnecessary laparotomies. When possible, staging laparoscopy is advantageous in allowing the detection of disseminated small nodules not apparent on conventional imaging [24, 25].

19.7 Classification of Peritoneal Metastases from NENs

Two quantitative staging systems are currently in use: the Gilly PC staging system [26] and the Peritoneal Cancer Index (PCI) [27]. The Gilly PC staging format (Table 19.1) takes into account size and partially distribution, localized or diffuse, of malignant granulations. Studies focusing on GC, moreover, observed that in resectable

Table 19.1 Gilly classification system: It is based on nodule size and simplified extent of intraperitoneal involvement (localized or diffused) [26]

Stage 0	No macroscopic disease
Stage 1	Malignant granulations less than 5 mm in diameter, localized in one part of the abdomen
Stage 2	Malignant granulations less than 5 mm in diameter, diffused to the whole abdomen
Stage 3	Localized or diffused malignant granulations 5–20 mm in diameter
Stage 4	Localized or diffused large malignant (more than 2 cm in diameter) mm in diameter

Scores vary from 0 to 4; patients with Gilly stage 3 or 4 have advanced disease which is often associated with a prognosis

Table 19.2 Lesion size score

LS 0	No tumor seen
LS 1	Tumor up to 0.5 cm
LS 2	Tumor up to 5.0 cm
LS 3	Tumor >5.0 cm or confluence

neoplasia with carcinomatosis stages 1 and 2, the 1-year survival rates were 80% versus 10% for patients with unresectable primary tumors in carcinomatosis stages 3 and 4. The PCI classification system (Table 19.2, Fig. 19.13) grades lesion distribution on the peritoneal surface on the basis of their size, producing a quantitative score. PCI gives a threshold value for favorable versus poor prognosis and moreover allows estimation of the probability of complete cytoreduction. The abdomen and the pelvic regions are divided by lines into nine regions (0–8). The small bowel is then divided into four regions. Regions 9 and 10 define the upper and lower portions of the jejunum; regions 11 and 12 define the upper and lower portions of the ileum. The LS (i.e., the largest implant size) is scored in each abdominal region. Implants are scored as LS-0 to LS-3 [27].

LS-0 means no implants are seen throughout the region; this measurement is made after complete adhesiolysis, and complete inspection of all parietal and visceral peritoneal surfaces. LS-1 refers to implants that are visible up to 0.5 cm in greatest diameter. LS-2 identifies nodules greater than 0.5 cm and up to 5 cm. LS-3 refers to implants 5 cm or greater in diameter.

As PC rarely occurs isolated, the ENETS expert group proposed the GPS (Table 19.3) which incorporates the Gilly classification with the extent of lymph node and liver metastases.

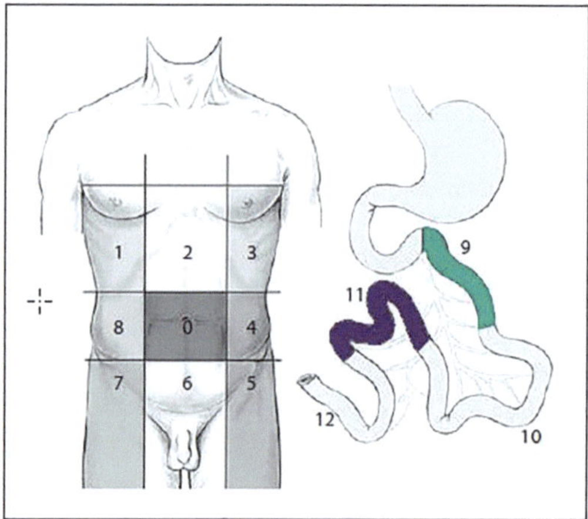

Fig. 19.13 Peritoneal Carcinomatosis Index (PCI) classification system [27]

Scores range from 0 to 9 (<3 points, GPS grade A deemed "low risk" of abdominal spread; 4–6 points, grade B considered as having an "intermediate risk"; and >7: grade C considered as having a "high risk" and usually unresectable). However, such a proposition requires prospective examination for validation [15, 16].

19.8 Management of Peritoneal Metastases Due to NENs

The management of peritoneal metastatic NENs is complex, and several therapeutic modalities exist aiming cure or treatment of complication in a curative or palliative mode. Therapeutic approaches for management of metastatic disease include surgical, medical, radiological, and nuclear medicine strategies. More recently, novel molecular targeted drugs have been introduced into the NET treatment armamentarium. Each of the management strategies exhibits potential therapeutic benefits and the indications [28].

19.9 Surgery/Surgery Combined Treatments

19.9.1 Surgery for Peritoneal Dissemination

Radical surgery with curative intent is the only potentially curative therapy leading to relatively good outcome. Surgery seems to be the most efficient tool among the different treatments of

Table 19.3 ENETS classification system: GPS grading system based on the lymph node and liver metastases [15, 16]

	0 point	1 point	2 points	3 points
Lymph node metastases	Local	Regional	Distant abdominal (retroperitoneal, hepatic pedicle)	Extra-abdominal
Liver metastases	No macroscopic nodule	One lobe less than five nodules	Both lobes five to ten nodules	Both lobes more than ten nodules
PC	No macroscopic nodule	Gilly I-II Resectable	Gilly III-IV Resectable	Gilly I-II-III-IV Unresectable

GPS grade A: 0–3 points, **GPS grade B**: 4–6 points, **GPS grade C:** 7–9 points. To avoid including patients with non-malignant ascites, patients with positive malignant cells obtained by peritoneal biopsies and/or positive cytology of the peritoneal fluid are considered as having proven PC. 1 Local: first (adjacent) to the primary tumor territory relay. 2 Regional: secondary tumor drainage territory relay

NENs, and it is suggested to be considered as first-line treatment. However, this is not a panacea, and patients' selection in order to offer them the most appropriate treatment remains a significant component of treatment success [29]. Peritoneal metastases are traditionally treated with skepticism as terminal stage disease with dismal prognosis and are regarded as contraindication for surgery precluding resection of other even resectable metastatic sites like the liver. One of the reasons is the recognized extremely high rate of recurrence (90–95%) following metastasis resection [30].

However, operative therapy although rarely curative in the setting of metastatic disease has an important role in achieving effective palliation from disease symptoms and in preventing further complications in selected patients. Particularly, peritoneal disease resection can protect from intestinal obstruction, ischemia, digestive hemorrhage, and segmental portal hypertension (left pancreas) leading to death in 40% of cases as well [14]. Hence, surgical resection of primary tumor should systematically be combined with excision of early locoregional peritoneal lesions (including extended lymphadenectomy), with the aim of preventing later complications associated with PC dissemination. For these reasons, the use of debulking surgery for peritoneal metastases has been developed.[1] Worth to notice that debulking surgery crucially improves symptom control in 91.5% of patients and extends 4-year overall survival in about 55%, compared with patients with unresected peritoneal disease (7.9 vs 4 years) [7, 10, 16, 31].

---

[1] The term "debulking surgery" describes a surgical technique that aims at reducing the cancerous burden, but not at its complete macroscopic eradication, primarily serving symptom relief and palliative care. There is limited removal of macroscopic tumor from the abdominal cavity avoiding extensive resections, especially from areas which can increase operation's morbidity and mortality, like surface of the upper abdomen (right and left upper quadrant, lesser omentum, and duodenal-hepatic ligament and "stripping" of diaphragmatic peritoneal coverage (Fig. 19.14) [32–35].

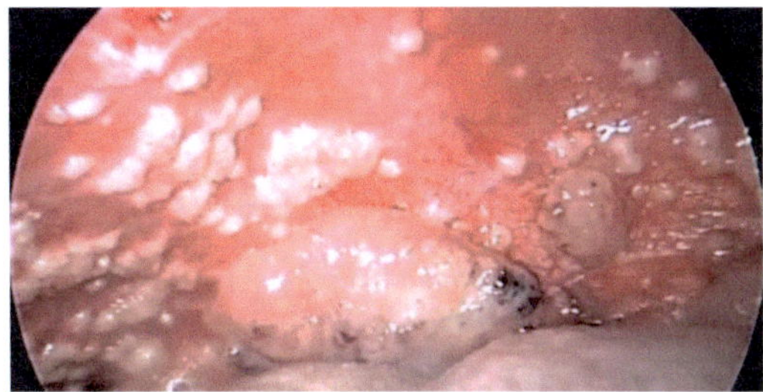

Fig. 19.14 Extensive involvement of sub-diaphragmatic peritoneum from peritoneal metastases due to NENs

19.9.2 Cytoreductive Surgery

Cytoreductive surgery (CRS) is a special kind of surgical manipulation incorporating a set of clearly defined and well-described surgical maneuvers that primarily target the "organ" that hosts metastases (i.e., the peritoneum) aiming complete resection of macroscopic disease with cure intent, known as peritonectomies (PRTs), according to Paul Sugarbaker [16, 36]. PRTs consist of a number of techniques, which can be used according to anatomical districts, aiming the complete removal of carcinomatosis with wide resection of parietal and visceral peritoneal areas in which the tumor is present, visceral and parenchymal exeresis, local excision, or in situ destruction of implants [37]. In brief, operation begins with abdominal incision and possible resection of previous scars as often old scars harbor cancer cells. A complete abdominal lysis of adhesions is performed to evaluate the possibility of surgical exeresis and carcinosis extension. Exeresis of parietal and visceral peritoneum represents the fundamental step of PRTs. Traditionally, wide peritoneal resection should be reserved to areas with extensive disease, whereas "à la demande" resection is suggested when implants are isolates with large areas of healthy tissue in between. If the healthy areas are limited, large peritonectomies—which can include entire anatomical sectors or even complete PRT—should be performed. Usually, PRT procedures include total anterior parietal peritonectomy (Fig. 19.15), omentectomy (Fig. 19.16), right and left subphrenic peritonectomy, pelvic peritonectomy, and lesser omentectomy with stripping of the omental bursa ±

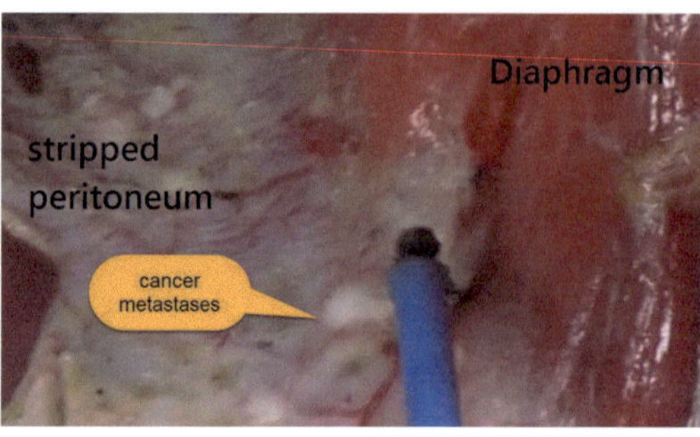

Fig. 19.15 "Stripping" for the resection of the subphrenic peritoneal cover. Whitish nodular cancer metastases are detached with peritoneal leaf

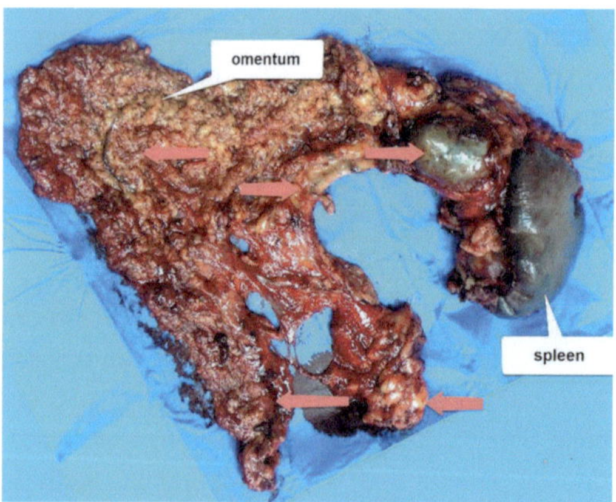

Fig. 19.16 Omentectomy en block with splenectomy (red arrows indicate omental metastases from NENs)

cholecystectomy [36]. When an organ or viscus is involved in massive carcinosis, it should be removed: cholecystectomy, hysterectomy, adnexectomy, splenectomy, and small- and large-bowel resection are the most common. Gastrectomy is most of the times unnecessary, while the colon can be sacrificed with minor functional impact and major advantages in terms of radicality. The extent of small-bowel resection must be well balanced to reduce surgical risk and preserve adequate digestive function, with a stoma (temporal or permanent) being necessary in about 30% of cases. Ovaries should be always removed, even if they appear macroscopically healthy, whereas the uterus should be removed only if directly involved. All sites and volumes of the residual disease following the cytoreductive surgery were prospectively recorded using the completeness of

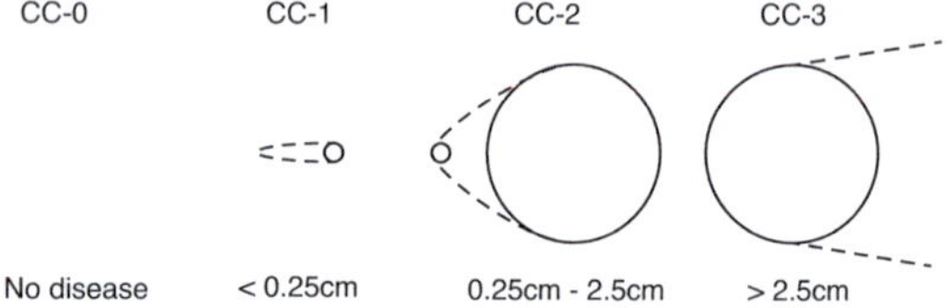

Fig. 19.17 Completeness of cytoreduction score (CCR score) [38]

cytoreduction score (CCR score). A CCR-0 indicates no visible evidence of residual tumors, CCR-1 residual tumors <2.5 mm in diameter, CCR-2 residual tumors between 2.5 mm and 2.5 cm in diameter, and CCR-3 residual tumors >2.5 cm in diameter or a confluence of tumors remaining at any site in the abdominopelvic cavity (Fig. 19.17) [38]. However, and despite such extensive surgical manipulation, the possibility of leaving behind vital cancer implants remains high. Microscopic residual disease has been identified in 23.3% of cases with normal looking peritoneum, indicating that total parietal peritonectomy (TPP) which comprised of removal of the entire parietal peritoneum and the greater and lesser omenta can be proved more beneficial compared to selective parietal peritonectomy (SPP, "à la demande resection") for patients with peritoneal metastases [39]. The experience in the 1_{st} Department of Surgery at Naval and Veterans Hospital of Athens, Greece, consists of 94 consecutive cytoreductive operations for peritoneal malignancies performed in a variety of primaries, between 2010 and 2019. In an effort to standardize the surgical approach of total parietal peritonectomy (TPP), we systematically apply this technique in our patients with the addition of special modifications. At the beginning prior laparotomy scar should be completely excised, while care is taken to avoid disruption of peritoneal membrane (Fig. 19.18). Next step includes detachment of the peritoneum from the posterior surface of the anterior abdominal wall in an anterolateral direction (Fig. 19.19). Laterally to the abdominal wall the extraperitoneal dissection is extended dorsally to the level of pericolic regions (anteroposterior extension), where it turns medially and is then facilitated by the medial traction of the ascending or descending colon propor-

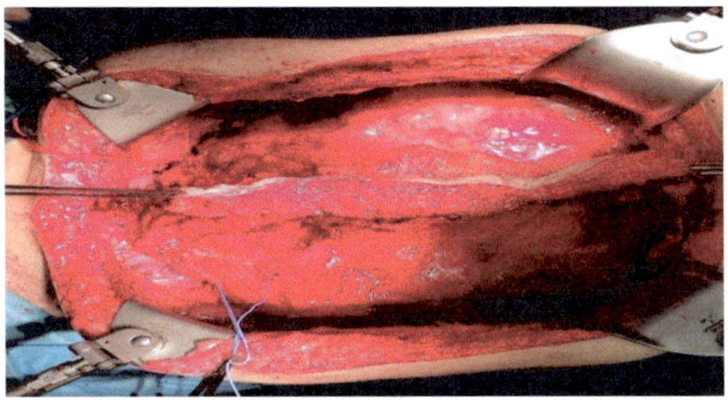

Fig. 19.18 Prior laparotomy scar should be completely excised, avoid disruption of peritoneal membrane

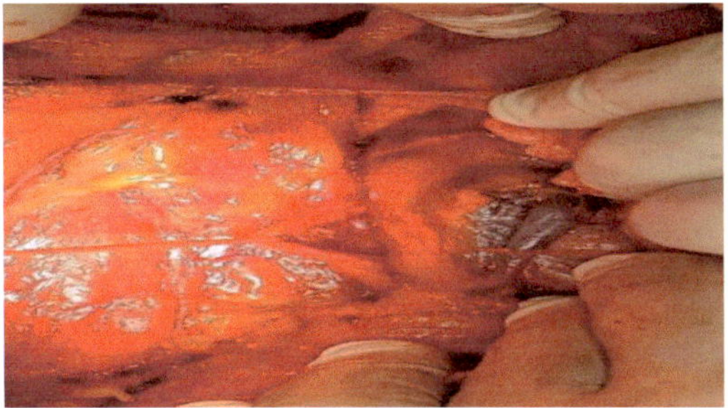

Fig. 19.21 Peritoneal detachment up to the retroperitoneal space; ureter identification

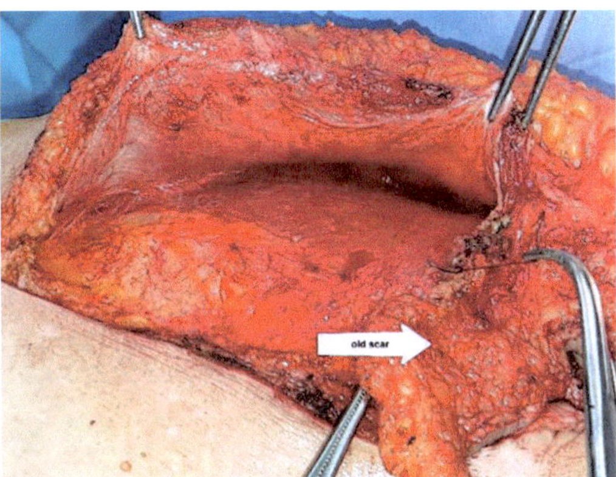

Fig. 19.19 Detachment of the parietal peritoneum form the anterior and lateral abdominal wall. Peritoneal leaf remains intact. Old scar is indicated by the arrow and re- remains attached to peritoneum (extra-peritoneal antero-lateral dissection)

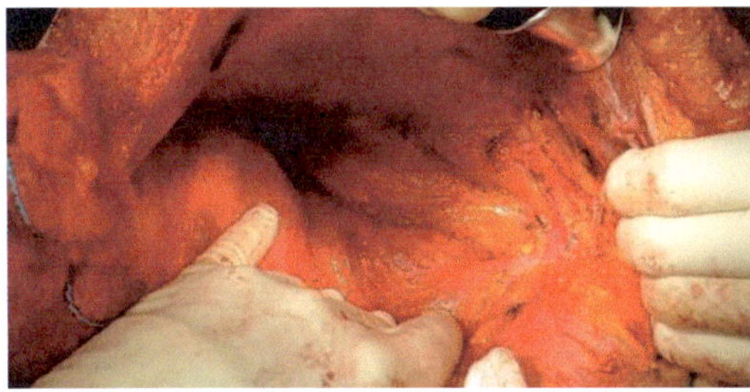

Fig. 19.20 Extension of lateral peritoneal detach-ment up to the retroperitoneal space/fat (extraperitoneal, antero-posterior dissection)

tionally, entering the retroperitoneal space and leaving behind the fascia of Toldt (Fig. 19.20). At this point it is necessary to strip out the loosely connected retroperitoneal fat from the peritoneum and leave it dorsally; otherwise the surgeon faces

the retro-renal space. The dissection deepens laterally identifying extraperitoneally—and with the peritoneum still intact—the ovarian and uterine vessels as well as both ureters (Fig. 19.21). Inferiorly, the extraperitoneal dissection continues with stripping of the peritoneum and the underlying fatty tissues away from the surface of the bladder. Following the above-described approach to pelvis entrance, with the peritoneum being still intact, dissection proceeds bilaterally in two different planes, one in front and one behind the pelvic organ complex (rectosigmoid in male, rectosigmoid and internal genitalia in female). The perirectal fat is dissected, and the rectal musculature is skeletonized in a way that permits the rectum and vagina being divided beneath the peritoneal reflection of the pouch of Douglas to complete the pelvic peritonectomy (Fig. 19.22). Surgical result is characterized by skeletonization of all anatomic elements (Figs. 19.23 and 19.24). Cranially detachment of the peritoneum from subphrenic areas terminates the peritoneal dissection. Using this surgical approach, a continuous leaf of closed peritoneum resembling a "cocoon" is created, containing all peritoneal organs, mucus ascites, and all peritoneal implants (Fig. 19.25). This operative technique represents a combination of the already described by de Vazquez and Sugarbaker "Total Anterior Parietal peritonectomy" [40] with the addition of elements from pelvic, left upper quadrant, and right upper quadrant PRTs. Therefore, it is described herein as total anteroposterior parietal PRT or total extraperitoneal parietal PRT ("cocoon") technique, facilitating all the necessary PRTs with the same

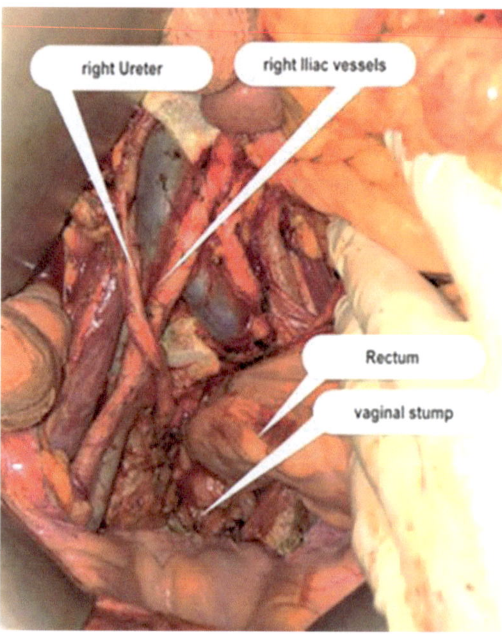

Fig. 19.22 Peritoneal detachment up to the retroperitoneal space; vaginal division extraperitoneally, beneath Douglas pouch

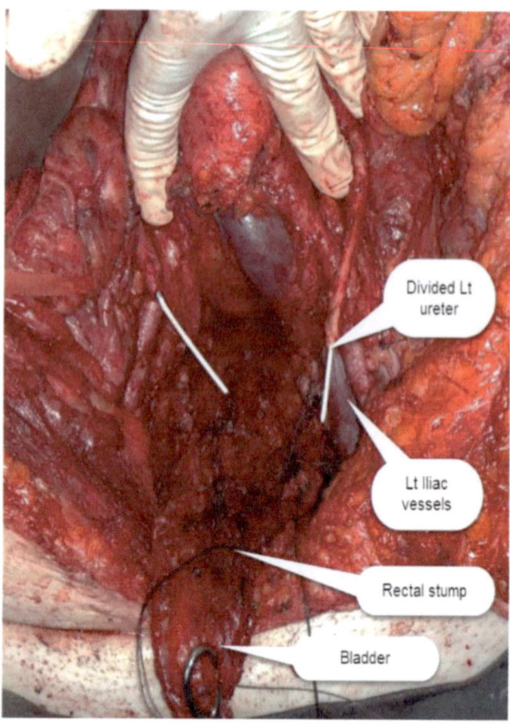

Fig. 19.24 Totally skeletonized pelvis, beneath Douglas pouch; both ureters are divided due to tumor invasion

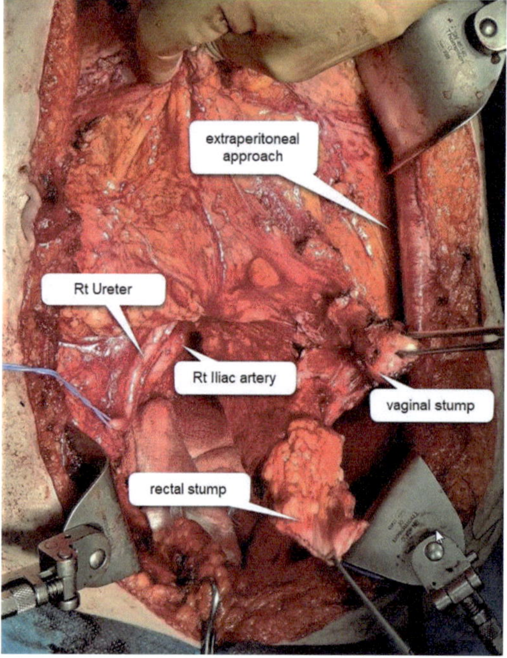

Fig. 19.23 Totally detached pelvic peritoneum intact; vaginal and rectal stumps have been divided extraperitoneally, beneath Douglas pouch detachment up to the retroperitoneal dissection

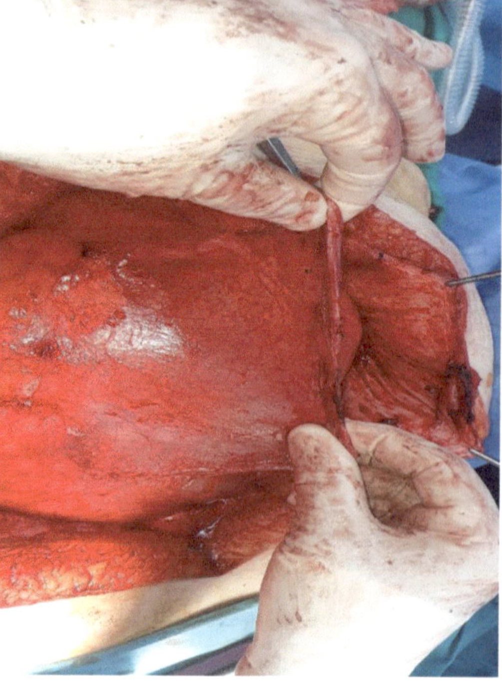

Fig. 19.25 A continuous leaf of closed peritoneum resembling a "cocoon" is created

surgical access and decreasing the total time of the surgical procedure [41].

19.9.3 Cytoreduction vs Debulking

The difference in the extent of resection between cytoreduction and debulking is well reflected in the study of Andréasson et al., where cytoreduction in 75% of patients resulted in higher rates of no residual macroscopic tumor (complete cytoreduction, R1) in comparison to 25% for patients who underwent debulking [31].

Advantages of extensive surgery have been concentrated in the hypothesis that reduction of tumor mass decreases the likelihood that cancer cell resistance develops, thereby making it less likely that new resistant cancer cell subclones will appear. Equally important, cytoreduction stimulates the remaining tumor cells to enter into a proliferative phase that is potentially more responsive to chemotherapy. Hence, the rationale underlying cytoreduction is that the fewer tumor cells left after it, the better they respond to chemotherapy [42].

Cytoreduction carries a survival benefit compared to palliative bypass or incomplete tumor removal. Thus, cytoreduction should be considered as the first treatment choice in patients with resectable peritoneal metastases in a good performance status [31].

19.9.4 Cytoreduction Combined with Intraperitoneal Chemotherapy or Peptide Receptor Radionuclide Therapy

Surgical approach to peritoneal metastases from NENs has been questioned once again during last decades mainly due to the development of new treatments for peritoneal malignancies generally. In the mid-1990s, thanks to Sugarbaker's pioneering efforts [19, 43], research began to develop integrated procedures for treating peritoneal surface malignancies based on a new therapeutic approach. This approach involved cytoreductive surgery (CRS) (peritonectomy procedures) combined with perioperative intraperitoneally administered chemotherapy in a hyperthermic (Hyperthermic Intraperitoneal Chemotherapy—HIPEC) or normothermic mode [19, 43] (Fig. 19.26). Furthermore, CRS combined with Peptide Receptor Radionuclide Therapy (PRRT) in OctreoScan positive peritoneal metastases, using the attractive ^{111}In-Octreotide Auger electron emission, in high activties, in tandem intraperitoneal/intravenous infusions, might be a keen and exceptional approach of these metastatic category.

The rationale of those applications is based on the theory that peritoneal carcinosis management apart from the use of cytoreductive surgery and peritonectomy procedures for macroscopic disease elimination needs further the addition of perioperative intraperitoneal chemotherapy

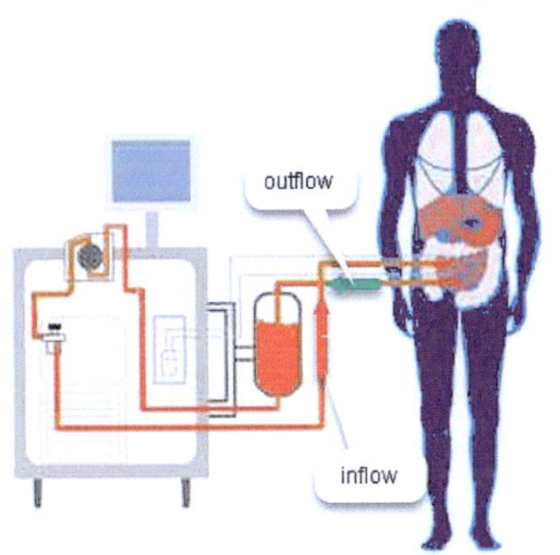

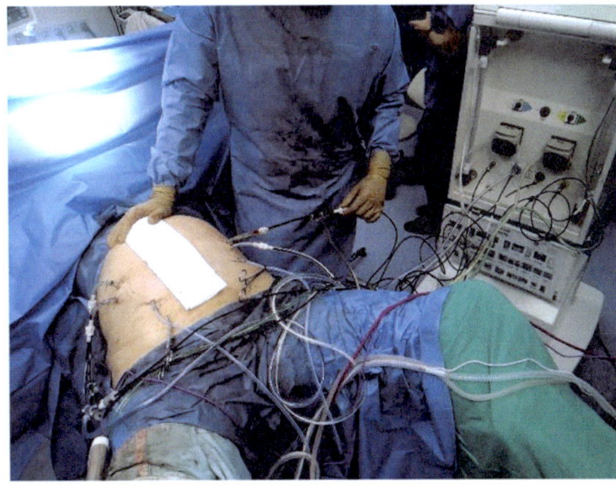

Fig. 19.26 System for hyperthermic intraperitoneal chemotherapy (HIPEC) administration adapted from https://www.yashodahospitals.com/blog/hipec-surgery-for-abdominal-cancer/#/

administration for microscopic residual disease control [21].

Hyperthermic Intraperitoneal Chemotherapy (HIPEC) represents intraoperative administration of chemotherapy in the abdominal cavity of the patient, with the use of a "closed" tube system connecting a "pump" device with the patient's abdomen, (up) schematic representation of HIPEC administration system, (down) operative theater application in our clinic.

Cytoreductive surgery in combination with HIPEC implementation significantly improves disease-free and overall survival in appropriately selected patients with peritoneal malignancies, generally. It is necessary to be emphasized that a maximum possible cytoreduction plays a crucial role in maximizing the possible efficacy of intraperitoneal chemotherapy. Its prognostic value has been confirmed for all forms of peritoneal cancer, both in primary and recurrent settings [36]. Completeness of cytoreduction is such a critical prognostic factor that any incomplete maneuver should discourage extensive surgical attempts which can increase morbidity.

19.9.5 Application of This Combined Treatment in Peritoneal Metastases Due to NENs

Resulted in contradictory results and has never been studied prospectively up-to-date. One of the factors responsible for these results remains the frequent association of peritoneal and liver metastases, making the management more comvdissemination. However, peritoneal metastases can be presented as the sole site of NENs metastases in about 33% of patients with peritoneal dissemination [44].

To the best of our knowledge, retrospective studies up-to-date demonstrate that the addition of intraperitoneal chemotherapy after complete surgical cytoreduction does not improve survival in patients with PM due to NENs [14, 16].

In studies comparing patients treated with or without the addition of intraperitoneal chemotherapy, similar 2-year overall survival rates have been reported (81 vs. 73%, respectively), reducing the potential impact of HIPEC in patient's prognosis. The improved 2-year disease-free survival in HIPEC cases with chemotherapy after cytoreduction (49 vs. 17%) was unfortunately attributed to decreased appearance of lung and bone metastases and not truly to reduced rate of peritoneal recurrence occurrence, which were similar between the two groups [45–49].

It is established that the more extensive the cytoreduction, the better the results of the method, and traditionally a total macroscopic clearance of the peritoneal metastases was the surgical target (CC-0).[2] This very aggressive management (in selected patients) leads to an overall survival of up to 60–80% with morbidity and mortality rate of 30% and 0–5%, respectively. Parameters playing significant role in decision making concerning surgical management with curative intent in patients with NENs peritoneal metastases (PMs) include:

(a) Origin of the primary tumor [48]
(b) Tumor differentiation [14, 50, 51]
(c) Extent of metastatic disease [16, 28, 52]
(d) Extent of peritoneal involvement

It has to be emphasized that PCI is the most powerful prognostic indicator for completeness of cytoreduction and for survival and especially for peritoneal metastases due to NENs; a score above 16 is a strong predictor for failure to accomplish complete cytoreduction [50, 53, 54].

History, regarding the management pharetra of NENs, proved that chemotherapy carries a restricted role, addressing to tumor aggressiveness and dedifferentiation. Thus, the benefit afforded by intraperitoneal chemotherapy addition to complete cytoreduction in patients with PMs due to NENs remains questionable.

---

[2]Completeness of Cytoreduction Score (CC Score) is discriminated according to the amount of residual tumor into three categories: CC-0, no macroscopic residual disease; CC-1, residual disease <2.5 mm; CC-2, residual disease 2.5 mm–2.5 cm; CC-3, residual disease >2.5 cm [47].

19.10 Conclusions and Perspectives

The ability to target and eradicate peritoneal tumor deposits (micrometastases) as small as 0.012 ± 0.009 g using a brief exposure of intraperitoneal tumor nodules to monoclonal antibodies and particularly peptides, radiolabeled with the Auger electron-emitting radionuclides as might be Indium-111, represents a promising new treatment approach to peritoneal carcinomatosis. The idea of this intraperitoneal implementation intraoperatively or laparoscopically (Pressurized Intraperitoneal Aerosol Chemotherapy, PIPAC) opens new horizons and perspectives for the patient's benefit. It appears that the "odyssey in the land of small tumors" still continues.

References

1. Yao JC, Manal H, Phan A, et al. One hundred years after "carcinoid": epidemiology of and prognostic factors for neuroendocrine tumors in 35,825 cases in the United States. J Clin Oncol. 2008;26(18):3063–72. https://i.pinimg.com/564x/fb/e3/cf/fbe3c-f14435a6902156add0a7993480c.jpg.
2. Hemminki K, Li X. Incidence trends and risk factors of carcinoid tumors: a nationwide epidemiologic study from Sweden. Cancer. 2001;92:2204–10.
3. Maggard MA, O'Connell JB, Ko CY. Updated population based review of carcinoid tumors. Ann Surg. 2004;240:117–22.
4. Van Cutsem E, Sagaert X, Topal B, et al. Gastric cancer. Lancet. 2016;388(10060):2654–64.
5. Riihimäki M, Hemminki A, Sundquist K, et al. The epidemiology of metastases in neuroendocrine tumors. Int J Cancer. 2016;139(12):2679–86.
6. Lawrence B, Gustafsson BI, Chan A, et al. The epidemiology of gastroentero-pancreatic neuroendocrine tumors. Endocrinol Metab Clin North Am. 2011;40:1–18, vii.
7. Singh S, Asa SL, Dey C, et al. Diagnosis and management of gastrointestinal neuroendocrine tumors: an evidence-based Canadian consensus. Cancer Treat Rev. 2016;47:32–45.
8. Modlin IM, Lye KD, Kidd M. A 5-decade analysis of 13,715 carcinoid tumors. Cancer. 2003;97:934–59.
9. Bhosale P, Shah A, Wei W, et al. Carcinoid tumours: predicting the location of the primary neoplasm based on the sites of metastases. Eur Radiol. 2013;23:400–7.
10. Chambers AJ, Pasieka JL, Dixon E, et al. The palliative benefit of aggressive surgical intervention for both hepatic and mesenteric metastases from neuroendocrine tumors. Surgery. 2008;144:645–53.
11. de Mestier L, Neuzillet C, Hentic O, et al. Prolonged survival in a patient with neuroendocrine tumor of the cecum and diffuse peritoneal carcinomatosis. Case Rep Gastroenterol. 2012;6(1):205–10.
12. Modlin IM, Oberg K, Chung DC, et al. Gastroenteropancreatic neuroendocrine tumours. Lancet Oncol. 2008;9:61–72.
13. Vasseur B, Cadiot G, Zins M, et al. Peritoneal carcinomatosis in patients with digestive endocrine tumors. Cancer. 1996;78:1686–92.
14. Elias D, Sideris L, Liberale G, et al. Surgical treatment of peritoneal carcinomatosis from well-differentiated digestive endocrine carcinomas. Surgery. 2005;137:411–6.
15. ENETS Newsletter Summer 2017. Neuroendocrinology. 2017;105(3):333–40.
16. Kianmanesh R, et al. ENETS consensus guidelines for the management of peritoneal carcinomatosis from neuroendocrine tumors. Neuroendocrinology. 2010;91:333–40.
17. Canbay E, Yonemura Y. Molecular mechanism of peritoneal metastases. In: Peritoneal surface malignancies. A curative approach. Cham: Springer International Publishing; 2015. p. 81–103.
18. Levy A. Peritoneal circulation: In: Robin Smithuis intraperitoneal fluid circulation, radiology assistant. 2009. https://radiologyassistant.nl/img/containers/main/peritoneum-and-mesentery-part-i-anatomy/a5097979751c5b_Afbeelding-6.jpg/734f6469bb1435 46d9e83d74c5626b0f.jpg.
19. Sugarbaker PH. Observations concerning cancer spread within the peritoneal cavity and concepts supporting an ordered pathophysiology, peritoneal carcinomatosis: principles and management. Boston: Kluwer Academic Publishers; 1996. p. 79–100.
20. Yonemura Y, Nojima N, Kawamura T, editors. Principles of the treatment of peritoneal carcinomatosis. Peritoneal dissemination. Molecular mechanisms and the latest therapy. Kanazawa: Maeda Shoten; 1998.
21. Glockzin G, Schlitt HJ, Piso P. Peritoneal carcinomatosis: patients' selection, perioperative complications and quality of life related to cytoreductive surgery and hyperthermic intraperitoneal chemotherapy. World J Surg Oncol. 2009;7:5.
22. Ruiz-Tovar J, Alonso HN, Morales CV, et al. Peritoneal carcinomatosis secondary to carcinoid tumour. Clin Transl Oncol. 2007;9:804–5.
23. Sundin A, Arnold R, Baudin E, et al. ENETS consensus guidelines for the standards of care in neuroendocrine tumors: radiological, nuclear medicine & hybrid imaging. Neuroendocrinology. 2017;105(3):212–44.
24. Seshadri RA, Hemanth RE. Diagnostic laparoscopy in the pre-operative assessment of patients undergoing cytoreductive surgery and HIPEC for peritoneal surface malignancies. Indian J Surg Oncol. 2016;7(2):230–5.

25. Carboni F, Federici O, Giofrè M, et al. An 18-year experience in diagnostic laparoscopy of peritoneal carcinomatosis: results from 744 patients. J Gastrointest Surg. 020;24(9):2096–103. https://doi.org/10.1007/s11605-019-04368-w.

26. Giacopuzzi S, Guerini F, Zanoni A. Giovanni de Manzoni classification of intraperitoneal spread Angelo Di Giorgio, Enrico Pinto treatment of peritoneal surface malignancies; state of the art and perspectives. Italia: Springer; 2015. p. 53.

27. Sammartino P, Biacchi D, Cornali T, et al. Computerized system for staging peritoneal surface malignancies. Ann Surg Oncol. 2016;23:1454–60. https://www.ncbi.nlm.nih.gov/books/NBK541114/figure/article-27027.image.f1/.

28. Pavel M, Baudin E, Couvelard A, et al. ENETS consensus guidelines for the management of patients with liver and other distant metastases from neuroendocrine neoplasms of foregut, midgut, hindgut, and unknown primary. Neuroendocrinology. 2012;95:157–76.

29. Kahan S, Teppara N, Babkowski R, et al. Isolated peritoneal carcinomatosis from gastrointestinal tract carcinoid tumor: two case reports and a review of the literature. Gastrointest Cancer Res. 2013;6(1):27–30.

30. Graff-Baker AN, Sauer DA, Pommier SJ, et al. Expanded criteria for carcinoid liver debulking: maintaining survival and increasing the number of eligible patients. Surgery. 2014;156:1369–76.

31. Andréasson H, Graf W, Nygren P, et al. Outcome differences between debulking surgery and cytoreductive surgery in patients with Pseudomyxoma peritonei. Eur J Surg Oncol. 2012;38(10):962–8.

32. Boudreaux JP, Putty B, Frey DJ, et al. Surgical treatment of advanced-stage carcinoid tumors: lessons learned. Ann Surg. 2005;241:839–45.

33. Makridis C, Ekbom A, Bring J, et al. Survival and daily physical activity in patients treated for advanced midgut carcinoid tumors. Surgery. 1997;122:1075–82.

34. Hellman P, Lundstrom T, Ohrvall U, et al. Effect of surgery on the outcome of midgut carcinoid disease with lymph node and liver metastases. World J Surg. 2002;26:991–7.

35. Steinmueller T, Kianmanesh R, Falconi M, et al. Consensus guidelines for the management of patients with liver metastases from digestive (neuro)endocrine tumors: foregut, midgut, hindgut, and unknown primary. Neuroendocrinology. 2008;87:47–62.

36. Sugarbaker PH. Peritonectomy procedures. Cancer Treat Res. 2007;134:247–64.

37. Angelo Di Giorgio peritonectomy techniques. In: Di Giorgio A, Pinto E, editors. Treatment of peritoneal surface malignancies, updates in surgery. Italia: © Springer; 2015. https://doi.org/10.1007/978-88-470-5711-1_9.

38. Jacquet P, Sugarbaker PH. Clinical research methodologies in diagnosis and staging of patients with peritoneal carcinomatosis. Cancer Treat Res. 1996;82:359–74.

39. Sinukumar S, Rajan F, Mehta S, et al. A comparison of outcomes following total and selective peritonectomy performed at the time of interval cytoreductive surgery for advanced serous epithelial ovarian, fallopian tube and primary peritoneal cancer—a study by INDEPSO. Eur J Surg Oncol. 2021;47(1):75–81. https://doi.org/10.1016/j.ejso.2019.02.031. pii: S0748-7983(19)30304-X.

40. de Lima Vazquez V, Sugarbaker PH. Total anterior parietal peritonectomy. J Surg Oncol. 2003;83(4):261–3.

41. Kyriazanos I, Papageorgiou D, Zoulamoglou M, et al. Total extraperitoneal access for parietal peritonectomy for peritoneal surface malignancy: The 'cocoon' technique. Eur J of Obstetrics, Gynecol Reprod Biol. 2020;251:258–62.

42. Tanaka K, Inoue Y, Toiyama J. The role of cytoreduction for metastatic and recurrent colorectal cancer in the era of multidisciplinary treatments. J Clin Oncol. 2010;28:14091.

43. Sugarbaker P. Peritoneal carcinomatosis: principle of management. Boston: Kluwer Academic Publisher; 1996.

44. Elias D, Lasser P, Ducreux M, et al. Liver resection (and associated extrahepatic resections) for metastatic well-differentiated endocrine tumors: a 15-year single center prospective study. Surgery. 2003;133:375–82.

45. Elias D, David A, Sourrouille I, et al. Neuroendocrine carcinomas: optimal surgery of peritoneal metastases (and associated intra-abdominal metastases). Surgery. 2014;155:5–12.

46. Elias D, Goéré D, Dumont F, et al. Role of hyperthermic intraoperative peritoneal chemotherapy in the management of peritoneal metastases. Eur J Cancer. 2014;50(2):332–40.

47. De Mestier L, Lardiere-Deguelte S, Brixi H, et al. Updating the surgical management of peritoneal carcinomatosis in patients with neuroendocrine tumors. Neuroendocrinology. 2015;101(2):105–11.

48. Madani A, Thomassen I, van Gestel YRBM, et al. Peritoneal metastases from gastroenteropancreatic neuroendocrine tumors: incidence, risk factors and prognosis. Ann Surg Oncol. 2017;24(8):2199–205.

49. Goéré D, Passot G, Gelli M, et al. Complete cytoreductive surgery plus HIPEC for peritoneal metastases from unusual cancer sites of origin: results from a worldwide analysis issue of the Peritoneal Surface Oncology Group International (PSOGI). Int J Hyperth. 2017;33(5):520–7. https://doi.org/10.1080/02656736.2017.1301576.

50. Au JT, Levine J, Aytaman A, et al. Management of peritoneal metastasis from neuroendocrine tumors. J Surg Oncol. 2013;108(6):385–6.

51. Radomski M, Pai RK, Shuai Y, et al. Curative surgical resection as a component of multimodality therapy for peritoneal metastases from goblet cell carcinoids. Ann Surg Oncol. 2016;23(13):4338–43.

52. Kianmanesh R, Sauvanet A, Hentic O, et al. Two-step surgery for synchronous bilobar liver metastases from digestive endocrine tumors: a safe approach for radical resection. Ann Surg. 2008;247:659–65.

53. Swellengrebel HA, Zoetmulder FA, Smeenk RM, et al. Quantitative intra-operative assessment of peritoneal carcinomatosis—a comparison of three prognostic tools. Eur J Surg Oncol. 2009;35:1078–84.

54. Kortylewicz B. Immunotherapy. 2011;3(4):491–4.

Yttrium-90 SIRT in NET

20

Sander C. Ebbers, Arthur J. A. T. Braat, and Marnix G. E. H. Lam

20.1 Introduction

During the past two decades, selective internal radiotherapy (SIRT, i.e., radioembolization) is being increasingly applied in patients suffering from unresectable hepatic metastases of neuroendocrine tumors (NET). Essentially, SIRT consists of administering microscopic spheres into the arterial vasculature of the liver. These microspheres are preloaded with the radioactive isotope yttrium-90 (^{90}Y), which decays with a half-life of 64.1 h, accompanied by the emission of high energy β-rays, of which the most abundant β has an energy of 2.4 MeV [1]. Due to preferential arterial blood flow to the tumors, the microspheres accumulate mainly in the tumors. The therapeutic effect is achieved by causing irreparable damage to the DNA of tumor cells by the ionizing radiation.

Currently, there are two types of ^{90}Y-microspheres commercially available: resin microspheres (SIR-Spheres®, Sirtex Medical Limited) and glass microspheres (TheraSpheres®, Bio-compatibles UK Ltd) [2, 3]. There are some

Table 20.1 Differences between the two types of ^{90}Y-microspheres currently available on the market

	Resin-microspheres	Glass-microspheres
Mean diameter (range)	32 (20–60) microns	25 (20–30) microns
Specific activity	50 Bq/sphere	1250–2500 Bq/sphere
Number of microspheres per 3 GBq	40–80 million	1.2–5 million
Density	1.6 g/mL	3.3 g/mL

differences between the two types of microspheres. These are described in Table 20.1 [2, 3]. However, both types of microspheres have been frequently utilized in the treatment of hepatic metastases from NET in the past decade.

20.2 Patient Selection

20.2.1 Indication

As a locoregional therapy for NET, SIRT currently can be considered in patients without extrahepatic disease or with highly symptomatic, hormone-related manifestations in which the majority of the tumor mass is situated in the liver [4].Due to the lack of comparative trials, it is highly recommended to discuss the feasibility of SIRT in a multidisciplinary tumor board. Actual

S. C. Ebbers (✉) · A. J. A. T. Braat
M. G. E. H. Lam
Departments of Radiology and Nuclear Medicine,
University Medical Center Utrecht,
Utrecht, The Netherlands
e-mail: s.c.ebbers-2@umcutrecht.nl

© Springer Nature Switzerland AG 2021
G. S. Limouris (ed.), *Liver Intra-arterial PRRT with ^{111}In-Octreotide*,
https://doi.org/10.1007/978-3-030-70773-6_20

treatment with ^{90}Y-SIRT should be decided based on individual patient characteristics.

The general work-up for patients with NET should include clinical and biochemical assessment. In general, ^{90}Y-SIRT can be considered in patients who have an Eastern Cooperative Oncology Group (ECOG) Performance Status of ≤2. The most important contraindication for treatment with ^{90}Y-SIRT is a compromised liver function, i.e., bilirubin level >34.2 μmol/L (>2 mg/dL) and an international normalized ratio (INR) >1.5, furthermore, a glomerular filtration rate <35 mL/min, a leukocyte count of <2 × 10^9/L, and a platelet count <50 × 10^9/L. Biliodigestive anastomosis and a biliary stent are considered relative contraindications. A biliodigestive anastomosis or biliary stent may give a higher chance of posttreatment abscess formation due to retrograde colonization of the biliary tree by intestinal bacteria. Treatment under prophylactic antibiotics can be considered, which prevents liver abscess formation [5]. ^{90}Y-SIRT is contraindicated in patients with a short life expectancy (i.e., <3 months) or an active hepatitis [6].

20.2.2 Work-Up

At baseline, at least an arterial-phase contrast-enhanced CT (CECT) or MRI should be performed. Special attention should be paid to the vascular anatomy of the liver, as many anatomical variants exist. Feasibility of the treatment greatly depends on the recognition of aberrant vessels and the understanding of the arterial supply of the tumors. In a standard anatomical situation, the celiac trunk divides into three main arteries, i.e., the splenic artery, the left gastric artery, and the common hepatic artery (CHA). Distal to this trifurcation, the gastroduodenal artery (GDA) branches off from the CHA, which then continues into the liver as the proper hepatic artery (PHA). At the hilar plate, the proper hepatic artery splits into the right hepatic artery (RHA) and the left hepatic artery (LHA). Both the RHA and the LHA can also arise from other vessels, either in isolation or in addition to the

normally present RHA and LHA (Fig. 20.1). Missing these arteries could potentially result in incomplete coverage of the tumor. Identification of local non-hepatic feeding vessels (i.e., culprit vessels) is important, as complications are likely to arise after infusion of microspheres into these arteries, either accidentally or due to retrograde flow (i.e., reflux) of microspheres. The most important is the right gastric artery (RGA), which provides arterial supply to the minor curvature of the stomach and originates from the PHA (45–57%), the LHA (23%), the GDA (3–12%), or the CHA (2.7–5%) [7]. Additionally, by acquiring this information using a CECT or CT angiography, the duration of the angiography procedure can be shortened.

20.2.3 Pre-treatment Angiography and Imaging

Maximizing the absorbed radiation dose in the tumor while keeping the absorbed dose in healthy liver tissue within safe limits is the key to a successful ^{90}Y-SIRT procedure. Additionally, a lung shunt radiation absorbed dose of less than 30 Gy in a single session or a cumulative dose of less than 50 Gy in multiple sessions based on planar imaging should be achieved to avoid a radiation pneumonitis after treatment. Also, any extrahepatic depositions should be avoided at all times. In order to inject a high dose of ^{90}Y-microspheres safely, a pre-treatment angiography is performed. During this angiography, a small amount of radioactive technetium-99m-macroaggregated albumin (^{99m}Tc-MAA) is infused into the vasculature of the liver from the proposed injection position. Before injecting the ^{99m}Tc-MAA, any culprit vessels should be identified and coil-embolized. Then, the desired injection position should be determined, so that all tumors are targeted completely and any extrahepatic deposition is avoided. A final check of the proposed micro-catheter position with the use of a C-arm cone beam CT (CBCT) is preferred above digital subtraction angiography (DSA) alone (Fig. 20.2) [8]. On post-injection planar scintigraphy, the lung

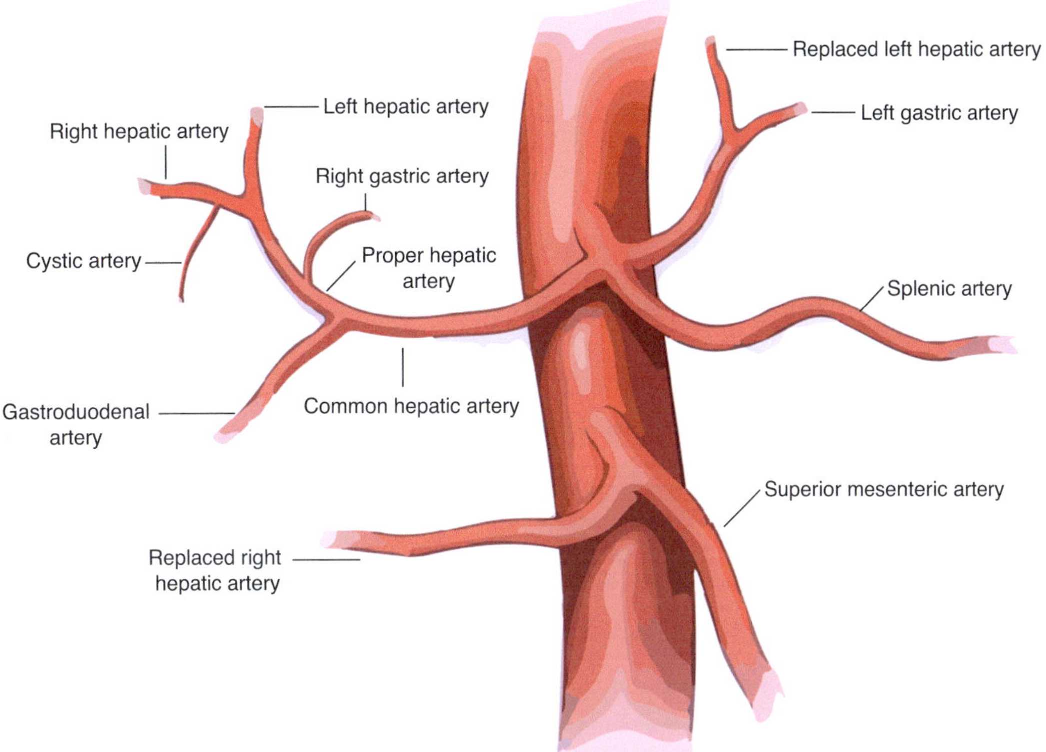

Fig. 20.1 Common anatomy of the arterial liver vasculature, showing the main branches of the celiac trunk, as well as the common origins of the replaced right and left hepatic arteries, if present

shunt fraction (LSF) can be measured. However, calculating the LSF on pre-treatment ^{99m}Tc-MAA planar imaging highly overestimates the true LSF of ^{99m}Tc-MAA, due to the absence of scatter and attenuation correction [9]. If a significant LSF is visualized on planar imaging, it is therefore preferable to quantify the lung absorbed dose on a ^{99m}Tc-MAA single-photon emission computed tomography (SPECT)/CT. However, this method also overestimates the predicted lung shunt of ^{90}Y-microspheres. This is due to the difference in particle size and behavior between the MAA particles and the microspheres. Additionally, any extrahepatic depositions of the ^{99m}Tc-MAA can be visualized using SPECT/CT, providing the interventional radiologist with the possibility to identify and coil-embolize any missed culprit vessels or modify the injection position. Finally, the ^{99m}Tc-MAA SPECT/CT provides an estimate for the predicted distribution of ^{90}Y-microspheres within the liver. An accurate assessment of the intrahepatic distribution of ^{90}Y-microspheres plays an important role in the dose calculation for the treatment session, as will be explained in the next section.

20.3 Treatment

20.3.1 Dose Calculation

After certainty has been obtained on adequate targeting of the liver metastases, and the absence of extrahepatic shunting, the treatment dose of ^{90}Y-microspheres can be ordered. When doing so, there are four different methods for calculating the desired activity for ^{90}Y-SIRT (Table 20.2). The empiric method only relies on the hepatic tumor load, without taking into consideration any other patient-related factors. Consequently, this has led to a large amount of toxicities and therefore its use is condemned [10].

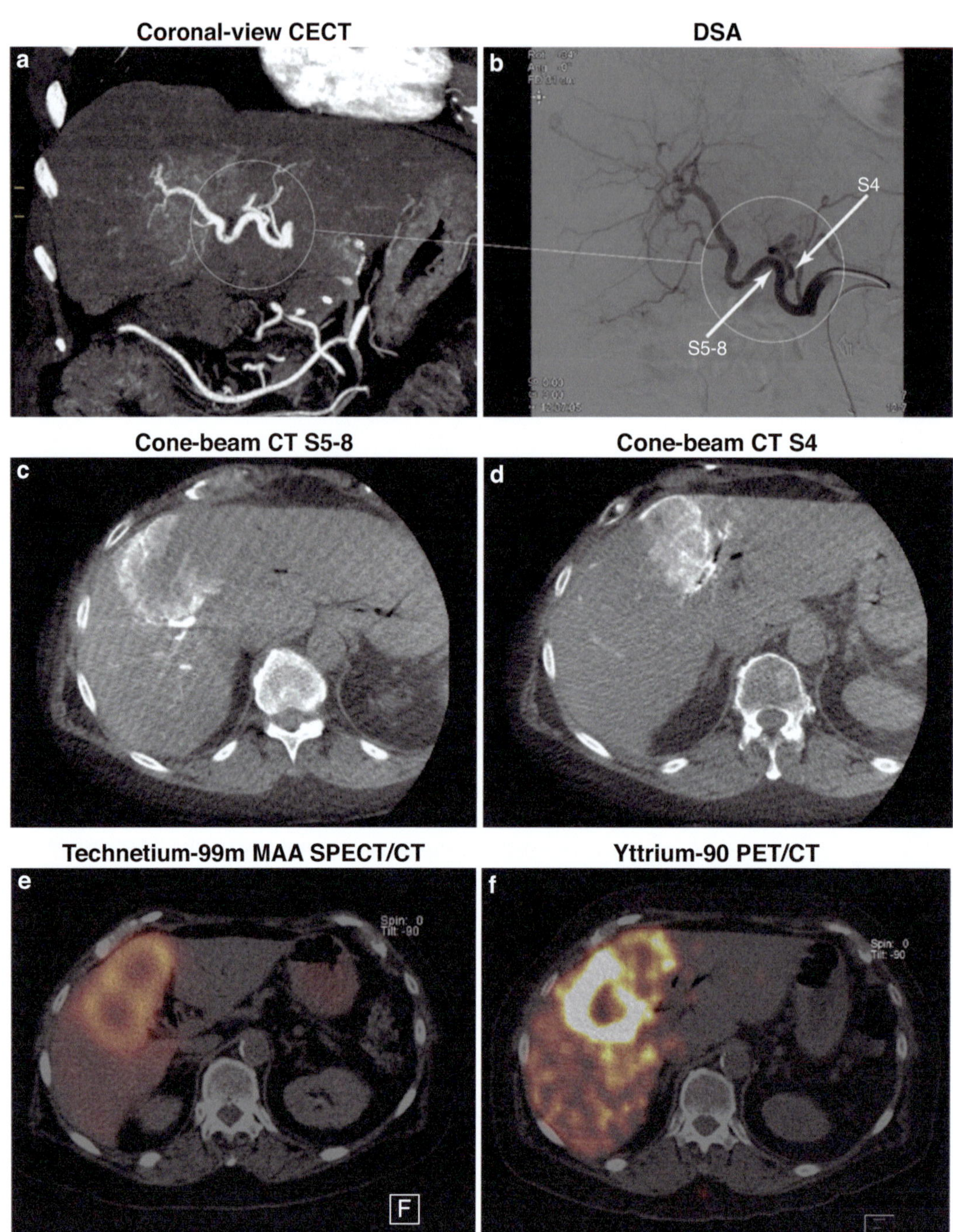

Fig. 20.2 Example of a radioembolization treatment with ⁹⁰Y glass microspheres in a 79-year-old woman with a grade 1 pancreatic NET in segment 4. Previously treated by primary tumor resection (pylorus preserving pancreaticoduodenectomy) and four cycles of ¹⁷⁷Lu-DOTATATE. (**a**) Pre-treatment contrast-enhanced CT showing normal arterial anatomy, (**b**) digital substraction angiography of the liver vasculature showing the two injection sites in the right hepatic artery (Couinaud segments 5–8) and the segment 4 artery, (**c, d**) cone beam CT after contrast injection from both injection sites, in which the complementary feeding of the tumor by both vessels can be acknowledged, resulting in a complete tumor coverage, (**e**) pre-treatment ⁹⁹ᵐTc-MAA SPECT/CT, (**f**) posttreatment ⁹⁰Y PET/CT

Table 20.2 Overview of the activity calculation methods used in ^{90}Y-SIRT

Method	Description
Empiric (not recommended)	Tumor load: $\leq$25%: 2.0 GBq 25–50%: 2.5 GBq $\geq$50%: 3.0 GBq
Body surface area (for resin-microspheres)	$A = \left(\text{BSA}-0.2\right) + \left(\dfrac{\text{tumor volume}}{\text{total liver volume}}\right)$
Partition model (should be preferred)	$A = \dfrac{D \times \left(\dfrac{T}{N} \times \text{mass}_{\text{tumor}} + \text{mass}_{\text{Liver}}\right)}{49.670 \times \left(1 - \text{LSF}\right)}$ where $\dfrac{T}{N} = \dfrac{A_{\text{tumor}} / \text{mass}_{\text{tumor}}}{A_{\text{healthy}} / \text{mass}_{\text{healthy}}}$
Glass-microspheres	$A = \dfrac{D \times \text{mass}_{\text{liver}}}{50 \times \left(1-\text{LSF}\right)}$

The most frequently used method for resin microspheres is the body surface area (BSA) method, due to its simplicity [11]. However, this method has many disadvantages. As with the empiric method, the size of the liver tissue is not taken into account. Additionally, the differential biodistribution of the microspheres in tumor and non-tumor tissue is not a factor in this calculation method. As tumors can be hypo- or hypervascular, this could lead to over- and undertreatment, respectively. In NET this is especially important, as these tumors are often hypervascular. This factor can be taken into account by using the pre-treatment ^{99m}Tc-MAA SPECT/CT. Based on the ^{99m}Tc-MAA SPECT/CT, a tumor-to-normal (T/N) absorbed dose ratio can be calculated, by drawing VOIs around the tumor and the healthy liver tissue. This method is implemented in the partition model, which is the third dose calculation method. For glass microspheres, the manufacturer proposed a specific dose calculation method, based on the desired dose in Gy for the entire targeted treatment volume. This method does not take the T/N ratio into account, therefore assuming a homogeneous distribution of ^{90}Y-microspheres. However, the partition model is now considered feasible for both resin and glass microspheres.

If multiple injection positions are used during treatment, the total treatment dose can be split according to the target volume per injection position. It is advocated to use multiple injection positions rather than one total-liver injection position, to avoid preferential flow of microspheres to one of the liver lobes (e.g., over treating one lobe, while under treating the other lobe) and avoid the risk of unexpected extrahepatic depositions.

20.3.2 Treatment Angiography

In a second angiography session, the prescribed dose of ^{90}Y-microspheres is injected from the exact same injection position(s) as during pre-treatment angiography, to avoid differences in intrahepatic distribution [12]. For both glass and resin microspheres, the manufacturer provides a dedicated administration set for the purpose of achieving a complete infusion of the microspheres, as well as shielding the nuclear medicine physician and the interventional radiologist from the high-energy radiation.

Due to the low specific activity of resin microspheres, the number of microspheres injected per treatment is much higher compared to glass microspheres. This may cause reflux or stasis of flow to happen more frequently during injection of resin microspheres. Injection of microspheres using a 5% glucose solution proves to be reducing stasis from occurring significantly [13]. Additionally, patients report less pain during the infusion. Abdominal pain during infusion is thought to be caused by the embolic effect of resin microspheres, even though this phenomenon rarely occurs in NET (<2%) [11]. Because the specific activity of glass microspheres is much higher, the embolic effect is less significant and post-embolization syndrome rarely occurs in general.

20.3.3 Posttreatment Imaging

Analyzing the distribution of ^{90}Y-microspheres after administration is paramount, as the predicted MAA distribution can differ from actual microsphere distribution [12]. Additionally, attention should be paid to the unexpected deposition of microspheres in the lungs or abdominal organs. Besides the high-energy β-radiation, ^{90}Y also emits a positron in one in every 31×10^3 decays [14]. With the use of modern time-of-flight PET/CT systems, it is feasible to image the ^{90}Y-distribution in the liver posttreatment. Furthermore, quantitative PET/CT images can be used for accurate dosimetry and dose-response calculations [15]. Alternatively, since ^{90}Y does not emit any γ-radiation on its own, bremsstrahlung SPECT/CT can be used to visualize the intra- and extrahepatic deposition of ^{90}Y-microspheres. However, bremsstrahlung SPECT/CT images are limited in resolution and are blurry.

20.4 Efficacy and Safety

20.4.1 Clinical Outcome

In the period shortly after ^{90}Y-SIRT, patients usually tolerate the treatment very well. In some cases, fatigue, nausea, or abdominal pain is reported by the patient. These side effects occur in approximately 56% of treated patients within the first 3 months after radioembolization [11]. Almost all symptoms resolve in the 6 months after treatment. Other complications occur in less than 4% of patients. Known complications that should be anticipated are radioembolization-induced liver disease (REILD), radiation-induced gastric or duodenal ulcer/gastritis, and liver abscess. During angiography, complications such as an arterial dissection, pain, and reflux should be anticipated, as well as NET-specific complications, such as a carcinoid crisis, caused by a sudden release of serotonin by the tumor. Even though these complications are rare, they can have a considerable effect on the patient's quality of life.

Multiple studies have shown that ^{90}Y-SIRT is safe and effective in reducing symptoms and establishing disease control in patients with progressive NET [11, 16, 17]. An example case is given in Fig. 20.3. In a meta-analysis, disease control was established in approximately 86% of patients (range 62–100%), while objective response to treatment was seen in 50% (range 12–80%) [17]. The meta-analysis however included predominantly smaller retrospective studies, with a very high between-study heterogeneity. In the meta-analysis, the percentage of pancreatic NET seemed to be associated with a lower objective response rate. Furthermore, the median overall survival after ^{90}Y-SIRT reported was 28½ months (range 14–70). In a large multicenter retrospective study, 244 patients were analyzed after having received ^{90}Y-SIRT [11]. A disease control rate of more than 90% was observed after 3–6 months, while the best objective response rate was 28.5%. The study also showed that a delayed treatment response can be seen in some patients, so that it may be beneficial to evaluate treatment at a later time point than at 3 months. Response rates were independent of the grading of the tumor. The median overall survival was 31 months (range 51 days–12 years) and was significantly dependent on tumor grading, intrahepatic tumor load, and the presence of extrahepatic disease. Finally, the study showed that after ^{90}Y-SIRT, 44% of patients had improvement and 35% of patients had complete resolution of tumor-related symptoms.

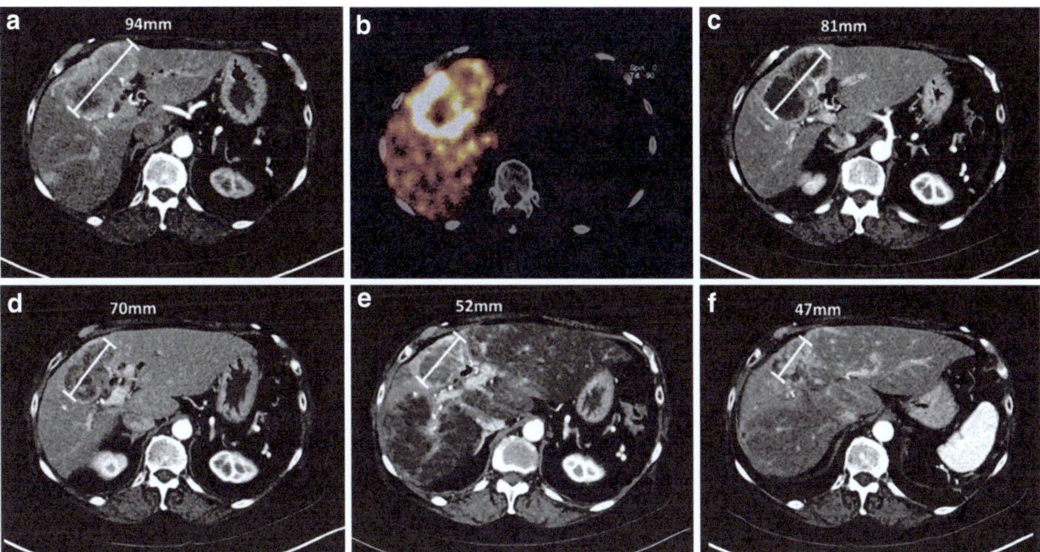

Fig. 20.3 Enduring partial response after a single ⁹⁰Y-SIRT session of the right liver lobe, in the same patient as illustrated in Fig. 20.2. (a) Baseline contrast-enhanced CT, (b) post-treatment ⁹⁰Y-PET/CT showing adequate targeting of the tumor, (c–f) contrast-enhanced CT scans at 3, 6, 9, and 13 months posttreatment, respectively, showing complete tumor necrosis at 3 months (c), and tumor necrosis resorption and size reduction in the months thereafter (d–f)

The mentioned response rates compare well to other embolic therapies, such as transarterial chemoembolization (TACE) or bland embolization (TAE) [18]. Side effects occur less frequent after ⁹⁰Y-SIRT, most likely due to the lesser embolic effect of the ⁹⁰Y-microspheres [16].

20.4.2 Future Perspectives

Unfortunately, at this moment there have been no comparative trials on the efficacy of ⁹⁰Y-SIRT in NET. This makes comparison with other treatment modalities difficult. Also, selecting patients for treatment with ⁹⁰Y-SIRT is still very much opinion-based, as it is not clear which patients benefit from ⁹⁰Y-SIRT the most. Because of the hypervascular nature of most NETs, and the likely presence of liver metastases, many patients seem to be good candidates to undergo ⁹⁰Y-SIRT.

However, some issues still need to be addressed, in order to improve outcome and reduce toxicity. There has been debate about the best timing to perform ⁹⁰Y-SIRT in NET patients, to achieve maximum treatment effect without any significant adverse effects. Currently, because of the limited evidence, ⁹⁰Y-SIRT is usually performed in the salvage setting. However, in selected patients it may be of added benefit to perform ⁹⁰Y-SIRT at an earlier stage of disease progression. For example, in patients with liver-only disease, it has been advocated as a bridge to surgery or liver transplantation [19, 20]. In addition to sole ⁹⁰Y-SIRT, the treatment can also be combined with systemic therapies. In a cohort of 19 grade II NET patients, ⁹⁰Y-SIRT was combined with capecitabine-temozolomide (CapTem) [21]. An objective response rate of 74% was objectified after liver-specific assessment, including three cases with complete response. Concerning overall response assessment, an objective response rate of 55% was seen in 11 patients who also had extrahepatic disease. Toxicity of combining both therapies in this cohort was equivalent to what could be expected from each therapy alone. Another treatment frequently utilized in patients with grade I and II NET, peptide receptor radionuclide therapy (PRRT) using the radiopharmaceutical ¹⁷⁷Lu-DOTATATE, has proved to be highly effective in prolonging progression-free survival [22].

Sequential treatment with PRRT and ^{90}Y-SIRT does not yield any significant added toxicity [23]. In theory, ^{90}Y-SIRT can also be used to boost outcome after PRRT, as has already been shown for holmium-166 radioembolization after PRRT in the HEPAR PLUS study [24].

A lot of research is currently being done to improve patient-specific dosimetry. As pointed out earlier, the key to boosting patient outcome while tempering the incidence of irreversible toxicity is obtaining an excellent tumor targeting during ^{90}Y-SIRT. This means that a high radiation absorbed dose should be achieved in the tumors while keeping healthy liver tissue doses at a minimum. For example, further improvements can be made in therapy planning [25]. Currently, pre-treatment angiography using ^{99m}Tc-MAA poorly predicts the microsphere distribution after ^{90}Y-SIRT [12]. Furthermore, the activity calculation methods prior to treatment, most frequently used by treatment centers today, still utilize a one-compartment model, as shown previously. Pre-treatment dosimetry based on predicted microsphere distribution should eventually lead to a more personalized dosimetry-based treatment planning. These new methods should also be validated in large prospective comparative studies.

In conclusion, ^{90}Y-SIRT is already widely and successfully deployed in the treatment of hepatic NET. Not only in patients with liver-only disease but also in patients with extrahepatic disease, ^{90}Y-SIRT should be considered to prolong patient survival while maintaining quality of life.

References

1. Selwyn RG, Nickles RJ, Thomadsen BR, et al. A new internal pair production branching ratio of 90Y: the development of a non-destructive assay for 90Y and 90Sr. Appl Radiat Isot. 2007;65(3):318–27. https://doi.org/10.1016/j.apradiso.2006.08.009.
2. Biocompatibles UK Ltd. Package Insert—TheraSphere® Yttrium-90 Glass Microspheres—Rev. 14.; 2014. https://www.btg-im.com/BTG/media/TheraSphere-Documents/PDF/TheraSphere-Package-Insert_USA_Rev-14.pdf. Accessed 26 Oct 2017.
3. Sirtex Medical Limited. Package Insert—SIR-Spheres ® Y-90 Resin Microspheres (Yttrium-90 Microspheres); 2017. https://www.sirtex.com/media/155126/ssl-us-13.pdf. Accessed 26 Oct 2017.
4. Pavel M, O'Toole D, Costa F, et al. ENETS consensus guidelines update for the management of distant metastatic disease of intestinal, pancreatic, bronchial neuroendocrine neoplasms (NEN) and NEN of unknown primary site. Neuroendocrinology. 2016;103(2):172–85. https://doi.org/10.1159/000443167.
5. Cholapranee A, van Houten D, Deitrick G, et al. Risk of liver abscess formation in patients with prior biliary intervention following yttrium-90 radioembolization. Cardiovasc Intervent Radiol. 2015;38(2):397–400. https://doi.org/10.1007/s00270-014-0947-5.
6. Braat AJAT, Smits MLJ, Braat MNGJA, et al. Y Hepatic radioembolization: an update on current practice and recent developments. J Nucl Med. 2015;56(7):1079–87. https://doi.org/10.2967/jnumed.115.157446.
7. Vesselle G, Petit I, Boucebci S, et al. Radioembolization with yttrium-90 microspheres work up: practical approach and literature review. Diagn Interv Imaging. 2015;96(6):547–62. https://doi.org/10.1016/j.diii.2014.03.014.
8. Louie JD, Kothary N, Kuo WT, et al. Incorporating cone-beam CT into the treatment planning for yttrium-90 radioembolization. J Vasc Interv Radiol. 2009;20(5):606–13. https://doi.org/10.1016/j.jvir.2009.01.021.
9. Elschot M, Nijsen JFW, Lam MGEH, et al. 99mTc-MAA overestimates the absorbed dose to the lungs in radioembolization: a quantitative evaluation in patients treated with 166Ho-microspheres. Eur J Nucl Med Mol Imaging. 2014;41(10):1965–75. https://doi.org/10.1007/s00259-014-2784-9.
10. Kennedy A, Nag S, Salem R, et al. Recommendations for radioembolization of hepatic malignancies using yttrium-90 microsphere brachytherapy: a consensus panel report from the radioembolization brachytherapy oncology consortium. Int J Radiat Oncol. 2007;68(1):13–23. https://doi.org/10.1016/j.ijrobp.2006.11.060.
11. Braat AJAT, Kappadath SC, Ahmadzadehfar H, et al. Radioembolization with 90Y resin microspheres of neuroendocrine liver metastases: international multicenter study on efficacy and toxicity. Cardiovasc Intervent Radiol. 2019;42(3):413–25. https://doi.org/10.1007/s00270-018-2148-0.
12. Wondergem M, Smits MLJ, Elschot M, et al. 99mTc-macroaggregated albumin poorly predicts the intrahepatic distribution of 90Y resin microspheres in hepatic radioembolization. J Nucl Med. 2013;54(8):1294–301. https://doi.org/10.2967/jnumed.112.117614.
13. Ahmadzadehfar H, Meyer C, Pieper CC, et al. Evaluation of the delivered activity of yttrium-90 resin microspheres using sterile water and 5 % glucose during administration. EJNMMI Res. 2015;5(1):54. https://doi.org/10.1186/s13550-015-0133-z.

14. Gates VL, Esmail AAH, Marshall K, et al. Internal pair production of 90Y permits hepatic localization of microspheres using routine PET: proof of concept. J Nucl Med. 2011;52(1):72–6. https://doi.org/10.2967/jnumed.110.080986.
15. Elschot M, Vermolen BJ, Lam MGEH, et al. Quantitative comparison of PET and Bremsstrahlung SPECT for imaging the in vivo yttrium-90 microsphere distribution after liver radioembolization. Villa E, ed. PLoS One. 2013;8(2):e55742. https://doi.org/10.1371/journal.pone.0055742.
16. Jia Z, Wang W. Yttrium-90 radioembolization for unresectable metastatic neuro-endocrine liver tumor: a systematic review. Eur J Radiol. 2018;100:23–9. https://doi.org/10.1016/j.ejrad.2018.01.012.
17. Devcic Z, Rosenberg J, Braat AJA, et al. The efficacy of hepatic 90 Y resin radioembolization for metastatic neuroendocrine tumors: a meta-analysis. J Nucl Med. 2014;55:1404–10. https://doi.org/10.2967/jnumed.113.135855.
18. Do Minh D, Chapiro J, Gorodetski B, et al. Intra-arterial therapy of neuro-endocrine tumour liver metastases: comparing conventional TACE, drug-eluting beads TACE and yttrium-90 radioembolisation as treatment options using a pro-pensity score analysis model. Eur Radiol. 2017;27(12):4995–5005. https://doi.org/10.1007/s00330-017-4856-2.
19. Braat MNGJA, Samim M, van den Bosch MAAJ, et al. The role of 90Y-radioembolization in downstaging primary and secondary hepatic malignancies: a systematic review. Clin Transl Imaging. 2016;4(4):283–95. https://doi.org/10.1007/s40336-016-0172-0.
20. Mafeld S, Littler P, Hayhurst H, et al. Liver resection after selective internal radiation therapy with yttrium-90: safety and outcomes. J Gastrointest Cancer. 2020;51(1):152–8. https://doi.org/10.1007/s12029-019-00221-0.
21. Soulen MC, van Houten D, Teitelbaum UR, et al. Safety and feasibility of integrating yttrium-90 radio-embolization with capecitabine-temozolomide for grade 2 liver-dominant metastatic neuroendocrine tumors. Pancreas. 2018;47(8):980–4. https://doi.org/10.1097/MPA.0000000000001115.
22. Strosberg J, El-Haddad G, Wolin E, et al. Phase 3 trial of 177 Lu-dotatate for midgut neuroendocrine tumors. N Engl J Med. 2017;376(2):125–35. https://doi.org/10.1056/NEJMoa1607427.
23. Ezziddin S, Meyer C, Kahancova S, et al. 90Y radioembolization after radiation exposure from peptide receptor radionuclide therapy. J Nucl Med. 2012;53(11):1663–9. https://doi.org/10.2967/jnumed.112.107482.
24. Braat AJAT, Kwekkeboom DJ, Kam BLR, et al. Additional hepatic 166Ho-radio-embolization in patients with neuroendocrine tumours treated with 177Lu-DOTATATE; a single center, interventional, non-randomized, non-comparative, open label, phase II study (HEPAR PLUS trial). BMC Gastroenterol. 2018;18(1):84. https://doi.org/10.1186/s12876-018-0817-8.
25. Smits MLJ, Dassen MG, Prince JF, et al. The superior predictive value of 166Ho-scout compared with 99mTc-macroaggregated albumin prior to 166Ho-micro-spheres radioembolization in patients with liver metastases. Eur J Nucl Med Mol Imaging. 2020;47(4):798–806. https://doi.org/10.1007/s00259-019-04460-y.

Holmium-166 Radioembolization in NET Patients

Martina Stella, Arthur J. A. T. Braat,
and Marnix G. E. H. Lam

Abbreviations

[166]Er	166-Erbium
[166]Ho	166-Holmium
[177]Lu	177-Lutetium
[90]Y	90-Yttrium
[99m]Tc	99-Metastable-Technetium
CECT	Contrast-enhanced computed tomography
CT	Computed tomography
DSA	Digital subtraction angiography
MAA	Macroaggregated albumin
NET	Neuroendocrine tumor
PET	Positron emission tomography
RECIST	Response evaluation criteria in solid tumors
SIRT	Selective internal radiation therapy
SPECT	Single-photon emission computed tomography

21.1 Introduction

The term radioembolization (or selective internal radiation therapy, SIRT) defines a treatment procedure used for chemoresistant and/or unresect-able primary or secondary liver tumors. Radioactive microspheres are injected via a microcatheter into the hepatic artery. Through the bloodstream, they will preferentially lodge in small arterioles that feed tumor, irradiating it. The treatment relies on the fact that blood supply to the tumors is mainly provided by the hepatic arterial vasculature (~90%), while the portal vein feeds the normal liver parenchyma [1].

Until a few years ago, yttrium-90 (^{90}Y) was the only radionuclide used for this procedure, with two types of microspheres commercially available: SIR-Spheres® (Sirtex Medical Ltd, Woburn, MA, United States) and TheraSpheres® (Boston Scientific, Marlborough, MA, United States). These two devices, both loaded with ^{90}Y, differ with respect to the matrix in which the radionuclide is embedded, microsphere diameter and density, activity per microsphere (i.e., specific activity), and number of microspheres per GBq unit (Table 21.1). Recently, a third device, QuiremSpheres® (Quirem Medical BV, Deventer, The Netherlands), became commercially available and can be used as an alternative to ^{90}Y, from which it differs by multiple features, summarized in Table 21.1. The main characteristic of QuiremSpheres® is that they are loaded with holmium-166 (^{166}Ho), an isotope of ^{165}Ho, which is partially activated to ^{166}Ho by neutron activation in a nuclear reactor. The radioactive isotope ^{166}Ho has a half-life of 26.8 h, much shorter than ^{90}Y, and decays by β^- emission to stable erbium-166 (^{166}Er). The most probable transition is the

M. Stella · A. J. A. T. Braat · M. G. E. H. Lam (✉)
Departments of Radiology and Nuclear Medicine,
University Medical Center Utrecht,
Utrecht, The Netherlands
e-mail: M.Lam@umcutrecht.nl

© Springer Nature Switzerland AG 2021
G. S. Limouris (ed.), *Liver Intra-arterial PRRT with ^{111}In-Octreotide*,
https://doi.org/10.1007/978-3-030-70773-6_21

Table 21.1 Microsphere characteristics. Comparison between SIR-Spheres®, TheraSpheres®, and QuiremSpheres®

	SIR-Spheres®	TheraSpheres®	QuiremSpheres®
Matrix	Resin	Glass	Poly-L-lactic acid
Diameter (mean, range)	32μm (20–60μm)	25μm (20–30μm)	30μm (25–35μm)
Density	1.6 g/mL	3.3 g/mL	1.4 g/mL
Isotope	^{90}Y	^{90}Y	^{166}Ho
β-energy mean/max	0.9/2.28 MeV	0.9/2.28 MeV	0.7/1.81 MeV
β penetration mean/max	2.5/11 mm	2.5/11 mm	2.5/8 mm
γ-energy mean/max	–	–	81 keV (6.7%)
Half-life	64.1 h	64.1 h	26.8 h
Number of microspheres for 3 GBq	40–80 million	1.2–5 million	7.5–15[a] million
Activity per microsphere	50 Bq	1250–2500 Bq	200–400 Bq
Imaging technique	• Bremsstrahlung SPECT • PET	• Bremsstrahlung SPECT • PET	• SPECT • MRI
Surrogate/scout	^{99m}Tc-MAA	^{99m}Tc-MAA	• QuiremScout® • ^{99m}Tc-MAA

[a]For a typical treatment, the amount of microspheres will be in the range of 15–25 million due to higher administered activity (see different ^{166}Ho half-time compared to ^{90}Y)

1.77 MeV β emission with a 49.9% probability (highest endpoint energy: 1.85 MeV β⁻ emission, 48.8% probability). β⁻ emission of 1.85 MeV is followed by a γ emission at 81 keV (6.56% probability) that can be imaged with single-photon emission computed tomography (SPECT). The isotope ^{166}Ho, together with its decay product ^{166}Er, is a paramagnetic metal, also known as lanthanides, and thus can be visualized using magnetic resonance imaging (MRI). In addition, ^{166}Ho microspheres density, equal to 1.4 g/cm^3, is comparable to the density of blood, and this could be beneficial for their intravascular flow dynamics and thus their biodistribution.

21.2 Clinical Workflow

Patient selection for ^{166}Ho radioembolization treatment is similar to ^{90}Y eligibility criteria (see chapter *Yttrium-90 SIRT in NET*). When eligible for ^{166}Ho radioembolization, a patient undergoes a procedure that encompasses three phases that can be summarized as follows:

- Pre-treatment evaluation/planning
- Treatment
- Treatment evaluation and follow-up

21.2.1 Pre-treatment Evaluation/Planning

During the pre-treatment phase, a scout procedure is performed. It consists of the injection of a small batch of ^{166}Ho microspheres (~250 MBq), the same particles used for treatment, to assess intrahepatic distribution and to exclude any extrahepatic shunting. These scout microspheres, called QuiremScout® (CE mark since 2019), have the advantage of sharing the same biophysical characteristics of microspheres used for treatment and thus are expected to better mimic the treatment while being clinically safe [2, 3]. In their study [2], Braat et al. showed that ^{166}Ho scout is a safe clinical alternative to ^{99m}Tc-MAA for radioembolization work-up. No adverse events related to the use of ^{166}Ho scout were recorded, while the maximum extrahepatic deposition related to ^{166}Ho scout dose was 14 Gy (below the limit suggested by a previous study [4, 5]). The theoretical assumption on superior predictive value of ^{166}Ho scout was confirmed, both qualitatively and quantitatively [3]. Based on a qualitative analysis, Smits et al. found ^{166}Ho scout to be superior to ^{99m}Tc-MAA (median score 4 vs. 2.5, $p < 0.001$). Quantitative analysis endorsed these results, confirming the superior predictive value of ^{166}Ho for intrahepatic distribution in comparison with ^{99m}Tc-MAA. ^{166}Ho presents narrower 95% limits of agreement compared to ^{99m}Tc-MAA with respect to both lesion and normal liver absorbed dose. In addition, since only 60 mg of QuiremScout® is injected, corresponding to approximately three million particles, with ^{166}Ho scout, the embolization effect is limited. Concurrently, both a digital subtraction angiography (DSA) and a cone beam CT image are performed, to verify catheter position, to assess liver perfused volume, and to verify complete targeting. After the ^{166}Ho scout injection, a SPECT/CT is acquired, which allows for the assessment of ^{166}Ho biodistribution. After the assessment of potential inadvertent extrahepatic activity and the assessment of intrahepatic distribution, the need for (additional) coiling, more appropriate injection positions, or different catheter (e.g., antireflux) can be evaluated by the treatment team. ^{166}Ho microspheres scout is a valuable alternative to ^{99m}Tc-macroaggregated albumin (^{99m}Tc-MAA), used as a surrogate for ^{166}Ho (or ^{90}Y). ^{99m}Tc-MAA has been demonstrated to be a poor predictor for both treatment activity distribution and lung shunt [3, 6]. ^{99m}Tc-MAA particles indeed represent a different size and morphology with respect to ^{166}Ho (and ^{90}Y) microspheres. They are randomly shaped (asymmetrical protein clumps), and because of the broad range in particle size (10–90μm), as a result of particle size reduction over time by erosion and fragmentation (<20μm) [7], they are prone to physiological arteriovenous shunting. On the contrary, ^{166}Ho-microsphere size is consistent and unaffected by erosion and fragmentation, which allows for a more proper treatment prediction (see Fig. 21.1).

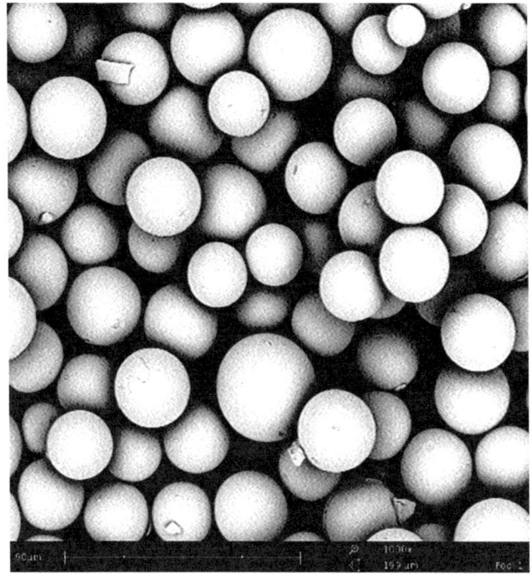

Fig. 21.1 Scanning electron microscope image of holmium microspheres. Content licensed under a Creative Common Attribution 2.0 Generic License. Publisher: Springer Nature. Content attributed to M. L. Smits et al., "Holmium-166 radioembolization for the treatment of patients with liver metastases: design of the phase I HEPAR trial," J. Exp. Clin. Cancer Res., vol. 29, no. 1, p. 70, Jun. 2010

After the scout procedure, the prescribed activity for radioembolization is currently calculated based on the Medical Internal Radiation Dose (MIRD) model, which assumes a homogenous microspheres distribution (even though it is known to be an oversimplification). The target whole-liver average absorbed dose is recommended to be equal to 60 Gy, based on the results of the initial dose-escalation study for ^{166}Ho radioembolization [8].The amount of activity for the treatment can be easily calculated according to the following formula:

$$A_{Ho166}\left[\text{MBq}\right] = 3781\left[\frac{\text{MBq}}{\text{kg}}\right] * \text{Liver Target Volume Weight}\left[\text{kg}\right]$$

Liver target volume weight is computed based on the target volume delineated on the pretreatment CECT/MRI or cone beam CT multiplied by the liver density [9] (1.06 g/cm^3).

21.2.2 Treatment and Follow-Up

Following the scout procedure, the radioembolization therapy is performed. The interventional radiologist, in the angiography room, places the catheters in the same position as they were placed for the scout procedure. The correct and identical positioning for the administration is paramount and needs to be verified using DSA [10]. Subsequently the ^{166}Ho microsphere prescribed activity is administered.

Once the therapeutic activity has decayed to a value below the saturation point of the gamma camera used for post-treatment imaging (i.e., 2–4 days after treatment, depending on administered activity), a SPECT/CT is acquired to verify the ^{166}Ho distribution and check for adequate targeting of the tumor lesions. Every few months, as per the institution's follow-up protocol, contrast-enhanced CT (CECT) is performed to assess the outcome of the radioembolization procedure. The maximum tumor reductive effect attained differs per tumor type and tumor biology. In a multicenter retrospective study in neuroendocrine neoplasms, most patients achieve the best imaging response after 3 months. However, in 20–26% of patients, the objective response is even better after 6 months. Periodic follow-up imaging every 3 months during the first year following radioembolization is advised [11].

21.3 Radiation Safety

As for any procedure that involves the use of radioactive material, the radiation exposure for personnel should be reduced as much as possible based on the ALARA (As-Low-As-Reasonably-Achievable) principal. During treatment, measurements indicated that the additional radiation exposure to staff caused by the ^{166}Ho microspheres procedure is negligible compared to the scattered X-rays from the X-ray tube prior and throughout the procedure [12]. Similar to ^{90}Y procedures, precautionary measures, such as the use of a new microcatheter for each injection position and a fluid-absorbing drape, should be considered in order to prevent radioactive contamination. Regulation concerning treatment administration and the release of the angiography suite after a ^{166}Ho treatment vary between centers and countries. Unforeseen ^{166}Ho radioactive con-

taminations may be more easily detected than ^{90}Y microspheres, because of the primary gamma photon emitted by ^{166}Ho. Finally, depending on the amount of administered therapeutic activity and the timing of release, patients can be released after treatment with minimal contact restrictions (2 days), based on reduction of radiation by distance and time and in consensus with the instructions by the Nuclear Regulatory Commission for patients with permanent implants [13].

21.4 Imaging

The most innovative feature of ^{166}Ho microspheres is their imaging potential. Because of 81 keV γ emission, a SPECT(/CT) can be used to visualize the microspheres within the patient. When using ^{166}Ho microspheres for both scout and treatment, the imaging modality is identical for both pre- and post-treatment assessment, making comparison a lot easier (compared to ^{99m}Tc-MAA SPECT and ^{90}Y-PET or Bremsstrahlung SPECT). Photons interacting with the patient and the detector cause some image-degrading effects. To cope with this issue, proper collimator selection (medium energy or high energy recommended) and reconstruction parameters to improve image quality and reduce scatter are required. Additional image-degrading effects are caused by patient breathing [14], which could be improved by adding breath gating to the SPECT/CT acquisition. However, on commercially available SPECT/CT systems, this is currently not available.

It is advised to correct for the downscatter using a double energy window approach, as an addition to the main ^{166}Ho photopeak window (centered at 81 keV) [15]. The imaging reconstruction model with iterative methods (e.g., 3D OSEM), already present in the clinical imaging system, leads to sufficient resolution and quality of the reconstructed images. When a quantitative reconstruction is required, more advanced reconstruction methods like the Monte Carlo simulation can be considered. This model simultaneously compensates for attenuation, scatter, and collimator-detector response and therefore improves quantification. Nonetheless, a quantitative approach using clinical images reconstructed with both attenuation and scatter correction has been assessed, giving promising results.

Because of the relatively short [166]Ho half-life (26.8 h), SPECT images have to be acquired within 6 days after administration, as otherwise the number of gamma photons is limited. However, an upper limit for the activity, depending on the SPECT system, is also present. Above a certain activity value, detector dead time will saturate, playing a negative role in imaging quality [16]. This issue can be taken into account with a proper calibration of the system [22].

SPECT may also be used after administration of ^{90}Y microspheres; Bremsstrahlung photons can be captured by SPECT as well, but due to the broad spectrum of energies released by the ^{90}Y photons and relatively low yield, acquisition quality is limited and often results in blurred images, which makes quantitative imaging more challenging. To allow for a quantitative approach, ^{90}Y PET imaging has emerged as a new image modality. Unfortunately, the low true coincidence rate has a major drawback, which leads to noisy images, long scan times, and background noise from scintillator decay.

Since [166]Ho and [166]Er are both lanthanide elements, they can be imaged with MRI. Indeed, this technique utilizes the paramagnetic nature of the microspheres rather than the radioactivity. This imaging modality has higher in plane resolution and can easily be combined with anatomical scans without the burden of breathing motion. Since a linear relationship between T2* times and holmium concentration was proven [17], this visualization method presents many new possibilities, as it has been shown in a study conducted by van de Maat et al. [18]. This could be an alternative to scintigraphy and an advantage in comparison to ^{90}Y imaging. MRI data could provide a quantitative measure of the intrahepatic microsphere biodistribution, thereby enabling radiation absorbed dose estimation on a tumor level. Thus, combination of magnetic resonance imaging and [166]Ho radioembolization has the potential to increase safety and efficacy of radioembolization and paves the way to image-guided therapy.

21.5 [166]Ho Radioembolization for Neuroendocrine Tumors

Neuroendocrine tumor (NET) patients often have metastases in the liver. Due to the hypervascular nature of these liver metastases, NET patients are good candidates for a radioembolization procedure, as was described for ^{90}Y microspheres in the chapter *Yttrium-90 SIRT in NET*. [166]Ho radioembolization was recently introduced as an alternative. It was tested in NET patients in two clinical trials, HEPAR II (NCT01612325) and HEPAR PLuS (NCT02067988). The former was a phase II study conducted between 2012 and 2015 and assessed tumor response after [166]Ho radioembolization and, among others, included two patients with liver metastases of neuroendocrine origin. The latter study entirely focused on efficacy and toxicity of adjuvant [166]Ho radioembolization after systemic lutetium-177-dotatate (^{177}Lu-dotatate) in NET patients with liver metastases. This study was recently completed, after the recruitment of 34 patients, and it showed that [166]Ho-radioembolization, as an adjunct to peptide receptor radionuclide therapy in patients with NET liver metastases, is safe and efficacious. In addition, it proved that radioembolization can be considered in patients with bulky liver disease, including after peptide receptor radionuclide therapy [23].

21.5.1 Clinical Case

To better understand [166]Ho radioembolization in liver disease of NET origin, a clinical case will be presented as an example of the current clinical workflow. A 58-year-old patient with metastatic small intestine NET (grade 1) with residual liver disease after ^{177}Lu-dotatate treatment was included in the HEPAR PLuS study [19]. On diagnostic CT examination (baseline, after ^{177}Lu-dotatate and prior to [166]Ho radioembolization), massive liver metastasis was acknowledged (Table 21.2, baseline column and Fig. 21.2a, b), mainly in the right liver. Evaluation of the hepatic vasculature showed a replaced right hepatic artery originating from the superior

Table 21.2 Lesion size and location

Liver segment	Baseline	3 months FU	6 months FU	9 months FU	12 months FU
Segment 2	32 mm	22 mm	19 mm	19 mm	17 mm
Right lateral Hemiliver	122 mm	108 mm	108 mm	108 mm	106 mm

Baseline CECT

1 year follow-up CECT

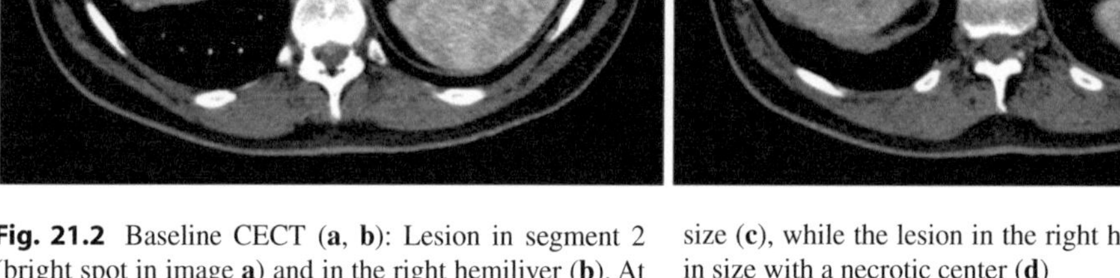

Fig. 21.2 Baseline CECT (**a**, **b**): Lesion in segment 2 (bright spot in image **a**) and in the right hemiliver (**b**). At the 1-year follow-up, the lesion in segment 2 decreased in size (**c**), while the lesion in the right hemiliver decreased in size with a necrotic center (**d**)

mesenteric artery. As per the study protocol, the patient underwent a ^{166}Ho scout procedure. After a selective catheterization of the tumor feeding vessel, originating from the left hepatic artery, 37 MBq of ^{166}Ho scout dose was injected, and in segments 5–8, 192 MBq was administered following catheterization of the right hepatic artery via the superior mesenteric artery. The scout procedure confirmed the absence of lung shunt and extrahepatic deposition while confirming a favorable tumor targeting (as depicted in Fig. 21.3a, b). The same day, the patient received ^{166}Ho treatment: 6774 MBq of QuiremSpheres® were successfully administered at the same injection positions as the scout procedure. The post-treatment SPECT/CT 3 days later confirmed the absence of extrahepatic uptake and adequate tumor targeting in the known metastases with relatively little activity in the healthy liver parenchyma, as predicted by the scout SPECT/CT (Fig. 21.3c, d). No activity was present in the caudate lobe and segment 3, in accor-

Pre-Treatment SPECT/CT

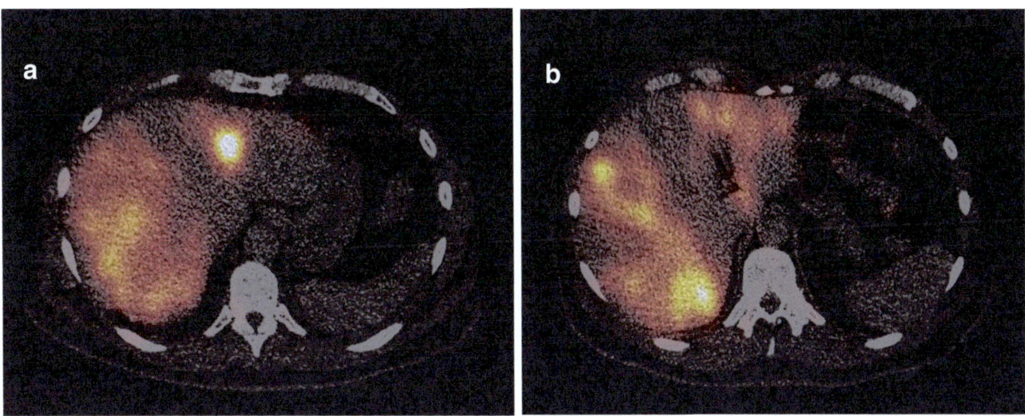

Post-Treatment SPECT/CT

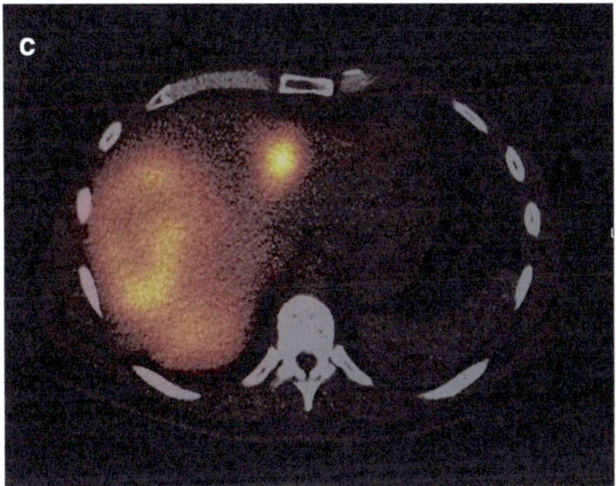
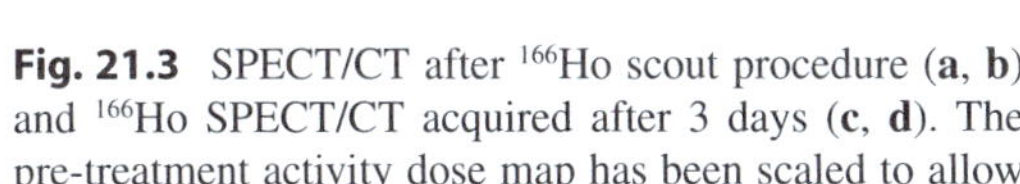
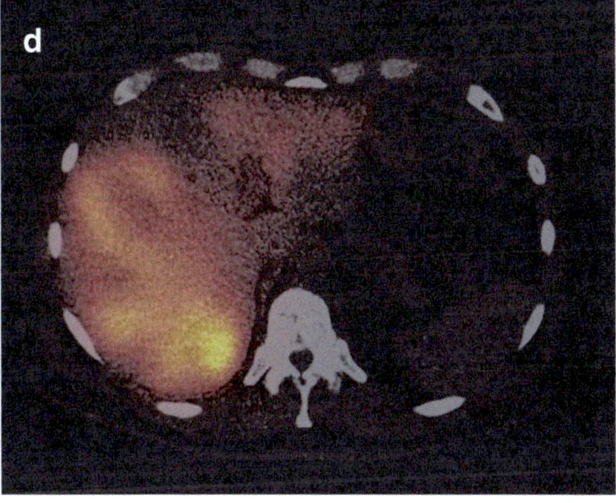

Fig. 21.3 SPECT/CT after ^{166}Ho scout procedure (**a, b**) and ^{166}Ho SPECT/CT acquired after 3 days (**c, d**). The pre-treatment activity dose map has been scaled to allow for a visual comparison between pre- and post-treatment acquisition. Note the match between the scout and treatment microsphere distribution

dance with the treatment plan. CECT at 3 months follow-up showed a tumor size reduction in segment 2 equal to 30%, while tumors in segments 5–8 reduced with 12% and 2%, respectively. For a quantitative assessment of tumor lesion sizes, measured according to RECIST 1.1 criteria (Response Evaluation Criteria In Solid Tumors), baseline and follow-up (3–12 months) measurements were reported in Table 21.1. In the following months after ^{166}Ho radioembolization, an ongoing decrease in size of all liver metastases was acknowledged (Table 21.2 and Fig. 21.2c, d). After 1 year, a substantial decrease in tumor size was observed, with a mean decrease of 30% (Fig. 21.2).

21.6 Future Perspectives

Radioembolization relies on the unique dual hepatic blood supply of the liver. However, liver vasculature differs among patients. Accurate assessment of microsphere distribution is fundamental, with a need to target tumor lesions with radioactive microspheres while sparing healthy liver tissue. This makes dosimetry paramount for any radioembolization treatment. To this end, based on the combined results of the quantitative and qualitative analyses, ^{166}Ho scout seemed superior to ^{99m}Tc-MAA in predicting the intrahepatic distribution [3]. Since ^{99m}Tc-MAA may overestimate the lung shunt fraction up to 170% when compared to [166]Ho microspheres [6], [166]Ho scout is also a superior alternative for lung shunt assessment. As already established for mCRC tumors, absorbed dose plays a significant role in lesion response in [166]Ho radioembolization [20]. An objective response was observed in 55% of the considered lesions, for which the recovered absorbed dose was significantly higher compared to lesions that did not present with an objective response (Mann-Whitney $U = 604.0$, $z = -2.983$, $p = 0.003$). A dose-response relationship likely also exists in NET patients, providing a dose threshold needed for a reliable tumor response. Additional dosimetric analysis of the HEPAR PLuS data may lead to more insights. The possibility to use clinically reconstructed SPECT/CT images for quantitative evaluation of absorbed dose was already proven. Currently, the estimate of lung shunt absorbed dose, resulting from [166]Ho radioembolization in NET patients, is under investigation, using the clinically available SPECT/CT.

Recently, the possibility to combine [166]Ho with another radionuclide labeled with a colloid, technetium-99m phytate (^{99m}Tc-phytate), was exploited [25] on both phantom [21] and patient data [24]. ^{99m}Tc-phytate accumulates in Kupffer cells, present in healthy liver tissue and absent in tumorous tissue, and may be imaged using SPECT/CT (Fig. 21.4). This dual isotope (DI) approach would enable the automatic segmentation of the tumors and healthy liver, enabling the estimate of absorbed dose in the healthy liver, considered to be the major dose limiting factor for radioembolization. Moreover, an automatic segmentation of the two compartments (tumor and healthy liver) would also pave the way to the clinical use of the partition model (see chapter on ^{90}Y radioembolization), which incorporates tissue masses and a measurement of the tumor-to-normal tissue (TN) ratio. This dose calculation method is more personalized, compared to the currently used technique (MIRD), and thus believed to be a better approach in terms of treatment accuracy. It allows for the selection of a prescribed activity that maximizes the absorbed dose to the tumor tissue while not exceeding toxicity thresholds for the healthy parenchyma. This approach could ultimately optimize treatment outcome.

Lastly, it is worth mentioning that the large magnetic susceptibility of holmium may enable MRI-based dosimetry and MR-guided treatments in the future. Once MRI-based dosimetry is adequately developed, the scout dose may even-

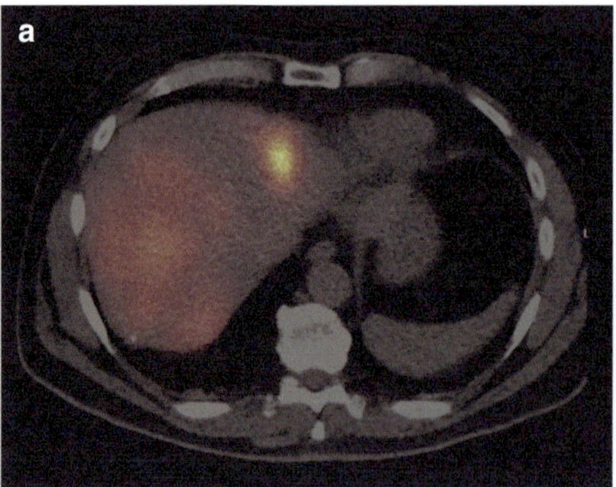

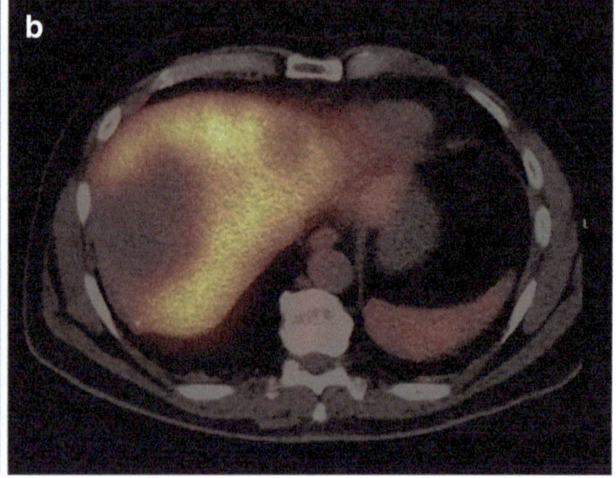

Fig. 21.4 Dual isotope protocol: [166]Ho (**a**) and ^{99m}Tc-phytate (**b**) uptake distribution visualized on a SPECT/CT. During the [166]Ho radioembolization treatment, the patient was administered with 6774 MBq of holmium-166. Three days after, when the activity was compatible with the dead time of the gamma camera, a SPECT/CT was acquired, following the administration of 50 MBq of [99m]Tc. To compensate for ^{99m}Tc downscatter, its influence in the [166]Ho photopeak window was accounted for in the DI image reconstruction using energy window-based scatter correction methods

tually be replaced for the stable, non-radioactive ^{165}Ho microspheres.

To conclude, ^{166}Ho radioembolization in NET patients has been demonstrated to be a feasible clinical practice. Even though more evidence has to be gained, the promising results show the potentialities of ^{166}Ho radioembolization in the treatment of metastases in the liver, commonly related to neuroendocrine tumors. Future steps can be made to obtain an optimized treatment and achieve a true personalized dosimetry in the treatment planning.

References

1. Ackerman NB, Hechmer PA. The blood supply of experimental liver metastases: V. Increased tumor perfusion with epinephrine. Am J Surg. 1980;140(5):625–31. https://doi.org/10.1016/0002-9610(80)90044-6.
2. Braat AJAT, Prince JF, van Rooij R, et al. Safety analysis of holmium-166 microsphere scout dose imaging during radioembolization work-up: a cohort study. Eur Radiol. 2018;28(3):920–8. https://doi.org/10.1007/s00330-017-4998-2.
3. Smits MLJ, Dassen MG, Prince JF, et al. The superior predictive value of 166Ho-scout compared with 99mTc-macroaggregated albumin prior to 166Ho-microspheres radioembolization in patients with liver metastases. Eur J Nucl Med Mol Imaging. 2020;47(4):798–806. https://doi.org/10.1007/s00259-019-04460-y.
4. Kao Y-H, Steinberg JD, Tay Y-S, et al. Post-radioembolization yttrium-90 PET/CT—part 2: dose-response and tumor predictive dosimetry for resin microspheres. EJNMMI Res. 2013;3(1):57. https://doi.org/10.1186/2191-219X-3-57.
5. Kao Y, Steinberg JD, Tay Y-S, et al. Post-radioembolization yttrium-90 PET/CT—part 1: diagnostic reporting. EJNMMI Res. 2013;3(1):56. https://doi.org/10.1186/2191-219X-3-56.
6. Elschot M, Nijsen JFW, Lam MGEH, et al. 99mTc-MAA overestimates the absorbed dose to the lungs in radioembolization: a quantitative evaluation in patients treated with 166Ho-microspheres. Eur J Nucl Med Mol Imaging. 2014;41(10):1965–75. https://doi.org/10.1007/s00259-014-2784-9.
7. Zhou XY, Jeffris KE, Yu EY, et al. First in vivo magnetic particle imaging of lung perfusion in rats. Phys Med Biol. 2017;62(9):3510–22. https://doi.org/10.1088/1361-6560/aa616c.
8. Smits MLJ, Nijsen JFW, van den Bosch MAAJ, et al. Holmium-166 radioembolisation in patients with unresectable, chemorefractory liver metastases (HEPAR trial): a phase 1, dose-escalation study. Lancet Oncol. 2012;13(10):1025–34. https://doi.org/10.1016/S1470-2045(12)70334-0.
9. White DR, Booz J, Griffith R V, et al. Report 44. J Int Comm Radiat Units Meas. 1989;os23(1):NP. https://doi.org/10.1093/jicru/os23.1.Report44.
10. Wondergem M, Smits MLJ, Elschot M, et al. 99mTc-macroaggregated albumin poorly predicts the intrahepatic distribution of 90Y resin microspheres in hepatic radioembolization. J Nucl Med. 2013;54(8):1294–301. https://doi.org/10.2967/jnumed.112.117614.
11. Braat AJAT, Kappadath SC, Ahmadzadehfar H, et al. Radioembolization with 90Y resin microspheres of neuroendocrine liver metastases: international multicenter study on efficacy and toxicity. Cardiovasc Intervent Radiol. 2019;42(3):413–25. https://doi.org/10.1007/s00270-018-2148-0.
12. Reinders MTM, Smits MLJ, van Roekel C, et al. Holmium-166 microsphere radioembolization of hepatic malignancies. Semin Nucl Med. 2019;49(3):237–43. https://doi.org/10.1053/j.semnuclmed.2019.01.008.
13. Prince JF, Smits MLJ, Krijger GC, et al. Radiation emission from patients treated with holmium-166 radioembolization. J Vasc Interv Radiol. 2014;25(12):1956–1963.e1. https://doi.org/10.1016/j.jvir.2014.09.003.
14. Bastiaannet R, Viergever MA, De Jong HWAM. Impact of respiratory motion and acquisition settings on SPECT liver dosimetry for radioembolization. Med Phys. 2017;44(10):5270–9. https://doi.org/10.1002/mp.12483.
15. De Wit TC, Xiao J, Nijsen JFW, et al. Hybrid scatter correction applied to quantitative holmium-166 SPECT. Phys Med Biol. 2006;51(19):4773–87. https://doi.org/10.1088/0031-9155/51/19/004.
16. Elschot M, Nijsen JFW, Dam AJ, et al. Quantitative evaluation of scintillation camera imaging characteristics of isotopes used in liver radio-embolization. Boswell CA, ed. PLoS One. 2011;6(11):e26174. https://doi.org/10.1371/journal.pone.0026174.
17. Nijsen JFW, Seppenwoolde J-H, Havenith T, et al. Liver tumors; MR imaging of radioactive holmium microspheres—phantom and rabbit study. Radiology. 2004;231(2):491–9. https://doi.org/10.1148/radiol.2312030594.
18. Van De Maat GH, Seevinck PR, Elschot M, et al. MRI-based biodistribution assessment of holmium-166 poly(L-lactic acid) microspheres after radio-embolisation. Eur Radiol. 2013;23(3):827–35. https://doi.org/10.1007/s00330-012-2648-2.
19. Braat AJAT, Kwekkeboom DJ, Kam BLR, et al. Additional hepatic 166Ho-radioembolization in patients with neuroendocrine tumours treated with 177Lu-DOTATATE; a single center, interventional, non-randomized, non-comparative, open label, phase II study (HEPAR PLUS trial). BMC Gastroenterol. 2018;18(1):84. https://doi.org/10.1186/s12876-018-0817-8.
20. Bastiaannet R, van Roekel C, Smits M, et al. First evidence for a dose-response relationship in patients treated with 166ho radioembolization: a prospective study. Journal of nuclear medicine: official publica-

tion, society of nuclear medicine. 2020;61(4):608–12. https://doi.org/10.2967/jnumed.119.232751.

21. van Rooij R, Braat A, de Jong H, et al. Simultaneous 166Ho/99mTc dual-isotope SPECT with Monte Carlo-based down scatter correction for automatic liver dosimetry in radioembolization. EJNMMI Physics. 2020;7(1):13. https://doi.org/10.1186/s40658-020-0280-9.

22. Stella M, Braat A, Lam M, et al. Gamma camera characterization at high holmium-166 activity in liver radioembolization. EJNMMI Physics. 2021;8(1):22. https://doi.org/10.1186/s40658-021-00372-9.

23. Braat A, Bruijnen R, van Rooij R, et al. Additional holmium-166 radioembolisation after lutetium-177-dotatate in patients with neuroendocrine tumour liver metastases (HEPAR PLuS): a single-centre, single-arm, open-label, phase 2 study. The Lancet. Oncology. 2020;21(4)561–70. https://doi.org/10.1016/S1470-2045(20)30027-9.

24. Stella M, Braat A, Lam M, et al. Quantitative 166Ho-microspheres SPECT derived from a dual-isotope acquisition with 99mTc-colloid is clinically feasible. EJNMMI Physics. 2020;7(1):48. https://doi.org/10.1186/s40658-020-00317-8.

25. Lam MG, Banerjee A, Goris ML, et al. Fusion dual-tracer SPECT-based hepatic dosimetry predicts outcome after radioembolization for a wide range of tumor cell types. European Journal of Nuclear Medicine and Molecular Imaging. 2015;42(8):1192–201. https://doi.org/10.1007/s00259-015-3048-z.

Complications and Side Effects on the Course of Liver Radio-Infusions with ^{111}In-Octreotide

Victor Ralph McCready, Athanasios G. Zafeirakis, and Georgios S. Limouris

22.1 Introduction

Peptide receptor radionuclide therapy (PRRT) has been used for more than 20 years as a systemic treatment approach in inoperable or metastatic somatostatin receptor (SSTR)-positive tumors. The acute side effects, generally adverse events, are usually mild; most of them are related to the co-administration of amino acids, such as nausea and vomiting. Others are due to the radiopharmaceutical ^{111}In-Octreotide, such as abdominal discomfort, hypotony, diarrhea, and fatigue. The exacerbation of endocrine syndromes, reported rarely, occurs only in patients with functional tumors and a large tumor burden. Chronic and permanent damage can affect target organs, particularly the kidneys and the bone marrow, but these are generally mild. Currently, when ^{177}Lu DOTATATE is used, the potential risk to kidney damage is significantly reduced, compared with the previous use of ^{90}Y-labeled analogues. Specifically with ^{111}In-Octreotide, the only subacute side effect is bone marrow toxicity that might limit the dose of radioactivity or require a temporary discontinuation of the PRRT procedure.

22.2 Side Effects

22.2.1 Acute Side Effects

The adverse reactions to radiopeptide therapies (PRRTs) are usually mild if the necessary precautions are taken. Adverse reactions may be acute (related either to the administration of amino acids or to the radiopharmaceutical itself), subacute, or chronic. The co-administration of amino acids extends the safety margin that allows a higher administered activity treatment. However, in the majority of patients, it is usually associated with side effects such as nausea and headache, whereas, rarely, metabolic acidosis can be observed [1, 2]. Care should be taken to avoid possible electrolyte disturbances with subsequent metabolic oxidation, which can lead to moderate nausea and vomiting. The management of the latter is hydration of the patient with normal saline and possibly the administration of antiemetics or corticosteroids. Radiopeptide therapy (PRRT) can aggravate the syndromes associated with the corresponding functional tumor due to abrupt mass release of hormones and stimulation of the receptors. The clinical event depends on the particular hormone involved. Vital signs (at least

V. R. McCready (✉)
Royal Sussex County Hospital, Brighton, UK
e-mail: ralph.mccready@nhs.net

A. G. Zafeirakis
Nuclear Medicine Department, Army Share Fund Hospital of Athens, Athens, Greece

G. S. Limouris
Nuclear Medicine, Medical School, National and Kapodistrian University of Athens, Athens, Greece

© Springer Nature Switzerland AG 2021
G. S. Limouris (ed.), *Liver Intra-arterial PRRT with ^{111}In-Octreotide*,
https://doi.org/10.1007/978-3-030-70773-6_22

blood pressure and pulse) should be monitored before and after the infusion of radiopeptides, especially in symptomatic patients. Therapeutic interventions should be undertaken to treat functional syndromes (e.g., carcinoid/hypotension syndrome, hypoglycemia, hypergastrinemia, hypertension, WDHA syndrome[1], electrolytic disorders) or their exacerbation [3]. In patients with small or without metastatic liver involvement, no significant liver toxicity has been reported. In the literature, however, in patients with massive hepatic metastases and impaired hepatic function, liver toxicity may occur, and this should be considered together with preexisting conditions affecting the liver in order to select the appropriate administered activity. Particularly after treatment, patients should avoid pregnancy for at least 6 months.

22.2.1.1   Carcinoid Crisis

"Carcinoid crisis" is a rare, life-threatening medical emergency involving cardiac and vasomotor instability probably due to the release of large amounts of vasoactive peptides from carcinoid tumors [4]. Carcinoid crisis is usually precipitated after mechanical stimulation of the tumor, stress, hypercapnia, hypothermia, hypotension, hypertension, initiation of chemotherapy, or drugs that cause a release of histamine [5, 6].

[1]WDHA (watery diarrhea, hypokalemia, and achlorhydria) syndrome is an unusual paraneoplastic condition caused by excess vasoactive intestinal polypeptide (VIP) secreted by certain tumors. The onset of the syndrome is insidious, and diagnosis is usually delayed by months to years. Morbidity and mortality from untreated WDHA syndrome are related to long-standing dehydration and electrolyte and acid-base disturbances resulting in chronic renal failure. Diagnosis requires documentation of large volumes of secretory diarrhea, elevated serum VIP levels, and localization of the VIP-secreting tumor. Treatment includes correction of volume, electrolyte, and metabolic abnormalities, pharmacotherapy to decrease gastrointestinal secretion and increase absorption, and ultimately surgical resection or debulking of the vipoma [8].

22.2.2   Chronic Side Effects

22.2.2.1   Renal Toxicity

In radiopeptide therapies, the kidneys are the critical organs that might limit the desired administered activity. Adequate kidney protection (not if ^{111}In-Octreotide but where ^{90}Y- or ^{177}Lu-labeled peptides are infused), as mentioned, is currently mandatory. However, despite renal protection, renal impairment may occur after PRRT [7].

22.2.2.2   Bone Marrow Toxicity

Severe (grade III and IV), mostly reversible, acute bone marrow toxicity is observed in 8/88 (9.1%) of patients as a persistent hematological dysfunction. In 2/88, hairy cell leukemia was diagnosed and died shortly afterward, whereas in 2/88, a persistent slightly elevated creatinine after ^{111}In-Octreotide treatment was noticed. The same acute bone marrow toxicity was observed in 10–13% after ^{90}Y-DOTATOC treatment and about 2–3% after treatment with ^{177}Lu-DOTATATE with sporadic cases of myelodysplastic syndrome or acute myeloid leukemia [9–11].

22.2.2.3   Endocrine Organs

Despite the existence of somatostatin receptors in the pituitary, thyroid, adrenal, and islets of Langerhans, no significant changes in their endocrine hormonal function have been reported [12].

22.3   Radiobiological Properties

The use of the pentetreotide carrier molecule, a somatostatin analogue, which binds with high affinity to the surface receptors, subtype 2, subtype 3, and subtype 5, presupposes that the therapeutic radionuclide selected must have an appropriate path length (range) to attack the DNA of the nucleus and cause cell death (Fig. 22.1). The length as well as the energy of the Auger and internal conversion electrons, emitted by the ^{111}In, is not ideal. They are extremely short in length which does not exceed the diameter of 2–3 cells nor can they affect adjacent cells because they are not capable of producing the crossfire effect. In addition, the 0.5–25 keV energy of Auger electrons and the 145–245 keV for internal conversion electrons is low compared to ^{90}Y or ^{177}Lu β-radiation.

However, these seemingly limiting features of ^{111}In emission have their benefits. Comparing the S values of the Auger and internal conversion electrons, ^{111}In delivers an impressive high dose [13] to the target, which explains the cellular damage caused. The possible renal, hepatic, and

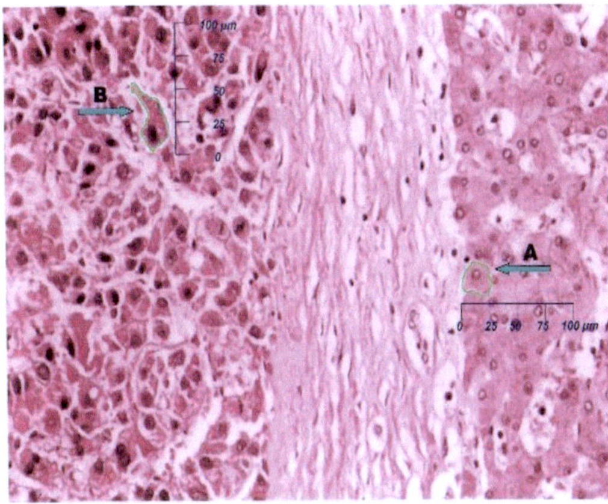

Fig. 22.1 Schematic representation of two scales (in blue) superimposed on a histologic sample of normal (**A**) and tumor liver cells (**B**). Cellular membrane is delineated by green line. Nuclei of normal and tumor cells are well distinguished. When comparing cell dimensions and distances between cell surface and nuclei, it obviously can be seen that DNA lies within the micrometer range of ^{111}In emissions (adapted and modified from Limouris et al. [22])

myeloid toxicity that strongly concerns almost all authors dealing with ^{111}In (Table 22.1) does not exist in practice. In fact, the relative biological activity (RBE) of Auger electrons is the predominant factor responsible for DNA damage, while the involvement of internal conversion electrons is essentially of minor importance. In addition, Coster-Kronig and super-Coster-Kronig electrons have some involvement, but they are negligible. All of the abovementioned emissions are cited as Auger electron emission, under the broad umbrella of their therapeutic efficacy, without being individually defined [23]. In addition, upon a thorough observation of ^{111}In decay [24], its two γ-photo-peaks emitting in 171 and 245 keV cover an abundance of 0.902 and 0.940 keV, respectively, which should not be overlooked. Consequently, we can conclude that to a large extent, the relative biological activity of ^{111}In is directly related to the burden induced by the γ-radiation on tissues in addition to that derived from Auger electrons. The DNA damage-cataract is due to both types of radiation, mentioned previously. With regard to apparent hepatotoxicity, according to our dosimetry calculations [25–29], the healthy hepatic parenchyma is surprisingly not at risk, although this was to be expected. This is directly linked to the route of administration, where, upon the first pass through the tumor's arterial supply network, the greater part of the radiopharmaceutical is attracted and taken up by the overexpressed tumor receptors; this results in

Table 22.1 Experteers working with ^{111}In-Octreotide

Author	No. of pts	Cumulative activity (GBq)	CR	PR	SD	PD
Krenning et al. (1994) [14]	1	20.3	–	1 (100%)	–	–
Tiensuu Janson et al. (1999) [15]	5	18.00	–	2 (40%)	3 (60%)	–
Caplin et al. (2000) [16]	8	3.10–15.200	–	–	7 (87.5%)	1 (12.5%)[a]
Nguyen et al. (2004) [17]	15	21.00	–	–	13 (87%)	2 (13%)
Valkema et al. (2002) [18]	26	4.7–160.0	–	2 (8%)	15 (58%)	9 (35%)
Anthony et al. (2002) [19]	26	6.7–46.6	–	2 (8%)	21 (81%)	3 (11%)
Buscombe et al. (2003) [20]	12	3.1–36.6	–	2 (17%)	7 (58%)	3 (25%)
Delpassand et al. (2008) [21]	29	35.3–37.3	–	2 (7%)	16 (55%)	11 (38%)[b]
Limouris et al. (2008)[c] [22]	17	13.0–77.0	1 (6%)	8 (47%)	3 (18%)	5 (29%)

[a]Unrelated to the tumor cause
[b]Not clearly reported
[c]Exclusive intra-arterially

Table 22.2 Tumor-absorbed dose comparison between i.v. and i.a. administration of ^{111}In-Octreotide

	Intra-arterial infusion	Intravenous infusion
Liver dose	0.14 (mGy/MBq)	0.40 (mGy/MBq)
Kidney dose	0.41 (mGy/MBq)	0.51 (mGy/MBq)
Tumor dose	15.20 (mGy/MBq)	11.20 (mGy/MBq)
Spleen dose	1.40 (mGy/MBq)	1.56 (mGy/MBq)
Bone marrow dose	0.0035 (mGy/MBq)	0.022 (mGy/MBq)
Tumor/liver dose ratio	108.57[a]	28.00
Tumor/kidney dose ratio	37.07	21.96

[a]The average absorbed dose per session to a tumor for a spherical mass of 10 g was estimated to be 10.8 mGy/MBq, depending on the histotype of the tumor

a lower distribution in the peritumoral healthy and comparatively poor in somatostatin receptor hepatic parenchyma, leading to a lower rate of absorbed radiation compared to that calculated after intravenous infusion (Table 22.2). However, it has to be noted that a recent study of Bergsma et al. [30] reported that a myelodysplastic syndrome (MDS) or leukemia was observed in half of the NET patients who received a very high administered activity (>100 GBq) of ^{111}In-Octreotide, intravenously.

On possible nephrotoxicity, recent research by de Jong et al. [31] have shown that the concentration of radiopharmaceuticals is distributed in the inner zone of the renal cortex, whereas the glomerular delicate coils are in the outer zone, and therefore the range of ^{111}In electrons cannot in practice affect them.

To date according to the latest follow-up data, no patient has developed any degree of renal toxicity.

References

1. Jamar F, Barone R, Mathieu I, et al. (86YDOTA0)-DPhe1-Tyr3-octreotide (SMT487)—a phase 1 clinical study: pharmacokinetics, biodistribution and renal protective effect of different regimens of amino acid co-infusion. Eur J Nucl Med Mol Imaging. 2003;30:510–8.
2. Rolleman EJ, Valkema R, de Jong M, et al. Safe and effective inhibition of renal uptake of radiolabelled octreotide by a combination of lysine and arginine. Eur J Nucl Med Mol Imaging. 2002;30:9–15.
3. de Keizer B, van Aken MO, Feelders RA, et al. Hormonal crises following receptor radionuclide therapy with the radiolabeled somatostatin analogue [177Lu-DOTA0,Tyr3]octreotate. Eur J Nucl Med Mol Imaging. 2008;35:749–55.
4. Yadav SK, Jha CK, Patil S, et al. Lutetium therapy-induced carcinoid crisis: a case report and review of the literature. J Can Res Ther. 2020;16(Suppl S1):206–8.
5. Vaughan DJ, Brunner MD. Anesthesia for patients with carcinoid syndrome. Int Anesthesiol Clin. 1997;35:129–42.
6. Mehta AC, Rafanan AL, Bulkley R, et al. Coronary spasm and cardiac arrest from carcinoid crisis during laser bronchoscopy. Chest. 1999;115:598–600.
7. Valkema R, Pauwels SA, Kvols LK, et al. Long-term follow-up of renal function after peptide receptor radiation therapy with 90Y-DOTA0,Tyr3-octreotide and 177Lu-DOTA0,Tyr3-octreotate. J Nucl Med. 2005;46:83S–91S.
8. Grier JF. WDHA (watery diarrhea, hypokalemia, achlorhydria) syndrome: clinical features, diagnosis, and treatment. South Med J. 1995;88(1):22–4.
9. Kwekkeboom DJ, Mueller-Brand J, Paganelli G, et al. Overview of results of peptide receptor radionuclide therapy with 3 radiolabeled somatostatin analogs. J Nucl Med. 2005;46(Suppl 1):62S–6S.
10. Bushnell DL Jr, O'Dorisio TM, O'Dorisio MS, et al. 90Y-Edotreotide for metastatic carcinoid refractory to octreotide. J Clin Oncol. 2010;28:1652–9.
11. Imhof A, Brunner P, Marincek N, et al. Response, survival, and long-term toxicity after therapy with the radiolabeled somatostatin analogue [90Y-DOTA]-TOC in metastasized neuroendocrine cancers. J Clin Oncol. 2011;29:2416–23.
12. Teunissen JJ, Krenning EP, de Jong FH, et al. Effects of therapy with [177Lu-DOTA0, Tyr3]octreotate on endocrine function. Eur J Nucl Med Mol Imaging. 2009;36:1758–66.
13. Goddu SM, Budinger TF. MIRD: cellular S values. Reston: SNM; 1997.
14. Krenning EP, Kooij PPM, Bakker WH, et al. Radiotherapy with a radiolabelled somatostatin analogue, [111In-DTPA-D.Phe1]-octreotide; a case history. Ann N Y Acad Sci. 1994;733:496–506.
15. Tiensuu Janson E, Eriksson B, Oberg K, et al. Treatment with high dose [(111)In-DTPA-D-PHE1]-octreotide in patients with neuroendocrine tumors—evaluation of therapeutic and toxic effects. Acta Oncol. 1999;38(3):373–7.
16. Caplin ME, Mielcarek W, Buscombe JR, et al. Toxicity of high-activity in-111 octreotide therapy in

patients with disseminated neuroendocrine tumours. Nucl Med Commun. 2000;21:97–102.

17. Nguyen C, Faraggi M, Giraudet A-L. Long-term efficacy of radionuclide therapy in patients with disseminated neuroendocrine tumors uncontrolled by conventional therapy. J Nucl Med. 2004;45:1660–8.

18. Valkema R, De Jong M, Bakker WH, et al. Phase I study of peptide receptor radionuclide therapy with [111In-DTPA°] octreotide: the Rotterdam experience. Semin Nucl Med. 2002;32(2):110–22.

19. Anthony LB, Woltering EA, Espanan GD, et al. Indium-111-pentetreotide prolongs survival in gastroenteropancreatic malignancies. Semin Nucl Med. 2002;32(2):123–32.

20. Buscombe JR, Caplin ME, Hilson JW. Long-term efficacy of high-activity 111In-pentetreotide therapy in patients with disseminated neuroendocrine tumors. J Nucl Med. 2003;44:1–6.

21. Delpassand ES, Samarghandi A, Zamanian S, et al. Peptide receptor radionuclide therapy with 177Lu-DOTATATE for patients with somatostatin receptor–expressing neuroendocrine tumors: the first US phase 2 experience. Pancreas. 2014;43(4):518–25. Lippincott Williams & Wilkins.

22. Limouris GS, Chatziioannou A, Kontogeorgakos D, et al. Selective hepatic arterial infusion of In-111-DTPA-Phe-octreotide in neuroendocrine liver metastases. Eur J Nucl Med Mol Imaging. 2008;35:1827.

23. Buchegger F, Perillo-Adamer F, Dupertuis YM, et al. Auger radiation targeted into DNA: a therapy perspective. Eur J Nucl Med Mol Imaging. 2006;33(11):1352–63.

24. Health Physics J. RADAR. 2008. http://www.doseinfo-radar.Com/RADAR Soft.html.

25. Limouris GS, Dimitropoulos N, Kontogeorgakos D, et al. Evaluation of the therapeutic response to In-111-DTPA octreotide-based targeted therapy in liver metastatic neuroendocrine tumours according to CT/MRI/US findings. Cancer Biother Radiopharm. 2005;20(2):215–7.

26. Kwekkeboom DJ, Mueller-Brand J, Paganelli G, et al. Overview of results of peptide receptor radionuclide therapy with 3 radiolabeled somatostatin analogs. J Nucl Med. 2005;46(Suppl 1):62–6.

27. Bodei L, Cremonesi M, Zoboli S, et al. Receptor-mediated radionuclide therapy with 90YDOTATOC in association with amino acid infusion: a phase I study. Eur J Nucl Med. 2003;30:207–16.

28. Waldherr C, Pless M, Maecke HR, et al. Tumor response and clinical benefit in neuroendocrine tumors after 7.4 GBq 90Y-DOTATOC. J Nucl Med. 2002;43(5):610–6.

29. Cremonesi M, Ferrari M, Bodei L. Dosimetry in peptide radionuclide receptor therapy: a review. J Nucl Med. 2006;47(9):1467–75.

30. Bergsma H, van Lom K, Raaijmakers MHGP, et al. Therapy-related hematological malignancies after peptide receptor radionuclide therapy with 177LuDOTATATE: incidence, course & predicting factors in patients with GEP-NETs. J Nucl Med. 2018;59(3):452–8.

31. De Jong M, Valkema R, Van Gameren A, et al. Inhomogeneous localization of radioactivity in the human kidney after injection of [111In-DTPA]octreotide. J Nucl Med. 2004;45(7):1168–71.

Progression-Free Survival and Response Rate in Neuroendocrine Liver-Metastasized Patients, Treated with ^{111}In-Octreotide

Georgios S. Limouris, Maria I. Paphiti, and Athanasios G. Zafeirakis

23.1 Introduction

The role of the tumor proliferation indexes (Ki-67 proliferation index and mitotic index)[1], in previewing and in some way "predicting" the efficacy

---

[1] **Ki-67** is a *nuclear antigen* expressed in proliferating cells and is expressed during the GI, S, G2, and M phases of the cell cycle. Cells are then stained with a Ki-67 *antibody*, and the number of stained nuclei is then expressed as a percentage of total tumor cells. The name is derived from the city of origin (Kiel, Germany) and the "67" number from the original clone in the 96-well plate.

The **mitotic index**, expressed *as the number of cells per microscopic field*, is determined by counting the number of cells undergoing mitosis through a light microscope on hematoxylin and eosin (H and E)-stained sections. Usually the number of mitotic figures is expressed as the total number in a defined number of high-power fields, i.e., 10 mitoses in 10 high-power fields. Since the field of vision area can considerably vary between different microscopes, the exact area of the high-power fields should be defined in order to compare results from different studies.

G. S. Limouris (✉)
Nuclear Medicine, Medical School, National and Kapodistrian University of Athens, Athens, Greece
e-mail: glimouris@med.uoa.gr

M. I. Paphiti
National Health System, Athens, Greece

A. G. Zafeirakis
Nuclear Medicine Department, Army Share Fund Hospital of Athens, Athens, Greece

of peptide receptor radionuclide therapy (PRRT) in NENS, still remains undetermined. This chapter is dealing with the evaluation of the response rate and progression-free survival of a cohort of neuroendocrine liver-metastasized patients, treated with high activities of ^{111}In-Octreotide as first-line therapy. Worldwide, there is little information related to the efficacy and response rate of this radiopharmaceutical beyond the normal 6-month assessment period. Our assumption proved that such treatment was beneficial for NEN patients, as expected based on the physicochemical properties of the radiopeptide ^{111}In-Octreotide. Focusing on the impact on tumor behavior, *in* liver-metastasized NEN patients, the correlation between their *expression patterns* and *patients' survival* leads to interesting results. These two parameters are briefly evaluated in this chapter analyzing their impact on ^{111}In-Octreotide prognosis, therapy response, and patients' survival.

23.2 Response Rate and Progression-Free Survival

Focusing on liver-metastasized neuroendocrine disease, progression-free survival and response rate contribute to their treatment final response and prognosis. In our institution, in a recently,

---

© Springer Nature Switzerland AG 2021
G. S. Limouris (ed.), *Liver Intra-arterial PRRT with ^{111}In-Octreotide*,
https://doi.org/10.1007/978-3-030-70773-6_23

Table 23.1 Patients' characteristics treated with ^{111}In-Octreotide

Patient no.	Patient's acronym	Age/sex	Primary origin
1	GA.KO	69//m	Small int exe
2	XA. VA	31/m	Pancreas exe
3	SI. PA	54/m	Pancreas exe
4	MP.NA	67/f	Small intest exe
5	DE. AN	71/f	Stomach exe
6	MP. NI	60/m	Pancreas exe
7	TS.GR	58/m	Small int exe
8	THE.KY	49/m	Sigmoid exe
9	BI.THE	72/m	Lung exe
10	SO/ST	76/f	Small int exe
11	XR.PA	52/m	Mesentery exe
12	BA.AL	53/f	Lung exe
13	KA.AN	61/f	Pancreas exe
14	PO.AR	63/m	Small intest exe

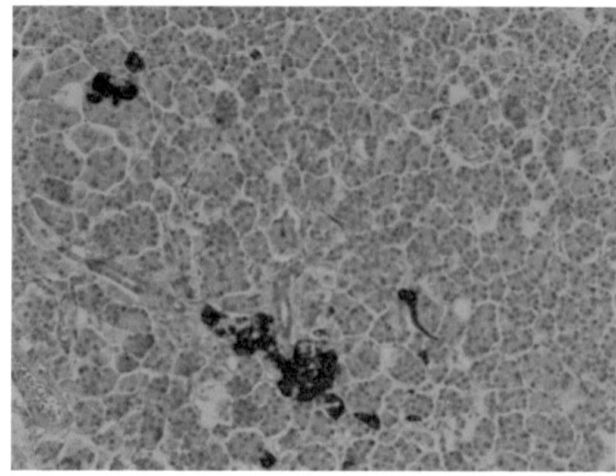

Fig. 23.1 Histological section of a low-grade pancreatic NET, showing positive immunoreaction to synaptophysin (immunostain ×10)

retrospectively evaluated sample check, in a cohort of 14 patients with nonfunctional, unresectable liver-metastatic NENs, treated with non-carrier-added ^{111}In-Octreotide after catheterization of the hepatic artery [with an injecting activity of precisely 5.92 GBq (160 mCi) per session, at standard intervals of 6–7 weeks], interesting findings were emerged (Table 23.1).

Patients (4, originated from pancreas, 5 from small intestines, 2 from lung cancer, 1 from mesentery, 1 from stomach, 1 from sigmoid) graded as G1/G2 and G3 were under long-acting somatostatin analog treatment (Fig. 23.1). The included patients were classified in two groups, as follows: group A, with Ki-67 < 20%, and group B with Ki-67 > 20%. Response was evaluated according to RECIST 1.1 criteria, and survival was analyzed based on Kaplan–Meier curve method. Cr-A was radio-immunologically measured and correlated with Ki-67 results.

In group A, partial response was observed in 5/7 (71.4%) patients and stable disease in 2/7 (28.6%), whereas in group B, stable disease was seen in 3/7 (42.9%) and progressive disease in 4/7 (57.1%). The median time of progression-free survival (PFS) for ^{111}In-Octreotide, in groups A and B, was 60 months and 12 months, respectively, whereas the mean OS accounted 64 months and 32 months, accordingly (Table 23.2). Cr-A values showed parallel to Ki-67 value level (Fig. 23.2). Besides these two parameters, i.e., response rate (RR) and progression-free survival (PFS), the proliferative factor Ki-67 emerges as a third acting determiner in the course of the therapeutic response, which, as a dominant response parameter, decisively defines both RR and even more PFS.

23.2.1 Response Rate

Referring to the international literature, the obtained results are limited because an extremely small number of authors (Table 23.3) have used ^{111}In-Octreotide for therapeutic purposes; thus reports on response rates are few whereas concerning PFS or OS in the majority of them were not referred.

In 2008, in a first preliminary study published in EJNMMI [14], of a 17-patient cohort, treated in our institution with ^{111}In-Octreotide (Table 23.3), 1 of 17 (6%) patients achieved a complete response (CR), 8 of 17 (47%) showed partial response (PR), and 3 (18%) achieved a

Table 23.2 Patients' results treated with ^{111}In-Octreotide

No.	Patient's acronym	No. of sessions	G, Ki-67	Response	Therapy course (months)	PFS (months)	OS (months)
1	GA.KO	7	G3, >20%	PD	8	6	25
2	XA. VA	3!	G3, >20%	PD	5	3	14
3	SI. PA	7	G3, >20%	PD	12	10	22
4	MP.NA	13	G3, >20%	PD	13	12	32
5	DE.AN	9	G2, <20%	SD	16	28	33
6	MP. NI	8	G2, <20%	SD	13	26	32
7	TS.GR	12	G1 <20%	PR	22	39	64
8	THE/KY	9	G3, >20%	SD	16	29	35
9	MPI.THE	16	G3, >20%	SD	27	84	>84
10	SO/ST	9	G3, >20%	SD	16	27	32
11	XR.PA	13	G1, <20%	PR	**24**	62	70
12	MPA.AL	19!	G1, <20%	PR	24	108	> 108
13	KA.AN	12	G1, <20%	PR	**18**	60	60
14	PO.AR	12	G1, <20%	PR	22	74	> 81

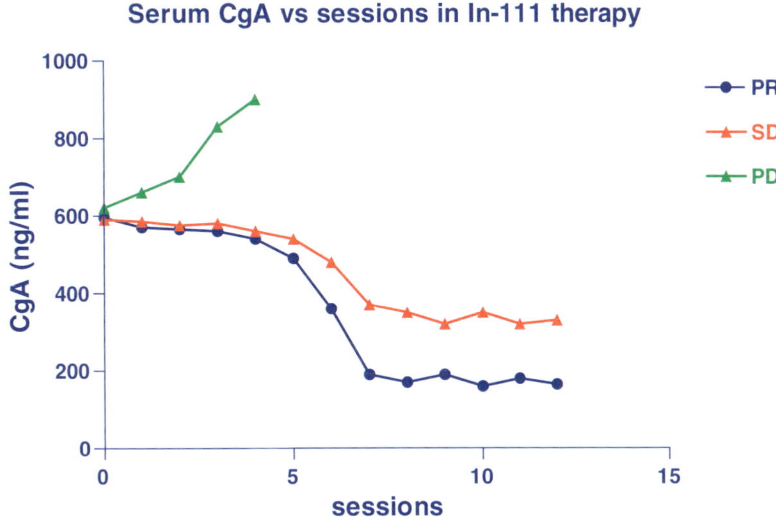

Fig. 23.2 Serum chromogranin-A levels during ^{111}In-Octreotide therapy in patients with PR, SD, and PD [1]

stable disease (SD), whereas in the remaining 5 (29%) patients, the disease progressed, the therapy was discontinued, and the patients died shortly thereafter. Consequently, 71% of these patients showed some radiological benefit (CR or PR or SD) from the treatment. Worldwide, only a limited number of authors reported on the efficacy of treatments in GEP-NET patients using high doses of ^{111}In-Octreotide. Our results in the CR/PR group (53%), compared to published data of other authors, were as follows: 2/26 patients (8%) of Valkema et al. [8], 2/12 patients (17.5%) of Buscombe et al. [11], 2/26 patients (8%) of Anthony et al. [10], and 2/29 patients (7.5%) of Delpassand et al. [15], whereas the radiological response initially assessed in another cohort of 80 patients [13] for an average of 29 months (1.26–60.2 months) following their last therapy was CR/PR in 6 patients (7.5%) and SD in 68 patients (85%), and the remaining 6 (7.5%) patients had PD.

Our observations for disease stabilization comparing our 18% (3/17 patients) data hardly

Table 23.3 Experteers working with ^{111}In-Octreotide

Authors	Patient's no.	Cumulative activity (GBq)	CR	PR	SD	PD	PFS (months)	OS (months)
Krenning et al. [2]	1	20.28	–	+	–	–	n.r.	n.r.
Kwekkeboom et al. [3]	30	Up to 74	–	6	8	16	n.r.	n.r.
Fjaelling et al. [4]	1	9.6	–	–	+	n.r	n.r	n.r
McCarthy et al. [5]	14	13.3	–	2	4	8	n.r.	n.r.
Meyers et al. [6]	1	53.3	–	–	+	–	n.r.	18
Tiensuu Janson E et al. [7]	3	24–48	–	–	2	1	n.r.	n.r.
Nguyen et al. [8]	14	13.1–22.5	–	–	12	2	16.1 ± 7.8	–
Valkema et al. [9]	40	20.0–160.0	–	7 (17.5%)	14 (35%)	19 (47.5%)	n.p.r.	n.p.r.
Anthony et al. [10]	26	6.7–46.6	–	2 (8%)	21 (81%)	3 (11%)	n.p.r.	18
Buscombe et al. [11]	16	3.1–36.6	2 (12.5%)	3 (18.75%)	7 (43.75%)	4 (25%)	9	n.p.r.
Kong et al. [12]	15	15.9–23.4	–	–	12 (80%)	3 (20%)	n.p.r.	n.p.r.
Delpassand et al. [13]	80	Up to 74	–	6 (7.5%)	68 (85%)	6 (7.5%)	n.p.r.	29
Limouris et al. i.a. [14]	17	17.76–112.48	1 (6%)	8 (47%)	3 (18%)	5 (29%)	32	>32
Limouris et al. i.v.[a]	10	5.92–53.28	–	–	3 (30%)	7 (70%)	8.5	17.5

n.r. non referred, *n.p.r.* non precisely referred

[a]Chapter 6 in this study

Table 23.4 Tumor-absorbed dose comparison between i.v. and i.a. administration of ^{111}In-Octreotide

	Intra-arterial infusion	Intravenous infusion
Liver dose	0.14 (mGy/MBq)	0.40 (mGy/MBq)
Kidney dose	0.41 (mGy/MBq)	0.51 (mGy/MBq)
Tumor dose	15.20 (mGy/MBq)	11.20 (mGy/MBq)
Spleen dose	1.40 (mGy/MBq)	1.56 (mGy/MBq)
Bone marrow dose	0.0035 (mGy/MBq)	0.022 (mGy/MBq)
Tumor/liver dose ratio	108.57[a]	28.00
Tumor/kidney dose ratio	37.07	21.96

[a]The average absorbed dose per session to a tumor for a spherical mass of 10 g was estimated to be 10.8 mGy/MBq, depending on the histotype of the tumor

differ from reports 35% (14/40 patients) of Valkema et al. [8], 43.75% (7/16 patients) of Buscombe et al. [11], 81% (21/26 patients) of Anthony et al. [10], and 85% (68/80 patients) of Delpassand et al. [13]. The superiority of our results compared to those of the aforementioned authors can be explained by the intra-arterial route of infusions almost exclusively performed as established protocol in our institution, where the tumor mean absorbed dose per session was estimated to be markedly higher compared to i.v. application (Table 23.4), a finding also reported by other authors [16, 17].

The results of the clinical evaluation of the Auger electron emitter ^{111}In conjugated to somatostatin analogues that target and exploit its receptor overexpression on neuroendocrine cells were encouraging, particularly as it was thereafter proven successful for the eradication of small volume tumors [14, 18]. Summarizing the results of the aforementioned studies, it might be concluded that the intravenous application of ^{111}In-pentetreotide particularly leads to disease stabilization (SD) in previously progressive tumors, clinical symptomatic improvement, and biochemical (Cr-A) decline [10].

23.2.2 Progression-Free Survival (PFS) and Overall Survival (OS)

Analyzing the beneficial impact on 86 NET patients treated with ^{111}In-Octreotide, the following results were obtained:

(α) *Meningiomas:* With a PFS of 29 months and 43 months OS in a meningioma case, ^{111}In-Octreotide may represent a promising PRRT option, *intra-arterially treated* (Chap. 17).

(β) *Colorectal tumors*: Kaplan–Meier curves in nine colorectal patients' study, intra-arterially treated with ^{111}In-DTPA[0]-Octreotide, showed a 36-month PFS ratio of 33.3%, in 3/9 patients, and a 36-month OS ratio of 55.6%, in 5/9 cases (Chap. 15).

(γ) *Paragangliomas:* According to the therapy response results in three paraganglioma patients' study, treated intra-arterially with ^{111}In-Octreotide, the 24-month PFS ratio was found to be 66.6%, in 2/3 patients, while the 24-month OS was 3/3 100% in 3/3 cases (Chap. 16).

(δ) *Bronchopulmonary neuroendocrine neoplasms:* In intravenously treated bronchopulmonary neuroendocrine (BPN) neoplasms (Chap. 14), five out of seven cases resulted in disease control, whereas the bronchopulmonary neuroendocrine (BPN) neoplasms' load in the two cases did not respond at all and died within 1 year after the initialization of the therapeutic scheme due to pulmonary aggravation. ^{111}In-Octreotide Auger electron emission achieves a rather insignificant disease control with a 42.9% 12-month median PFS and OS ratio, thus rendering ^{111}In-Octrerotide not promising for an objective outcome in that context of lacking established treatment alternatives.

(ε) *Intravenously treated neuroendocrine tumors:* Progression-free and overall survival (OS) ratio of ten NETs, *intravenously treated* with ^{111}In-Octreotide for a 12-month post-infusion period, was 3/10 (30.0%)

and 6/10 (60.0%), respectively. The mean PFS in months was 8.5 and for OS 17.5. These results advocated our concern and convicted us that the intravenous administration of ^{111}In-octreotide in high activities for PRRT is not indicated and not suggested as therapeutic treatment option in patients with neuroendocrine disease (Chap. 6).

(στ) *Drum-port system:* Finally, in nine patients, intra-arterially treated through an implanted drum-port system, the mean PFS in months was 49.0 and for OS 60.0 (Chap. 8).

23.3 Conclusions

Conclusively, taken into account that Ki-67 may (α) change throughout the disease course, (β) differ between primary tumor and metastases, and (γ) often behave more aggressive progressively, it would be inappropriate to draw hints regarding its "predictive" value and impact on therapy response and disease behavior. Even though Kaplan–Meir results of this study demonstrate a favorable match response in the long term, in cases with G1/G2 as well as with G3 GEP-NETs, patients with a Ki-67 index of greater than 20% seemed, even not concordant, to benefit from PRRT, with a notable long-term outcome. Thus, we should be very cautious, to draw hints regarding its "prediction" and even more its "prognosis," in NENs.

References

1. Limouris GS, Poulantzas V, Troumpoukis N, et al. Comparison of 111In-[DTPA0] octreotide versus non-carrier added 177Lu-[DOTA0, Tyr3]-octreotate efficacy in patients with GEP-NET treated intra-arterially for liver metastases. Clin Nucl Med. 2016;41(3):194–200.
2. Krenning EP, Kooij PP, Bakker WH, et al. Radiotherapy with a radiolabeled somatostatin analogue, [111In-DTPA-D-Phe1]-octreotide. A case history. Ann N Y Acad Sci. 1994;733:496–506.
3. Kwekkeboom D, Krenning EP, de Jong M. Peptide receptor imaging and therapy. J Nucl Med. 2000;41(10):1704–13.
4. Fjaelling M, Andersson P, Forssell-Aronsson E, et al. Systemic radionuclide therapy using indium-111-DTPA-D-Phe1-octreotide in midgut carcinoid syndrome. J Nucl Med. 1996;37:1519–21.
5. McCarthy KE, Woltering EA, Espenan GD, et al. In situ radiotherapy with 111In-pentetreotide: initial observations and future directions. Cancer J Sci Am. 1998;4:94–102.
6. Meyers MO, Anthony LB, McCarthy KE, et al. High dose indium 111In pentetreotide radiotherapy for metastatic atypical carcinoid tumor. South Med J. 2000;93:809–11.
7. Tiensuu Janson E, Eriksson B, Öberg K, et al. Treatment with high dose [111In-DTPA-D-PHE1]-octreotide in patients with neuroendocrine tumors: evaluation of therapeutic and toxic effects. Acta Oncol. 1999;38(3):373–7.
8. Nguyen C, Faraggi M, Giraudet A-L, et al. Long-term efficacy of radionuclide therapy in patients with disseminated neuroendocrine tumors uncontrolled by conventional therapy. J Nucl Med. 2004;45(10):1660–8.
9. Valkema R, De Jong M, Bakker WH, et al. Phase I study of peptide receptor radionuclide therapy with [111In-DTPA°]octreotide: the Rotterdam experience. Semin Nucl Med. 2002;32(2):110–22.
10. Anthony LB, Woltering EA, Espenan GD, et al. Indium-111-pente-treotide prolongs survival in gastroenteropancreatic malignancies. Semin Nucl Med. 2002;32:123–32.
11. Buscombe JR, Caplin ME, Andrew JW. Long-term efficacy of high-activity 111In-pentetreotide therapy in patients with disseminated neuroendocrine tumors. J Nucl Med. 2003;44(1):1–6.
12. Kong G, Johnston V, Ramdave S, et al. High-administered activity In-111 octreotide therapy with concomitant radio-sensitizing 5FU chemotherapy for treatment of neuroendocrine tumors: preliminary experience. Cancer Biother Radiopharm. 2009;24(5):527–33.
13. Delpassand ES, Sims-Mourtada J, Saso H, et al. Safety and efficacy of radionuclide therapy with high-activity In-111 pentetreotide in patients with progressive neuroendocrine tumors. Cancer Biother Radiopharm. 2008;23(3):292–300.
14. Limouris GS, Chatziioannou A, Kontogeorgakos D, et al. Selective hepatic arterial infusion of In-111-DTPA-Phe1-octreotide in neuroendocrine liver metastases. EJNMMI. 2008;35(10):1827–37.
15. Delpassand ES, Samarghandi A, Mourtada JS, et al. Long-term survival, toxicity profile, and role of F-18 FDG PET/CT scan in patients with progressive neuroendocrine tumors following peptide receptor radionuclide therapy with high activity In-111 pentetreotide. Theranostics. 2012;2(5):472–80.
16. Pool SE, Kam BL, Koning GA, et al. [(111)In-DTPA]octreotide tumor uptake in GEPNET liver metastases after intra-arterial administration: an

overview of preclinical and clinical observations and implications for tumor radiation dose after peptide radionuclide therapy. Cancer Biother Radiopharm. 2014;29(4):179–87.

17. Kratochwil C, Giesel FL, López-Benítez R, et al. Intraindividual comparison of selective arterial versus venous 68Ga-DOTATOC PET/CT in patients with gastroenteropancreatic neuroendocrine tumors. Clin Cancer Res. 2010;16(10):2899–905.

18. Reilly MN. Monoclonal antibody and peptide-targeted radiotherapy of cancer, Chapter 9. New Jersey: Wiley; 2010.

Therapy Response vs. Variability of Tumor Size, Absorbed Dose, and Ki-67 Index After ^{111}In-Octreotide Intra-arterial Infusions

Victor Ralph McCready, Maria I. Paphiti, and Georgios S. Limouris

24.1 Introduction

GEP-NETs are classified according to their Ki-67 proliferation index into three grades: G1 or low grade (mitoses <2/10 HPF or 2 mm^2, or Ki 67-labeling index of <3%), G2 or intermediate grade (mitoses of 2–20/HPF, or Ki 67-labeling index of 3–20%), and G3 or high grade (mitoses >20/10 HPF or Ki 67-labeling index >20%) [1]. Although the treatment between G1 and G2 is similar, some cases may present unexpected evolution, especially G2 cases with a proliferative index greater than 10% for Ki-67 [2]. Focusing on metastases to the liver, in addition to Ki-67 **proliferation index**, the variability of **tumor size** in liver parenchyma and the **absorbed dose** crucially determine and contribute to their prognosis. These three parameters are briefly evaluated in this chapter analyzing their impact on ^{111}In-Octreotide prognosis and therapy response.

V. R. McCready (✉)
Royal Sussex County Hospital, Brighton, UK
e-mail: ralph.mccready@nhs.net

M. I. Paphiti
National Health System, Athens, Greece

G. S. Limouris
Nuclear Medicine, Medical School, National and Kapodistrian University of Athens, Athens, Greece

24.2 Tumor Size, Absorbed Dose, and Ki-67 Index

Focusing on metastases to the liver, in parallel with the Ki-67 proliferation index, and absorbed dose, tumor size variability substantially affects its treatment response and prognosis. Furthermore, the correlation between volume pattern and patients' survival is a parameter that has to be taken into account, to be compared and analyzed. In our Institution, the retrospective, selective study in a cohort of 14 patients with nonfunctioning, unresectable liver-metastatic NENs, treated with non-carrier-added ^{111}In-Octreotide after catheterization of the hepatic artery [12 sessions each, with an administered activity of precisely 5.92 GBq (160 mCi) per session, at standard intervals of 2 months] showed interesting findings (Table 24.1).

Patients (three originated from the pancreas, five from the small intestine, three from the lungs, one from the mesentry, one from the rectum, one from the sigmoid) graded as G1/G2 and G3 were under long-acting somatostatin analog treatment. The included cohort was classified into three groups as follows: Group A, with liver metastases tumor-size (LMTS) maximum diameter of less than 20 mm; Group B, with LMTS from 20 up to 40 mm; and Group C, with LMTS larger than 40 mm. Response was evaluated based on RECIST 1.1 criteria, and overall survival (OS)

© Springer Nature Switzerland AG 2021
G. S. Limouris (ed.), *Liver Intra-arterial PRRT with ^{111}In-Octreotide*,
https://doi.org/10.1007/978-3-030-70773-6_24

Table 24.1 Patients' characteristics treated with ^{111}In-Octreotide

Patients name	Age/sex	Primary origin	No. of sessions	Initial no. of liver lesions	Final no. of liver lesions	Response	Overall survival (months)
1. G.K	69//m	Small int exer	7	5	5	PD	17
2. X.V	31/m	Pancreas exer	3!	2	2	PD	8
3. S.P	54/m	Pancreas exer	7	3	3	PD	20
4. M.N	67/f	Small int exer	13	6	6	PD	32
5. D.I	46/m	Rectum pgl exer	12	3	2	SD	156
6. P.I	56/m	Lung exer	12	3	3	SD	72
7. T.G	58/m	Small int exer	12	5	1	PR	96
8. T/K	49/m	Sigmoid/exer	9	4	4	SD	17
9. B.T	72/m	Lung exer	16	6	6	SD	84
10. S/S	76f	Small int exer	9	5	5	SD	82
11. X.P	52/m	Mesenterium exer	13	5	3	PR	93
12. B.A	53/f	Lung exer	19!	5	2	PR	192
13. K.A	61/f	Pancreas exer	12	6	2	PR	41
14. P.A	63/m	Small intest exer	12	6	3	PR	**81**

m male, *f* female, *small int* small intestine, *exer* surgically removed, *pgl* paraganglioma

was analyzed according to Kaplan-Meier curve method. Chromogranin-A (Cr-A) was radio-immunologically measured and correlated with Ki-67 levels.

Our results (Tables 24.2 and 24.3) showed a partial response in 3/6 (50.0%) patients of Group A (mean absorbed dose of 450 Gy) and in 2/3 (66.7%) patients of Group B (mean absorbed dose of 150 Gy), whereas a stable disease was noticed in 1/5 (20.0%) patients of Group C (mean absorbed dose of 450 Gy). The median overall survival in Group A was 85 months, in Group B 81 months, and in Group C 20 months. On follow-up, Cr-A values showed parallel with the Ki-67 levels.

In parallel, it is worth noting to correlate the data obtained after non carrier added (n.c.a.) ^{177}Lu-DOTATATE implementation in another cohort of 12 cases. In Table 24.3, Group A with the smallest diameter of liver lesions but with a Ki-67 > 20% up to 40% showed a partial response (PR) in two out of five (40%) patients; in Group C, with the largest tumor diameter and with a Ki-67 > 40%, no patient achieved a PR; finally, in Group B with a medium tumor diameter but with a Ki-67 < 20%, a PR was observed in two out of three (66.7%) patients. Besides these two param-

eters, i.e., the tumor size and absorbed dose, the proliferative factor Ki-67 emerges as a third prognostic predictor of the course of the therapeutic response. Accordingly, this leads to the hypothesis that the proliferation index Ki-67, as a response parameter, overrides the effect of the absorbed dose and even more than that of tumor volume. The Cr-A values were similar to Ki-67 value level (Fig. 24.1).

24.2.1 Tumor Size

The Auger emission path length of ^{111}In is more suitable for the treatment of micro-metastases and small-sized tumors up to 20 mm due to the best uniformity of irradiation and the best expected response. That is why ^{111}In is not currently used as a candidate for peptide receptor radionuclide therapy (PRRT), as can be seen in the analysis of the results from the study. Based on the observations of Capello et al. [3] in rats but not in humans, as was the case in our study, "curative" outcomes occurred in the small-sized tumors (≤ 1 cm^2) after at least three injections of 111 MBq or a single intravenous injection of

Table 24.2 Patients' post-therapy outcome with ^{111}In-Octreotide

Patient's name	No. of foci	ø ≤ 2 cm	ø > 2 cm up to 4 cm	ø > 4 cm	Post-treatment foci/response	Ki-67
1. G.K	5	–	–	4.8, 4.2, 6.8, 4.1	5/PD	>20%
2. X.V	2	–	–	4.1, 7.2	2/PD	>20%
3. S.P	3	–	–	4.6, 5.0, 5.2	3/PD	>20%
4. M.N	2	–	–	5.4, 6.3	2/PD	>20%
5. D.I	3	–	–	4.2, 5.0, 5.2	3/SD	>2% <20%
6. P.I	3	–	2.8, 3.4, 3.2	–	3/SD	>2% <20%
7. T.G	5	0.8, 1.2, 1.1, 1.6, 1.9	–	–	1/PR	<2%
8. T/K	4	0.8, 1.6, 1.9, 1.0	–	–	4/SD	>20%
9. B.T	6	1.8, 1.1, 1.4, 0.8, 1.0, 1.6	–	–	6/SD	>20%
10. S.S	5	1.4, 1.8, 1.6, 08., 1.2	–	–	5/SD	>20%
11. X.P	5	0.9, 1.2, 1.4, 1.8, 1.0	–	–	3/PR	<2%
12. B.A	5	–	2.0, 2.1, 3.1, 2.8, 3.5	–	2/PR	<2%
13. K.A	5	1.2, 0.8, 1.5, 1.8, 1.0	–	–	1/PR	<2%
14. P.A	6	–	2.4, 2.0, 2.8, 3.0, 3.4, 3.8	–	3/PR	<2%

Table 24.3 Patients' post-therapy outcome with n.c.a. [177]Lu DOTATATE

Patients	Initial ø in mm	Final ø in mm	% tumor reduction	Accumulated absorbed dose (Gy)
Group A	Tumor size ø 20–30 mm	Ki-67 > 20% up to 40%	Partial response	Tumor dose
TE	21	<10	>52.38	450
GE	30	20	33.33	270
K1	20	14	30	265
B	27	19	29.63	259
P	14	9	35.71	238
Group B	Tumor size ø >30 mm–40 mm	Ki-67 < 20%	Partial response	Tumor dose
F	30.6	<10	>67.32	178
M1	39	8	79.48	245
F	40	27	32.5	234
Group C	Tumor size ø >40 mm	Ki-67 > 40%	Stable disease	Tumor dose
K2	65	52	20	392
F1	64	55	14.06	139.6
F2	67	51	23.88	128.6
M2	49	46	6.12	87.2

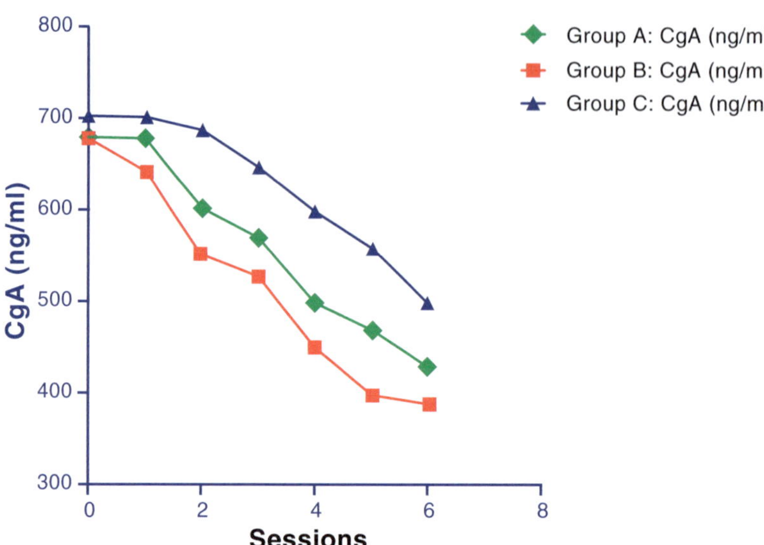

Fig. 24.1 Comparison of Cg-A changes on the course in therapy of patients treated with n.c.a. ^{177}Lu-DOTATATE

370 MBq of ^{111}In-Octreotide, leading to a dose of 6.3–7.8 mGy/MBq (1–10 g tumor). Regarding the larger ($\geq$8 cm^2) tumors, the effects are much less pronounced, and only partial responses are achieved. According to O'Donoghue et al. [4], based on a mathematical model, the tumor curability was examined in relation to the tumor size, and it was found that the optimal tumor diameter was 34.0 mm and 2.0 mm if ^{90}Y and ^{177}Lu were employed, respectively, without mentioning anything about ^{111}In-Octreotide. The authors reported further that tumors smaller than the optimal size would not absorb all the energy of the β-emitting radionuclides. This can be expected, since it is obvious, that, in large-sized tumors, more hypoxic areas due to the poor vascularization, enhancing the interstitial pressure, are present, thereby limiting the "radionuclide curability" [5], resulting from less accessible areas to the radionuclide irradiation.

24.2.2 Absorbed Dose

Understanding the relation between tumor-absorbed dose and response, either as lesion shrinkage, degeneration, or both, leads to the optimization of the treatment procedure by individualizing the amount of injected radioactivity.

Evaluating the preliminary results of the therapy, a direct analogy between absorbed dose and responding tumor can be observed, i.e., the higher the tumor absorbed dose, the more obvious the resulting lesion shrinkage and/or degeneration degree. In parallel, there is a great necessity to protect the critical organs, bone marrow, and kidneys, reducing, as much as possible, by appropriate procedures the absorbed dose to them. Importantly, the maximum acceptable dose to these organs, adopted from external-beam radiation therapy, is still under discussion [6–9].

However, this direct dilation between administered activity and absorbed dose is not a precept, since some tumors expected to have a high absorbed dose persistently showed limited or minor response (shrinkage or degeneration). These findings of a lack of correlation between cumulative activity and absorbed dose produces for the nuclear physician a dilemma which should act as an incentive to analyze the main parameters which lead to this outcome.

The wide range of absorbed doses found is likely to be related to factors such as heterogeneity in binding affinity and receptor density, hypoxia, proliferation rate, interstitial pressure, necrosis, and the aforementioned differences in tumor volume. All these factors potentially influence the tumor-specific radiosensitivity and the overall outcome of the therapy.

Cremonesi et al. [10] and Pauwels et al. [11] presented the first correlation between absorbed dose and tumor reduction in a study of 13 patients diagnosed with gastro-entero-pancreatic NETs and treated with ^{90}Y-DOTATOC PRRT. Quantitative ^{90}Y-DOTATOC imaging was used for dosimetry and CT for tumor response without mentioning anything about ^{111}In-Octreotide. The correlation was not high but was significant (Pearson coefficient $R^2 = 0.5$), confirming the value of tumor dosimetry and demonstrating the necessity to irradiate tumors with absorbed doses higher than 120 Gy in order to improve responses. In agreement with the results of this study, Del Prete et al. [12] found that, with ^{177}Lu DOTATATE therapy, tumor lesions exposed to absorbed doses exceeding about 130 Gy did not progress; however no significant correlation between the radiological response and the cumulative lesion absorbed dose was found [12]. Interestingly, a strong inverse correlation was found between the biochemical response (change in chromogranin A level) and the tumor absorbed dose (Pearson $R^2 = -0.84$), suggesting that PRRT has a significant effect on tumor secretory function that is independent of the tumor size response, especially at absorbed doses exceeding 100 Gy. The most recent study is that by Ilan et al. [9] in which 24 patients treated with ^{177}Lu-DOTATATE showed a correlation between the tumor-absorbed doses and tumor volume reduction, as assessed by CT, with a Pearson coefficient R^2 of 0.64 for tumors with diameter larger than 2.2 cm (higher uncertainty) and 0.91 for tumors with diameter larger than 4 cm. The most significant factor influencing outcome was the accuracy of the dosimetry which was based on SPECT with correction for attenuation, scatter, detector response, and the partial volume effect.

24.2.3 Ki-67 Proliferation Index

The role of the Ki-67 tumor proliferation index in predicting the efficacy of PRRT in NENs still remains undetermined. According to Ezzidin et al. [13] in G1/G2 tumors (Ki-67 $\leq 20\%$), the partial response (PR) was 40%, the minor response 15%, the stable disease (SD) 34%, and the progressive disease (PD) 11%. However, G3 tumors (Ki-67 > 20%) showed progression in 71% of patients. In 2018, Nicolini et al. [14] found that in a total of 33 patients with advanced NENs, only 2 patients (6%) achieved a PR and 21 (64%) showed SD. The median progression-free survival (PFS) was 23 months, and the median overall survival (OS) was 52.9 months. Progression-free survival was significantly better in patients with a Ki-67 index of $\leq 35\%$ than in those with a Ki-67 index of >35%. Recently, in a study of Zhang et al. [15] in 69 patients with a median follow-up of 94.3 months and G3 (Ki-67 > 20% up to 57%) tumors, treated with ^{177}Lu- and/or ^{90}Y-labeled DOTATATE or DOTATOC, the median PFS was 9.6 months and the median OS was 19.9 months. In the case of patients with G3 NENs with a Ki-67 of more than 55% ($n = 53$), the median PFS was 11 months and median OS 22 months. Patients with a Ki-67 > 55% ($n = 11$) had a median PFS of 4 months and a median OS of 7 months.

In conclusion, to the best of our knowledge, this is the first report, from a dedicated multidisciplinary team, of the results of liver metastases from NENs, after intra-arterial PRRT using the Auger and internal conversion electrons of ^{111}In emission, as the first-line therapy analyzing their tumoricidal effectiveness [16]. The final achievement of stabilizing (SD) GEP-neuroendocrine large-volume (~6 cm) liver metastases with an absorbed dose of 450 Gy compared with the partial response (PR) in patients with smaller volume liver metastases with 150 Gy absorbed dose undeniably indicates the negative impact that the tumor volume plays in PRRT response.

Thus, the surgical excision of these large volume tumors before peptide receptor radionuclide therapy should be a sine qua non.

References

1. Bosman FT, Carneiro F, Hruban RH, et al. WHO classification of tumours of the digestive system. 4th Ed. 2010. Vol. 3, pp.417.
2. Nuñez-Valdovinos B, Carmona-Bayonas A, Jimenez-Fonseca P, et al. Neuroendocrine tumor heterogeneity adds uncertainty to the World Health Organization 2010 classification: real-world data from the Spanish tumor registry (R-GETNE). Oncologist. 2018;23:422–32.
3. Capello A, Krenning E, Bernard B, et al. 111In-labelled somatostatin analogues in a rat tumor model: somatostatin receptor status and effects of peptide receptor radionuclide therapy. Eur J Nucl Med Mol Imaging. 2005;32(11):1288–95.
4. O'Donoghue JA, Bardies M, et al. Relationships between tumor size and curability for uniformly targeted therapy with beta-emitting radionuclides. J Nucl Med. 1995;36:1902–9.
5. Jain RK. Transport of molecules, particles, and cells in solid tumors. Annu Rev Biomed Eng. 2013;1:241–63.
6. Sandström M, Garske-Roman U, Granberg D, et al. Individualized dosimetry of kidney and bone marrow in patients undergoing 177Lu-DOTA-octreotate treatment. J Nucl Med. 2013;54:33–41.
7. Cremonesi M, Ferrari M, Bodei L, et al. Dosimetry in peptide radionuclide receptor therapy: a review. J Nucl Med. 2006;47:1467–75.
8. Barone R, Borson-Chazot F, Valkema R, et al. Patient-specific dosimetry in predicting renal toxicity with 90Y-DOTATOC: relevance of kidney volume and dose rate in finding a dose-effect relationship. J Nucl Med. 2005;46(Suppl 1):99S–106S.
9. Ilan E, Sandström M, Wassberg C, et al. Dose response of pancreatic neuroendocrine tumors treated with peptide receptor radionuclide therapy using 177Lu-DOTATATE. J Nucl Med. 2015;56(2):177–82.
10. Cremonesi M, Ferrari ME, Bodei L, et al. Correlation of dose with toxicity and tumor response to 90Y- and 177Lu-PRRT provides the basis for optimization through individualized treatment planning. Eur J Nucl Med Mol Imaging. 2018;45(13):2426–41.
11. Pauwels S, Barone R, Walrand S, et al. Practical dosimetry of peptide receptor radionuclide therapy with (90)Y-labeled somatostatin analogs. J Nucl Med. 2005;46(Suppl 1):92S–8S.
12. Del Prete M, Buteau FA, Beauregard JM. Personalized 177Lu octreotate peptide receptor radionuclide therapy of neuroendocrine tumours: a simulation study. Eur J Nucl Med Mol Imaging. 2017;44(9):1490–500.
13. Ezzidin S, Opitz M, Attassi M, et al. Impact of the Ki-67 proliferation index on response to peptide receptor radionuclide therapy. Eur J Nucl Med Mol Imaging. 2011;38(3):459–66.
14. Nicolini S, Severi S, Ianniello A, et al. Investigation of receptor radionuclide therapy with 177Lu-DOTATATE in patients with GEP-NEN and a high Ki-67 proliferation index. Eur J Nucl Med Mol Imaging. 2018;45(6):923–30.
15. Zhang J, Kulkarni H, Singh A, et al. Peptide receptor radionuclide therapy (PRRT) in patients with progressive grade 3 neuroendocrine neoplasms (NEN). J Nucl Med. 2019;60(11):560.
16. Paphiti M, Karfis I, Demetriadi EZ, et al. Best therapy response vs. variability of tumor size, absorbed dose and Ki-67 index after n.c.a. Lu-177 Dotatate intra-arterial infusions. Eur J Nucl Med Mol Imaging. 2017;44(Suppl 2):159. [abstract].